PERFORMING SEX

PERFORMING SEX

The Making and Unmaking
of Women's Erotic Lives

BREANNE FAHS

SUNY
PRESS

Cover art by Annie Buckley. Left image: Title: "Shirt." Media: Altered shirt, black sharpie. Dimensions: 33" high. Year: 2003. Right image: Title: "Slip." Media: Altered slip. Dimensions: 42" high. Year: 2003.

Published by
STATE UNIVERSITY OF NEW YORK PRESS, ALBANY

© 2011 State University of New York

For information, contact State University of New York Press, Albany, NY
www.sunypress.edu

Production, Laurie Searl
Marketing, Fran Keneston

Library of Congress Cataloging in Publication Data

Fahs, Breanne.
  Performing sex: the making and unmaking of women's erotic lives / Breanne Fahs.
    p. cm.
  Includes bibliographical references and index.
  ISBN 978-1-4384-3782-8 (pbk. : alk. paper)
  ISBN 978-1-4384-3781-1 (hardcover : alk. paper)
  1. Women—Sexual behavior. 2. Sex (Psychology) 3. Women and erotica. I. Title.
  HQ29.F34 2011
  306.7082—dc22

                                        2011003225

10 9 8 7 6 5 4 3 2 1

For my mother, Rebecca Elizabeth,
her mother, Rebecca Mae,
and her mother, Myrtle Elizabeth

CONTENTS

ACKNOWLEDGMENTS

I OFFER THANKS to the many people who have helped to see this book through to completion. To paraphrase Judith Butler, political change is only possible when we undergo a radical shift in our understanding of the possible and the real. I have encountered many who have shifted my notions of the possible and the real and who have made contributions to this book. First and foremost, I thank the long line of women in my life who broke the rules about gender, prioritized each other, and expected a great deal more than tradition would allow. Thanks especially to my mother and my sister, as both have provided immeasurable amounts of support, love, and graciousness throughout the writing of this book.

I wholeheartedly thank my interview participants, each of whom was brave enough to speak truth to power and to share intimate parts of her life with me. I spent many provocative hours talking one-on-one with a group of articulate and compelling women who were sincere, generous, and wise. This book has only been possible to the extent that these forty women provided a window into their lives.

Thank you to SUNY Press, who has been lovely to work with, and to my editor, Larin McLaughlin, for believing in the book and extending such unwavering support. Thanks to Annie Buckley for the cover art and Clint Van Winkle for indexing.

I owe much recognition to my research assistants and students, who have provided innumerable hours of research support as well as collegial encouragement, passion, and interest in the project. Special thanks to

Molly Armistead, Jennifer Bertagni, Kalen Brest, Mitchell Call, Emily Chaloner, Katie Courter, Natalie Das, Denise Delgado, Ashley Gohr, Alisha Herman, Christopher Liguori, Alyssa McAlister, Mary McCraw, Adrielle Munger, Jennifer Pryor, Maureen Rathkamp, April Sanford, Judith Sipes, Luke Slaeton, Jamie Starner, Cassandra Trevino, Jennifer Thompson, Theresa Williams, and Hilary Wolf. I have also benefitted from the enthusiasm, creativity, and feminist sensibilities of the students in the sexuality seminars I teach at Arizona State University, and though these students are too numerous to mention here, I thank them with gusto. My students have stood by this project from day one and have pushed me to constantly reimagine the problems young women face in their quest toward sexual liberation. I have benefitted enormously from our many conversations over the years.

I extend thanks to my fellow sex researchers who have provided mentorship, dialogued with me at conferences and meetings, conducted brave and cutting-edge research, and blazed forward in a field that continues to suffer from underfunding, underrecognition, and relentless attacks from conservative and regressive institutions. An extra special thanks to Sara McClelland, who, aside from being the most wickedly talented sex researcher I know, also happens to be a terrific friend, colleague, and confidant. Her comments added clarity, wisdom, and organization to early drafts of this book.

Many organizations have provided funding for parts of this research. This support facilitated the continued progress of the project and often arrived at precisely the right moment to ensure its continuation. I extend gratitude to the Foundation for the Scientific Study of Sexuality; Arizona State University's New College of Interdisciplinary Arts and Sciences; University of Michigan's Department of Women's Studies and Clinical Psychology; the Institute for Research on Women and Gender at the University of Michigan; and the Lesbian, Gay, Bisexual, and Transgender Summer Institute for their support of this work.

As a junior scholar, I extend heartfelt gratitude for the outstanding mentorship, political support, and personal encouragement I received from more senior scholars while writing this book. Leonore Tiefer's frank and funny advice has helped fuel the project along. Abby Stewart has provided support in every sense of the word, from critical and editorial support to emotional, social, and institutional support. Love and thanks to Elmer Griffin, who taught me new ways to see and think and who never made excuses for men behaving badly. Certainly, this manuscript benefitted from the razor-sharp critical eye and radical feminist sensibilities of Eric Swank, who waded through several drafts in painstaking detail and offered countless keen insights, well-timed (and incredibly funny) pep talks, thoughtful suggestions, careful revisions to words and concepts, and rigorous strategies for improvement along the way. I deeply appreciate the support and solidarity of many other colleagues and mentors as well, particularly Deborah Martinson, Sarah Stage, Monica Casper, Alejandra Elenes, Michelle Tellez, Stephanie Fink De Backer, Mary Bjork, Bertha Manninen, Kelly Rafferty, Mary Margaret Fonow, Valerie Kemper, Karin Martin, Chris Peterson, Jayati Lal, Sandra Graham-Bermann, David Winter, and Carroll Smith-Rosenberg.

Truly, I could never exhaust the many ways I am grateful for my friends and fellow travelers, all of whom have positively impacted this book. Thanks especially to Lori Errico-Seaman, Sean Seaman, Jan Habarth, Steve Du Bois, Garyn Tsuru, Wendy D'Andrea, Marcy Winokur, Jennifer Taylor, Megan Moore, Denise Delgado, David Frost, Joanna Martori, and Devaki Ramalingam. I give a humble and heartfelt thank you to Toby Oshiro, for his contagious love of words and his astute insights on just about everything. Finally, love and gratitude to M. L., for being there at the beginning, and to E. S., for being there at the end.

An earlier version of chapter 2 appeared in *Journal of Bisexuality* in 2009.

INTRODUCTION

> Bodies are not the brute effects of a pregiven nature, but are
> historically specific effects of forms of social and institu-
> tional production and inscription . . . Whatever (historical)
> identity the body has, this is the result of a play of forces
> unifying and codifying the different organs, processes and
> functions which comprise it. These forces are never capable
> of completely subduing the bodies and bodily energies they
> thereby produce, for there is a resistance to the imposition
> of discipline, and a potential for revolt in the functioning of
> any regime of power."
>
> —Grosz, *Sexual Subversions*

I RECENTLY SAW a photo of two women walking down a street in
small-town America, flanked on either side by a strip club and a Baptist
church. This image offered a poignant centerpiece to think about when
writing this book, which is, most centrally, an exposé about the unin-
tended consequences of the women's liberation movement and the
sexual revolution. More precisely, this book deals with the current *trappings of empowerment discourse*—the whiplash and contradiction inherent
to this peculiar moment in time, where women are wedged between
post-sexual revolution celebrations of progress and alarmingly aggressive new modes of disempowerment they encounter when trying to
reap the benefits of such progress.

In 2005, when I initially set out to interview women about their
sexuality, I had imagined that women would mostly discuss progress nar-

ratives about the ways they have moved *away from* histories of repression
that had plagued their mothers and grandmothers. Indeed, women in
the United States today suffer far less from constraints about their sexuality as inherently "dirty" or "wrong": they routinely have multiple
sexual partners; movements against sexual violence have become widespread and politically effective; women have wider access to representations of (and language about) sex; women's enjoyment of sex no longer
qualifies them as "insane" or nonnormative; and women face relatively
little resistance when seeking most forms of birth control, among other
things. Still, as I began to converse with women about their sexual lives,
it became clear that, despite many advances women have made with
sexuality, another set of daunting problems has taken root.

To illuminate these obstacles, consider this: over half of women
report having faked orgasm (Wiederman, 1997); nearly half of all
women report rape fantasies and many cite them as their favorite fantasies (Critelli & Bivona, 2008); pharmaceutical companies aggressively
campaign to create Viagra for women and drugs to induce women's
desire (Tiefer, 2004); women's same-sex experiences overwhelmingly
occur more and more often in the context of men demanding threesomes (Wilson, 1987); nearly half of all women apparently have "sexual
dysfunction" (Shifren et al., 2008); *Girls Gone Wild* netted over $90 mil-
lion in 2003, making it one of the most profitable forms of "pornography" in existence (De Solenni, 2003); women underreport or minimize
the occurrence of rape, in part because their husbands are the most
likely perpetrators against them (Martin, Taft, & Resick, 2007); women
describe body image problems so often that scholars now refer to
women's body dysmorphia as "normative discontent" (Silberstein et al.,
1988); when asked about their motivations for orgasm, women ranked
pleasing their partner over pleasing themselves as the reason they
wanted to orgasm (Nicolson & Burr, 2003); and so on. Although the
women's movement was a liberatory force that improved, and continues
to improve, women's lives in myriad ways, the stories women told me
about their sexuality indicated that much of the progress of the movement has stalled or regressed and therefore must be reevaluated and
reimagined given the current sexual climate.

Why, in an age characterized so often by *sexual progress* and *sexual
liberation*, do women struggle so intensely about their sexuality? Why do

women simultaneously claim that they feel empowered and disempowered by their sexuality? Further still, how are women—across all demographic groups, in a variety of social contexts, regardless of relationship status, length, or satisfaction—*performing* their sexuality?

While this book features 40 women as they discuss their experiences with sexuality, it is intended as a broader reflection about the sexual lives of women today. Metaphorically, the women whose voices appear in this book lead lives much like those women in the aforementioned photo, negotiating a confusing and contradictory path that tells them, on the one hand, that they must repress their sexuality and live "moral" lives based on silence and the reproduction of traditional gender roles. On the other hand, they simultaneously hear that sexually liberated women should have fun with their sexuality—they join other suburban moms by taking strip aerobics, watch *Sex and the City* with their girlfriends, orgasm (or pretend to orgasm) regularly and efficiently, and mold their sexuality based on the fantasies of powerful corporate and patriarchal interests. Despite the many political advances for women promoted in the past four decades in the United States, constructions of women have not strayed far from the virgin/whore paradigm (that is, women as either innocent or corrupt, pure or impure, sweet or nasty); in fact, the stories women offer about their sexuality in the following chapters indicate that the virgin/whore paradigm has simply been reinvented, repackaged, and reinvigorated.

In conversing with women during the past five years, one theme reappeared time and time again: women live in a state of contradiction, beholden to cultural scripts that lay down precise rules about how they can think, behave, and experience themselves, while they also struggle to define their sexuality on their own terms. As Audre Lorde (1993) argued:

When we live outside ourselves, and by that I mean on external directives only rather than from our internal knowledge and needs, when we live away from those erotic guides from within ourselves, then our lives are limited by external and alien forms, and we conform to the needs of a structure that is not based on human need, let alone an individual's. But when we begin to live from within outward, in touch with the power of the erotic within ourselves, and allowing that power to inform and illuminate our actions upon the world around us, then we begin to be responsible to ourselves in the deepest sense. For as we begin to recognize our deepest feelings, we begin to give up, of necessity, being satisfied with suffering and self-negation, and with the numbness which so often seems like their only alternative in our society. Our acts against oppression become integral with self, motivated and empowered from within. (p. 342)

This book is a meditation on this precise predicament: How do women negotiate the dual impulses to live *outside of themselves*—as they respond to pressures from partners, culture, media, parents, schooling, friends, institutions, patriarchy—while also living, as Lorde would say, "from within outward"?

Certainly, this is a staggering task, particularly when considering how much sexual baggage women inherit on a nearly daily basis. To say Americans "have issues" about sex would be a gross understatement. Whether in popular culture—filled with contradictory images and depictions of women as both oversexed vixens and undersexed virgins—or within institutions (e.g., government, workplaces, military, schools, families, etc.), discourse on, interest in, and concern about women's sexuality lunges forward and then pulls back. Of course, sex sells (and not just in a commercial sense, but also academically), yet something holds people back from having authentic and analytical conversations, public dialogues, and discussions about "dirty" themes. For example, in 1994 when Jocelyn Elders, then Surgeon General of the United States, suggested that teenagers should masturbate as a way to avoid riskier sexual behaviors and to curb the spread of AIDS and other STDs, Bill Clinton promptly fired her (Duffy, 1994). These sorts of incidents only got worse with the Bush administration. In 2007, Bush appointed Susan Orr as the head of Population Affairs; she argued that birth control was part of the "culture of death" and advocated for a "conscience clause" for pharmacists who did not want to dispense birth control to unmarried women (Morgan, 2007). As a culture, sex is talked about, sometimes ad nauseum, but ironically it often still feels like a transgression. Teenagers educate themselves about sex via pornography or their misinformed peers yet enter college classrooms without knowing anything about the technical workings of the clitoris (e.g., pornography teaches viewers to believe that merely *looking* at a woman's clitoris will inspire her to immediately have multiple orgasms). Women's studies curricula now include sexuality studies work, but universities are nervous about offering such classes. Women talk with each other about G-spots and Kegels, threesomes and blowjobs, and yet rarely criticize the social context that enforces the social norming of pubic hair removal, the backlash debates surrounding Gardasil, or the rigidity of sex education documents as heterosexual training manuals. Something of the "good girl" complex still pushes through.

To transcend these erotic silences, these "missing discourses," requires serious conversations about topics that inspire uneasiness and hesitation. As a women's studies professor and practicing clinical psychologist, I have had the pleasure of engaging in numerous conversations about women's sexuality with my students, interview participants, clinical psychology clients, friends, colleagues, family members, fellow activists, and scholars. This has happened formally, after presenting work at professional conferences, and informally, while working through and debating ideas with friends and family members. This has happened institutionally, while conducting interviews and reviewing the transcripts, and outside of institutions, while supporting demonstrations and mobilizing for women's rights. Again and again, symptoms appear to suggest that, regardless of age, race, class, body, or cohort, women experience their sexuality as not fully a product of the personal and sexual agency they purportedly gained following the women's movement. Women find themselves in new quandaries, puzzled by the difficulties of feeling simultaneously free and trapped.

While sexuality has many personal qualities, women are also beholden to broader societal contexts that dictate their relationships to their bodies, partners, and institutions. One central question of the book—and one not fully resolved but explored at length here—asks: *Can women possess their own desire if the terms of sexuality cater more to the desires of men?* In other words, if part of being an oppressed person means that you are *in reference to* the dominant ideologies of those in power—in this case, men's sexual fantasies, desires, wishes, wants, pleasures, representations, interests, needs—how do oppressed people construct themselves outside of the oppressor? If the terms of sexuality favor men's experiences, we must interrogate how this might affect women's sexuality. Case in point: definitions of when sex starts and stops, whose orgasm matters more, whose orgasm occurs more frequently, whose genitals are "clean" compared with whose genitals are "dirty" and "smelly," whose desires take up space in pornography, who is "served" and who "serves" (and so on) all lean toward a male-centered version of sex. This is not to suggest that men *want* it this way—or even that they truly benefit from such an arrangement (this remains an open question for future research)—but rather, that social scripts favor men's sexual pleasure over women's sexual pleasure. Even simple details—that penile-vaginal intercourse (PVI) does not consistently lead to orgasm for women, yet women describe PVI as their most pleasurable sexual activity—reveal women's orientation toward adopting sexual scripts that facilitate men's pleasure (Costa & Brody, 2007; Fugl-Meyer et al., 2006; Nicolson & Burr, 2003). Men's sexual subjectivities consistently trump women's sexual subjectivities, thereby transforming women into a kind of mirror for men's sexual experiences. In all likelihood, the neoconservative movement, most traditional social institutions, and the "moral majority" would not disagree with this as the *natural* order of gender roles. All argue, in essence, that women's bodies and sexualities should *service men's bodies and sexualities*, whether via traditional gender roles, an emphasis on sex that facilitates male pleasure (and reproduction), or the denigration of women as full sexual agents capable of sexual desire and pleasure just like men. No wonder, then, that women have to invent crafty and strategic measures to cope with this arrangement, resist it, and jockey for some sort of sexual power.

THE CONCEPT OF PERFORMANCE

To ground this book, theories of gender as performance (Butler, 1990; Lorber, 1994; West & Zimmerman, 1987) underlie much of the analysis. While fierce debates ensue about the specific definitions and mechanisms of gendered performances, these theories agree that people's social statuses are created, maintained, and challenged by socially-constructed gender distinctions between men and women. Much of the last two decades of feminist scholarship has suggested that certain kinds of performance—particularly the performances of gender that oppose biological essentialism—directly contribute to social justice for women. Since West and Zimmerman's (1987) essay on gender as a performance, most gender scholars have agreed that people construct their gender by acting out or resisting conventional scripts of how men and women should behave. Due to the power of social structures, and the various sanctions on gendered behavior that arise from these structures, most people conform to conventional definitions of masculinity and femininity in their everyday lives. While the pressures of conforming are strong, gender roles are not static or predetermined, and people can challenge and rebel against traditional constraints. In fact, the establishment of gender as performance sweepingly *rejected* the biological essentialist claim that sex, gender, and bodies are "natural," arguing instead that *everything* is beholden to social constructionism (or, more precisely, *culture* instead of nature). Women *become* women, and men *become* men, most often because of the social scripts they inherit and reproduce when internalizing appropriate gendered behavior. As Simone de Beauvoir (1989, originally published 1952) said, "One is not born, but rather becomes, a woman."

Competing tensions have arisen around the concept of 'performance' (or, as some say, "dramaturgical selves"). Symbolic interactionists, such as George Herbert Mead (1934) and Charles Cooley (1902), posited that selves are connected to "definitions of the situation" and that people derive meaning from social interactions, constantly modifying their interpretations of social life based on the cultural scripts they bring to those interactions (e.g., "the looking glass self"). Building on these claims, Erving Goffman (1956) famously argued that social interactions always require individuals to gauge the responses of others, "perform" to others' liking, and manage the self based on the impressions and desires of others. By deconstructing the binary between performance and authenticity, he claimed that people always performed when engaging in face-to-face interactions (e.g., "front regions") and that if individuals did retain an "authentic self" (a claim he debated even with himself) it only occurred in private where no social interactions occurred (e.g., "back regions"). Sexuality, then, represented a tricky intersection between typical "front region" settings, such as schools, churches, and government, and typical "back region" settings, such as families, private homes, or relationships to bodies. Later sociologists, such as Zimmerman and West (1987) and Judith Lorber (1994), have revised these arguments to suggest that *nothing* is behind the various masks people wear, but, rather, that *everything* entails performances that reflect the cultural norms of the day.[1]

Such theories opened up new possibilities for women subverting their roles as passive, subservient, and "naturally" good at domesticity (notably, though, symbolic interactionists rarely addressed sexuality). If gender and sexuality were simply performances of what culture demands, and nothing was True or Essential, then women could also perform *outside* of their traditionally feminine roles. In such performances, they could invent new ways of being women, thereby resisting their assigned roles as mothers, wives, and caretakers (if they chose to). Judith Butler (1990) asserted that understanding the entirety of gender as itself a performance opens up new avenues for all kinds of less traditional gender presentations: transgender identities, subversions of femininity, playing around with body norms, and a whole host of other possibilities. She asserted that *nothing* exists outside of the social. Women (and men) can always perform differently, try on new roles, provoke new questions. In *Gender Trouble*, Butler (1990) argued, "The purpose . . . is to expose the tenuousness of gender 'reality' in order to counter the violence performed by gender norms" (p. xxiv). Butler's concept of performance as something that opens up space for newness and subversion brought to light the possibilities of doing gender differently. If women could derive liberation and empowerment from nontraditional gender roles, what other possibilities did the concept of performance offer?

While Butler, Goffman, and Lorber's concept of performance offered hopeful possibilities for crafty subversions of traditional gender roles, their work also highlights the stranglehold of cultural norms in women's lives. Butler argued that individuals do not perform their individual needs, but rather, that gendered performances reflect larger discourses over which they have little control. Performance can, therefore, result either in subversive actions or in further solidifying the status quo. Case in point: If women can now perform as primary breadwinners in their family, does this free them of the burden of domestic labor (Hochschild & Manning, 2003)? If women can now join the military, urinate standing up, and eliminate their menstrual cycles to facilitate "better combat" (Oliver, 2007), does this make them equal to men? If women buy dildos and use them during sex, is this performance subversive or simply a recreation of traditional norms that mandate penises for women's sexual satisfaction (Findlay, 1992)? If everything references social constructionism, and everything is *produced* by social scripts, women face the enormous burden of interpreting these scripts, deciding how (and if) to subvert them, and making new, more empowering scripts. This has proven to be a Herculean task, particularly since, as this book outlines, empowerment discourses are swiftly appropriated and distorted.

Much attention has been paid to this quagmire of performance. Entire fields like "performance studies" take up questions about how performance has entered discourse (artistically, interpersonally, discursively, and so on). Scholars continually struggle with the idea of an "authentic self," with most arguing that authenticity cannot exist as long as cultural scripts dictate behavior. Others have questioned the progressive qualities of performance, noting that people's performances often reinforce oppressive ideologies (Butler, 1990). If gay, lesbian, and bisexual people can, for example, perform as heterosexual, this reinforces their invisibility. If women perform as men, this may erase the visibility or "otherness" of women. For this book, when speaking with women about their sexualities, women disclosed all sorts of performances, many of which *reinscribed* rather than unsettled traditional gender roles. Women discussed performing as a means to make their partners happy, to satisfy ideas of what women *should* do or *should* be, to mesh with cultural expectations that they felt they could not meet. These performances often came at the expense of asserting agency and equality. As such, the versions of performance described in this book fit closely with contemporary interpretations and criticisms of Butler that posit that, in order to maximally use Butler's concept of performance, one must, in essence, return Butler to the sociological realm of Goffman (Brickell, 2005; Denzin, 2002; Van House, 2009). In this book, these interviews favor "performance" over "performativity" by allowing some degree of subjective agency even if women generally remain in reference to larger discourses.

As *subjects* and *objects* of performance, women simultaneously, and paradoxically, exert power and agency over their sexuality even while they are stripped of power and rendered beholden to cultural norms. They create sexual scripts and *are created by* sexual scripts (Frith & Kitzinger, 2001; Jones & Hostler, 2002; Wiederman, 2005), as they enact roles created by larger discourses and norms over which they have little personal control. Women described events, feelings, motivations, and relationships with much confusion about how to negotiate sexual empowerment in this post-sexual revolution age. In short, women typically understood that this cultural moment (and this cultural context) valued men's sexual fulfillment and pleasure over their own, yet they often struggled to resist, respond, or make sense of their actions and feelings. Women struggle to negotiate, as Carole Vance (1984) has argued, "pleasure and danger." Thus, though Butler's notions of newness and subversion in performance are possible—particularly as actions in response to oppressive regimes and institutions—the stories of performance within this book do not always represent a hopeful or promising development in women's lives. Rather, these interviews showcase the growing number of questions raised as women navigate a culture that values men's desires and offers men greater rights, privileges, and rewards. Women know that they have more options than their mothers and grandmothers yet still report faking orgasm or performing bisexuality for their boyfriends or indulging in rape fantasies or wanting to medically induce sexual desire. In this age, when sexual liberation feels ephemeral to women, performance may have transitioned from a potentially liberatory action to a mere survival strategy, where women embrace discourses of disempowerment as a condition of "being women."

The central theme of this book—one explored in different ways throughout each chapter—offers this: contemporary performances of sexual liberation occur with considerable costs to women. As Anne Russo (1987) has said, even the *debates* about sexual liberation that occur in the feminist literatures emphasize and reinvigorate the virgin/whore dichotomy, as do women's mechanisms for finding sexual "liberation." During these conversations, I found it striking how often I heard the same themes: dissatisfaction with double standards, confusion about how to negotiate pleasure with their partners, disgust at how little space women had to express their desires, guilt and shame about not being fully authentic, sadness and anger surrounding the coercion they had faced, recognition of themselves as not "normal" in comparison to other women, perplexed feelings about why they could not orgasm efficiently enough, anger at witnessing younger generations of girls face the same problems reinvented anew. Women often performed to meet others' expectations, to cope with the complex problems they faced with their sexualities. As such, can women ever arrive at liberated sexuality? If everything is a performance, and performances are derived from social scripts and social norms, can women perform their way toward sexual empowerment? Indeed, this book serves as a kind of cautionary tale about what has happened to women in an age where sexual empowerment is expected, yet women face constant mechanisms of disempowerment. That said, the questions of *what performance is, whether women can escape from it*, and *whether performance can liberate women* all remain open for the reader to decide. Out of necessity, this book asks more questions than it answers.

To trace the workings of this tension between empowerment and disempowerment, the following six chapters address the kinds of performances women describe in their sexual lives, structured from the smallest and most literal version of performance and ending with the most abstract version of performance: expecting and/or pretending to orgasm, performing as bisexual in front of men, medicating women's sexual desire, performing pleasure and love, mislabeling or going along with coercive acts in the name of empowerment, and concocting sexual fantasies laden with inequalities and lopsided power relationships. While not all women experienced performance, and the tensions between empowerment and disempowerment, in the same way—some women internalized the pressure to orgasm far more intensely than the pressure to engage in dominance fantasies; some women internalized the idea that they should *want* more sex, while other women internalized the idea that rape wasn't really rape—women's sexual lives remained rife with contradiction and conflicts. Their stories complicate the notion of 'choice' and 'power,' for even when they *chose* to engage in S/M, have a threesome, watch sexually violent advertisements, hook up with female friends at a party, or participate in a porn film, these choices still referenced larger cultural scripts that had clear ideas about women, their bodies, and their sexualities. Individual choices never negate or erase the large contexts in which they occur. As Butler (1990) has shown, performances map onto larger discourses and do not always represent individual choices and decisions. For example, women do not "choose" to have a threesome without referencing the larger context of their bodies circulating in the media, law, schools, and families as, perhaps, "men's property." Women do not choose to have their breasts enlarged without that action referencing cultural norms that value women's large breasts and small bodies. An individual woman cannot "decide" such things without accessing these reservoirs of cultural discourse about women, their bodies, and their sexualities.

This leads to an important question: How are women's individual sexual lives informed by this particular cultural moment, where women straddle the leftover elements of repression, the newly regimented ideologies of sexual performance, and contradictory claims to sexual liberation? To address this question, people should consider the conversations about women's sexuality that *are not* happening as much as the conversations that *are* happening. Hegemonic worldviews reveal themselves via the topics and visions that are ignored, and by the enforcement of the status quo. Ideas about performance, sexuality, and empowerment are always emerging and under construction in politically interesting and relevant ways. Certain themes and topics push through into the foreground, while others fall into the background. When I refer to conversations people *are* currently having, what I mean more specifically is that certain discourses of sexuality have prominence, relevance, and even a bit of trendiness at times (the "it" topics). For example, it seems clear that scholars enjoy discussing the perils of abstinence-only sex education and the importance of fostering better sexual skill development early on in women's lives (Fine, 1988; Irvine, 2002; McClelland & Fine, 2008). There is lengthy talk about the influence of the religious Right, its stranglehold over the public conversations about sex in this country, and the importance of combating the hypocrisies of, say, restricting sexual information and then acting surprised when teenagers get pregnant (or contract STDs and AIDS). Informally, women talk amongst themselves, too. Women have made more spaces within their lives to discuss sex with their friends, to compare notes, to tell jokes, to discuss once-unmentionable things such as masturbation and anal sex. Women watch and enjoy *Sex and the City*, *Desperate House-wives*, and a host of sexuality themed reality shows (even if they miss the obvious limitations of the consumerism=liberated sex paradigm). In comparison to previous decades, people now seem fairly well versed in talking about the importance of women claiming sexuality on their own terms.

Media sources, preachers, grandmothers, yoga teachers, and every-body else, in all kinds of forums, gossip and rant about sex and politics. In the past 15 years alone, from the Bill Clinton and Monica Lewinsky scandal all the way through to the Ted Haggard scandal, the John Edwards affair, and Bristol Palin's pregnancy, people have learned how to speak in semisavvy ways about the relationship between public and private, the relevance of politicians' hypocrisies and slip-ups, and the role of sex in the legal system. Academically, sex has entered the college classroom, as disciplines ranging from women's studies to sociology, from communications to English, have started to take seriously the inclusion of queer theory, sexuality studies, and sex research into the mainstream framework of the disciplines. More and more students read Adrienne Rich and Audre Lorde, Michael Messner and Jackson Katz, much to the dismay of conservative anti-academic-freedom groups. Within the media, more and more queer-friendly spaces have opened up, and many more celebrities and public figures actively support the expansion of gay rights. Clinically, more individuals and couples talk meaningfully and openly about sex in the context of therapy. Clients express interest in improving their sexual relationships, connecting their sexuality to other aspects of their lives, and feeling less shame and guilt about their preferences and desires. In all of these spheres, people are *talking*, certainly.

There are also conversations that people are *starting* to have, even if punctuated by reluctance, doubt, and hesitation. For example, as Ameri-cans have become savvier at deconstructing media culture, reading blogs, and getting news from multiple sources (e.g., comedy shows, newspapers, websites, peer groups), different conversations (re)emerge. When *The New York Times* published an outrageous spread in the *NYT Magazine* in February 2009 about "new sex research" and the age-old question of what women want in bed, the feminist blogosphere responded mightily with specific and detailed critiques about the

importance of maintaining a plurality of feminist voices in the mainstream media. As these "alternative" modes of communication erupt,
different subjects garner more attention: people have begun talking
about the more awkward moments of a feminist politics—women selling their virginity online, women embracing the word *slut*, women
reconstructing their hymens, the problematics of "sport sex," and the
like. People have begun to familiarize themselves, especially within
feminist and academic circles, with the principles of sex positivity as a
basic and underlying premise of sexuality studies, particularly with regard
to questioning the divisions between "good" and "bad," "normal" and
"abnormal" sex. Scholars have moved away from the "biological essentialism" versus "social constructionism" debate as the primary debate in
sexology and have instead replaced that with a plurality of debates
about the meaning of sex and gender. Social constructionism has
stomped on biological essentialism in most sexological circles, even if
feminist voices are still marginalized and silenced far too often. Smart
sex researchers, witty sex journalists, and emerging men's and women's
studies scholars are selling books and doing speaking tours. These
voices, opinions, and perspectives are getting around.

Other progressive conversations have also begun to emerge. For
example, in feminist activist circles, people have started talking about
the problems of medicating sexuality, as new groups have sprung up
that deconstruct medical ideas of the "normal" and "abnormal" (e.g.,
The New View campaign). The medical field gets away with archaic
views about gender far less often, and perspectives about sex outside of
the tabloid circuits get more widespread coverage. That said, feminist
sexologists have been criticized harshly for failing to address the "realness" of women's distress about their lack of orgasms, lack of desire, or
lack of interest in sex. People are just starting to have conversations
about the interplay between an *activist* politics about sex (e.g., challenging women's Viagra) and a *clinical* model of sex (e.g., recognizing
women's distress as real and important). Similarly, in the classroom,
some emerging conversations add a fresh twist to conversations that
have been happening since the 1950s and 1960s pioneering sex
research work of Kinsey (1948; 1953) and Masters and Johnson (1966)
first materialized. Students demonstrate more comfort with the idea of
sexual fluidity, fundamental bisexuality, and multiple sexual identities; as

a related factor, they speak about queer theory and queer politics with increasing energy and rigor.

Along these lines, many have started to dialogue about the social justice potential of identity politics, particularly as the diversity of women's lived experiences takes center stage in discussions of the Big Themes: work, marriage, sex, love, romance, family, war, the environment, reproductive rights, bodies, globalization, activism, and the like. Discussions of the interplay between identity categories—most prominently, race, class, gender, sexual identity, and ability, and less prominently, size, age, cohort, religion, etc.—has infused sexuality studies in a major way. People have begun to discuss not only how different women are differently gendered female, but also, how different women experience sexuality in fundamentally different ways. Proximity toward and away from identity categories has become an emerging discussion at national conferences in women's studies and sexuality studies. Within the classroom, this concern for identity politics has also loomed large in the courses I teach (e.g., Race, Class, and Gender; Gender, Bodies, and Health; Critical Perspectives on Sexuality, etc.). Anecdotally, I have noticed increasing numbers of men "coming out" as feminists and encouraging other men to do the same, while more and more heterosexual students take fiercely antihomophobic positions with their homophobic classmates.

That said, the conversations people are *not* having also showcase the limitations and blocks to contemporary sexual politics. This book is concerned primarily with *those* conversations—the palpable silences, the pauses in our politics, the interruptions and backlashes to our (unquestionably controversial) collective ideas about progress. Of these noticeable silences, the lack of critical thinking about the political implications of pleasure *and* the general disregard for what women *say* about their sexual performances concern me most. Transitioning from theory to practice occurs far too infrequently. Scholars rarely ask people how they *feel* about sexuality, often because funding limitations mandate their interest in what people *do* instead. We know very little about women's subjective sensibilities about sex. As offshoots of this theme, silences about the political implications of sexual normality, imbalances in research funding about sex, the construction of women as "giving" away their bodily experiences (e.g., orgasm, childbirth, virginity, love, etc.), the troubling lack of common language about women's sexuality (e.g., no commonly used terms for women's masturbation), the pervasive attention to women as sexual victims in contrast to the nearly universal lack of regard for men as perpetrators of sexual violence, and feminist silences about sexual empowerment and broadening the scope of feminism all characterize this particular cultural moment. This is worrisome.

Related to these (non)conversations, some questions emerge: Why are psychologists so concerned with establishing frequent sex and frequent orgasm as the "sexually normal" thing to do? Why does research about pleasure and satisfaction rarely receive any funding, while research about disease, psychiatric drugs for sexuality, numbers and types of sexual partners, and teen pregnancy receives the majority of the limited amount of sex research funding? How can scholars teach critical thinking about sexuality when most students enter college without comprehensive sexual education? (I had one student ask me recently whether women *can* have orgasms, because she was taught that "only men do that.") How can people converse about sex when the people engaging in the conversations have drastically different frames of reference for what sex *is* and what it means? Why do some women conceptualize sex as a form of labor, while other women conceptualize sex as a representation of personal freedom? How can people negotiate a sexual politics that challenges hegemonic masculinity while also helping men to feel invested in challenging contemporary social scripts?

As women's narratives reveal throughout this book, women's capacity for full sexual liberation has become partially disabled by the conflicting pressures they endure. While sexual freedom and sexual expression are paramount to any kind of liberation politics—and the deconstruction of "good" and "bad," "right" and "wrong" sex sits at the center of these politics—one should be permanently nervous about the relationship between sex and liberation politics. While sexuality has the *potential* to empower women and help them access reservoirs of strength and knowledge, it remains fraught with contradictions, particularly as women struggle to simultaneously live "from within outward" while also attending to external pressures and demands. While sex can facilitate knowledge making, and while it can advocate for the importance of embodiment and the integrity of bodies themselves, sex can also further entrench people into the muck of violence, imbalanced power relations, cultural hang-ups, and the snarled interplay between our imperfect selves and our imperfect society.

Stepping back from these problems and looking at gender politics more broadly, it concerns me that, particularly at this historical moment, every time women claim something as *liberation*, it typically gets appropriated into something disempowering or oppressive. In other words, every subversion of gender can end up replicating and reinforcing the very politics it tries to subvert. This is true with work politics (e.g., women went to work outside the home, yet now work a "second shift" at home), education (e.g., women sought education, and the fields they entered have overwhelmingly lost their power and status), bodies (e.g., women fought for their rights to control their bodies, yet this line of thinking has been used to justify plastic surgery and Female Genital Mutilation in the name of "personal agency"), and, of course, sexuality (e.g., women fought for the orgasm in order to escape sexual repression but are now *required* to orgasm, which has resulted in increased incidences of faking orgasm). The conversations within this book take seriously this problem and, rather than providing answers for how to best liberate women from sexual oppression, these narratives show different ways women have become more shifty and strategic in *defining* liberation and resistance. Impulses toward resistance *do matter* and can exist in all sorts of ways, sexually and otherwise.

Given these constraints and contradictions, this book considers the question of how women negotiate the terms of their sexuality in a culture that simultaneously advocates for their empowerment and disempowerment. Women's performances of sex—and their internalization of the social scripts that dictate those performances—represent one of the major ways to trace the continued iteration of sexism, male dominance, hegemonic notions of gender, and lopsided power relations. (One can imagine, too, that similar research about men's performances could yield compelling information about how men face similar and different challenges in their sexualities). By listening to women, it is possible to better understand *why* women deny their experiences of coercion, perform bisexual behavior, fake their orgasms, and medicate their desire. These conversations offer insights about what these performances mean and how they might reinforce gender inequities while also offering a path away from such inequities. I hope that the narratives within this book can serve as a bridge into some of these conversations that people are *not* having, just as they can stimulate new ideas for areas of sex research that remain sorely understudied. Consequently, this book is designed to speak *across* audiences, both *academically*, as it targets scholars and students from women and gender studies, sociology, psychology, sexuality studies, health studies, critical theory, and cultural studies, and *interpersonally*, as it can provoke conversations between those within and outside of academia.

INTRODUCING 40 WOMEN

As a qualitative researcher indebted very much to my two main fields—women's studies and psychology—I interviewed 40 women who spoke about their sexualities in a multitude of ways. Throughout this book, not only do their voices help to illuminate certain arguments or present different categories of experience, but also, their stories can provoke deeper thinking about the multiplicity of women's sexual experiences. Some of these women appear more prominently within these chapters, and some hide on the margins; this fact is not insignificant, as it reveals the unevenness of how their sexual narratives speak to larger conversations about sexuality. Still more, I anticipate that readers may feel that certain voices sound more familiar or close to home than others; within those moments, I hope that these women's words can serve both as a testament to their own experience and as a mechanism for *representing* other women's experiences.

I interviewed 40 women over the course of three years (2005–2007) in both Ann Arbor, Michigan (N=20) and Phoenix, Arizona (N=20) (for full sampling techniques, see appendix 2). Because I wanted to speak to women from many different social backgrounds and statuses, I used a purposive sampling technique to select women from a variety of racial/ethnic backgrounds, sexual identities, and ages. All of these women participated in a tape-recorded, two-hour face-to-face interview where I asked them about their sexual histories, sexual practices, and feelings and attitudes about sexuality.[2] The group of women I interviewed included 58% heterosexual women, 18% lesbian women, and 24% bisexual women. For racial/ethnic background, the group of women included 65% white women and 35% women of color, with participants of color identifying as Asian American, African American, Indian American, Chicana/Latina, Native American, and biracial. A diverse group of ages was also represented, including 52% ages 18–31, 28% ages 32–45, and 20% ages 46–59. The women described a range of socioeconomic backgrounds, educational backgrounds, employment histories, presence/absence of children, and relationship statuses. That said, most worked outside of the home full time, and some had high-paying "white collar" jobs (e.g., administrator, engineer) while others had low-paying "pink collar" jobs (e.g., receptionist, waitress). Perhaps because the sample was recruited from entertainment and arts listings, and because Ann Arbor is an intellectual center of the Midwest, the sample was slightly more educated than the general population. Also, because people often do not converse about sexuality in public discourse, those women who volunteered for the study may have been more oriented toward articulate discussions of sexuality, gender, and their personal lives. Consequently, while this group was diverse in many ways—and generally quite articulate in both samples—voices that may have shied away from sex-themed research (or those more silent about sexuality) are likely not as well represented.

In terms of sexual frequency, I interviewed women who ranged from completely celibate since the 1980s to a working pornography actress (who reportedly had already had sex with hundreds of men and women), along with mostly everyone in between (e.g., highly sexed newlyweds, women who reported feeling bored by sex, those who occasionally dated, those with multiple partners, etc.). Women differed greatly in their partnered relationship status as well, as the group included married women, single women (some with no sexual partners, some with one partner, and some with multiple partners), cohabitating women, and divorced women. Most women had had multiple sexual partners in the past, yet most currently reported having one primary sexual partner at the present time. Women differently prioritized sexuality, as not all women enjoyed sex or were inclined to value it, while others described sex as a central part of their lives.

Most of the women explicitly mentioned their stated reasons for participating in the study, and this too represented a substantial range of motivations. For example, some women said that participating in a sex research study helped them to rebel against their repressed upbringings, while others said that they wanted to support sex-positive research. Some women felt it was an opportunity to talk about aspects of their sexuality they usually kept to themselves, while other women said they participated just for the money and because they were "broke." Nearly all participants mentioned that they were glad they had participated once the interview had finished, and some happily accepted their $20.00 payment while others tried to reject the payment. This suggests that self-selection for the study did not yield a particular *type* of woman who participated, but rather, that many different women participated for many different reasons.

That said, social identities such as race, class, age, size, religious background, socioeconomic status, geographical location, and sexual identity undoubtedly impacted their responses, though the particular ways that this occurred cannot be fully explored or known. I imagine many readers will ask about the various *differences* between women and how this affected their interpretations of sexuality. Women have inherited a long history of sexism (where women's bodies are labeled as "dirty," "disgusting," and less valuable than men's bodies), racism (in which women of color more often face accusations of sexual promiscuity and licentiousness), classism (in which poor women's sexuality has long been controlled by institutions such as the government and impoverished educational systems), ageism and sizeism (where older and fatter women rarely see representations of themselves as sexual in the media, and where their sexualities are frankly denied and denigrated), and homophobia (where sexual minorities face accusations of immorality and deviance on a routine basis). These legacies undoubtedly impacted women's responses, though I spend far too little time in each chapter analyzing these systematic differences between groups of women. This is a conscious choice on my part, for while such an omission runs the risk of privileging the middle-class white perspective in a seemingly unquestioning way, it also skirts the problem of constructing women's interpretations as a *causal outcome* of their social identities. It is impossible to know, for example, whether women's reticence about embracing sexual pleasure stems from their conservative religious upbringing, their fears of being seen as a "slut" by their friends, legacies of racism that prohibit active sexual desire, concerns about reproductive control resulting from ongoing medical intrusions, or internalized homophobia stemming from longstanding prohibitions against same-sex desire. I hope readers will not take the relative lack of social identity analysis as a gesture at *hiding* these complexities but rather, as a gesture of bringing forth the complexities of women's lived experiences without privileging certain social identities over others or overanalyzing these identities at the expense of their broader arguments. Still, in moments of obvious difference, I have provided analysis of how these differences may matter (e.g., pressures to perform bisexuality differently impact heterosexual women than lesbian or bisexual women, so each group has a different stake in these scenarios). In my quantitative work (Fahs & Swank, 2011), I better address the concrete ways that social categories influence women's sexual satisfaction and sexual activity.

The interviews provided semistructured open-ended questions in a variety of areas: sexual satisfaction, best and worst sexual experiences, sexual behavior, political socialization, body image, partnered relationships, sexual identity, and ideas about women's sexuality more broadly. The interviews were designed as a way for women to construct their own narratives about sexuality without the constraints of me imposing categories or frames as much as possible. In doing so, I could focus the book on discovering, highlighting, and delineating different themes that emerged from the interviews. For example, when asking about sexual identity, I specifically probed for their *stories* of how they came to understand themselves as bisexual, lesbian, or heterosexual, as well as their history of how these categories may have fluctuated in their lives. During our conversations, I made every effort not to interrupt or interject with affirmations, negations, or value judgments; instead, I let the women speak about each question until they had exhausted their thought processes. Our conversations took place within environments (e.g., a psychologist's office, women's center on campus) conducive both to privacy and openness.

To give a specific example of one of the questions, I asked the women, "Many women report that their feelings about their own bodies greatly affect their experience of sex. How do you feel your body image affects your sexual experiences?" Some questions included follow-up probing questions depending on the information they

provided. Some of the probes looked for greater clarity and elabora-
tions on what the women conveyed, while other probes explored the
topics that women ignored in their narratives. In the body image question mentioned above, if they did not discuss comfort with nudity or
comfort with having sex while menstruating, I asked about these issues
during our conversation about that question. This method allowed for
rich, textured, and vivid descriptions of women's thoughts and feelings
about their sexualities.

Subjectively, I felt that most of the interviews were characterized by
great ease, rapport, and frankness between the women and me. Most
women seemed comfortable and open enough to share stories about
their intimate lives during the interview. Since many of these narratives
included joyous and painful moments, many women (close to a third)
cried during the interviews, particularly when discussing sexual violence and/or abuse or when discussing an ex-partner no longer in their
lives, and many said that the interviews "brought things up" for them
that they wanted to think more about or even seek therapy for. The
interviews were designed to situate women's lived experiences of their
bodies into an open-ended conversational framework.

Once the interviews were completed, the interviews were tran-
scribed verbatim and analyzed through a process that allowed for a con-
tinual examination and reexamination of the transcripts until themes
and patterns emerged. The extraction and analysis of these themes went
through a long line of adjustments and verifications until the themes
became more refined and specific. This book relies upon a combination
of their words along with my analysis and framing in order to illuminate the concepts and themes presented in each chapter. In all, I felt,
and continue to feel, incredibly fortunate to have had such an interesting, diverse, forthcoming, and insightful group of women to speak with
in such intensity and detail.

CHAPTER DESCRIPTIONS

Because tensions between empowerment and disempowerment
appeared so frequently in women's narratives about their sexuality—
and because they enacted various performances in response to such

tensions—this book takes up the question of *how, why, and under what circumstances* women perform aspects of their sexuality in response to these tensions. Each chapter addresses a distinct symptom of this paradigm by asking, in a different way: What kinds of performances are women enacting, and how do they manifest themselves? How do these performances reflect scripts of empowerment and disempowerment? How do these performances deconstruct ideas about "authenticity"? How might performances limit and oppress women, and how do they reveal complex resistances and responses to oppression?

Importantly, these six chapters are meant both as contained analyses about particular subjects and as pieces of a larger conversation about the tensions outlined so far. By connecting data from popular culture, social science literatures, and cultural texts with women's own scripts and narratives (as gleaned in the qualitative interviews), the texture of the challenges women face sexually come alive. I conceptualize performance as a *paradigm* in women's lives, that is, a *concept* rather than a distinct *action*; as such, each of these chapters fits into this paradigm in a different manner. The chapters are ordered such that they progress from the smaller and more concrete examples of performance (e.g., orgasms, performing bisexuality, Viagra for women) to the more abstract examples of performance (e.g., constructing pleasure and love, minimizing the significance of coercion, concocting sexual fantasy). This ordering intentionally illustrates how performance snakes its way through women's lives in ways that one can immediately see (e.g., *Girls Gone Wild*) and in ephemeral and more invisible ways (e.g., internal workings of fantasy).

Chapter 1 examines orgasm—and specifically, faking orgasm—as it relates to the cultural mandate for women's sexual performance. In the context of the entire book, this chapter takes the most literal approach to the construction of performing sex as it interrogates several aspects of orgasm, including the construction of orgasm as a *gift* from a partner, similarities and differences in heterosexual and homosexual relationships with regard to orgasm, women's descriptions of themselves as "on stage" during sex, internal and external pressures to orgasm, and justifications for faking orgasm during sex. Key exploratory questions include: What are the effects of orgasm being constructed as something a partner "gives" to a woman? How do women experience themselves when performing a "fake" orgasm (and can one definitively distinguish a fake orgasm from a real one)? How do women negotiate the complexities of a partnered relationship in their performance of orgasm? What significance does orgasm have for women's sexual satisfaction? How is orgasm both personal and political?

Extending many of these themes from chapter 1, chapter 2 addresses the relatively new and rapidly proliferating phenomenon of heterosexual-identified women reporting that they engage in performative bisexuality. Unlike other forms of bisexual erotic behavior, performative bisexuality is defined primarily as engaging in homoerotic acts with other women, usually in front of men and in the context of *social* settings such as fraternity parties, bars, clubs, and other crowded, sexualized spaces. While more common among younger women (ages 18–35), older women also report an increase in pressures from their partners to participate in performative homoeroticism, often as pressures to engage in group sex or "threesomes." The chapter considers women's experiences with performative bisexuality, their responses to other women doing this, reactions to *Girls Gone Wild* and other mediated versions of performative bisexuality, and their conflicted feelings about same-sex attraction and sexual activity. Key questions include: Does performative bisexuality represent a progressive trend of increasing acceptance toward bisexuality for women? Or is performative bisexuality a reactionary manifestation of ever-increasing efforts to control and manipulate women's sexuality for the purpose of serving men's pleasure? Is performative bisexuality indeed (as Adrienne Rich suggested about heterosexuality) "compulsory," and if so, how does that translate into women's sexual consciousness? How does performative bisexuality *violate* compulsory heterosexuality while also referencing it?

The next chapter—chapter 3—explores corporate control over women's sexuality along with women's responses to such intrusions. In light of recent pharmaceutical attempts to develop Viagra for women—and thus medicalize women's sexual performance and their ability to orgasm and experience sexual desire—chapter 3 explores the symbolic implications of women's sexual enhancement drugs. Specifically, this chapter looks at mainstream newspaper articles about Viagra for women and other sexual pharmaceuticals, along with women's narratives about these drugs, to examine the interplay between the medical and social aspects of sexual performance. This chapter draws from the New View campaign, a feminist group that challenges corporate intrusions into women's sexuality, while more directly situating these issues within the specific narratives women have about their imagined relationship to sexual pharmaceuticals. This chapter is *prospective* in its examination, as women's narratives focus on their potential to medicate their sexuality. Key questions include: How do pharmaceutical companies manufacture women's need for a sexual enhancement drug, and how do women speak about this manufactured need? What might it mean in women's lives if drug companies successfully develop Viagra for women? Would women resist these drugs or comply with cultural expectations that they need them? How would the introduction of women's Viagra onto the marketplace change women's experiences of sex and/or complicate expectations of sexual performance? What do women's feelings about sexual pharmaceuticals say about the norms of sexual performance? What does medi(c)ated sexuality look like?

Chapters 4 and 5, though seemingly opposite in their approach to the study of sexual performance, address questions that parallel each other. Chapter 4 asks about the interplay among pleasure, satisfaction, and performance, while chapter 5 examines the relationships among coercion, sexual violence, and performance. Each of these chapters looks in depth at women's responses to their best and worst sexual experiences as the framework for examining the tensions between pleasure and coercion. Chapter 4 highlights women's descriptions of intense pleasure to discuss the relationships among power, agency, sexual performance, and emotional/physical satisfaction. Women's descriptions of love as a condition of pleasure, along with their ideas about how pleasure can be derived from a number of other sexual situations, form the crux of the chapter. Key questions include: What specific sexual experiences and stories stand out in women's narratives of pleasure? What do sexual memories of pleasure look like, and why do they matter? How might women's cultural status be communicated via their descriptions of pleasure and sexual satisfaction? How can pleasure simultaneously represent empowerment and disempowerment? Is pleasure even an appropriate site of cultural criticism?

Chapter 5, by addressing women's worst sexual experiences, illuminates the centrality of dominance, coercion, and power in women's sexual lives. The chapter makes a central claim that, when discussing coercion, it is not a matter of *if* women have experienced coercion, but rather a matter of *how, in what context,* and *what the coercion meant to them.* Women's varied descriptions of coercion reveal tensions between empowerment and disempowerment. This chapter delves into the ways women construct experiences of sexual aggression and how these different constructions affect women's personal agency. In doing so, women's negotiations of coercion, and their labeling of these experiences, might reveal some protective and destructive qualities of performance, as avoiding rape labels may protect women from psychological harm while also normalizing and mainstreaming the violence. Thus, by simultaneously encouraging women to perform as "liberated" and "empowered," yet barraging them with messages of fear about their physical, mental, and sexual vulnerability, women become indoctrinated into a kind of double consciousness. Key questions in this chapter include: How does coercion appear in women's lives, and how do women respond to it? What do women's stories about their worst sexual experiences reveal about the gendered aspects of power and performance? How is women's sexual access to men normalized and demanded by conventional scripts of gender? What does this "double consciousness" between empowerment and domination look like for women? How do women experience the conflation of repulsion and flattery while being sexually harassed or objectified? Finally, how is women's relationship to domination a *performative* relationship, particularly as they *construct meaning* from coercive sexual experiences?

Chapter 6 examines two groups of related material: narratives of pornography and the role of sexual fantasy in women's lives. Specifically, this chapter analyzes the precise qualities of women's sexual fantasies as they relate to mainstream pornographic representations of women in order to interrogate *how* and *to what extent* mainstream pornography narratives interact with women's sexual consciousness. This chapter offers insights about the internal colonization of women's mental space as it relates to what they fantasize about (chapter 6) and what they describe as sexually pleasurable (chapter 4). Sexual fantasy narratives, because they removed the partnered context of women's lives and represent such a literal version of the "unreal," offer a window into the conflicts, contradictions, and tensions in women's sexualities.

Key questions include: What are the different types of women's sexual fantasies, and how do these fantasies both collude with, and resist, the impositions of patriarchy? What does it mean that there is such an enormous amount of coercion in women's sexual fantasies? What does the distance between literal pleasure and sexual fantasy say about the gendered politics of performance? What emotional narratives and cultural scripts do women attach to their sexual fantasies? Are fantasies politically relevant, whimsically interesting, or primarily a reflection of deep-seated internalization of male fantasy narratives?

The concluding chapter ties together the book by reframing several of the questions that arose during the first seven chapters, including: What is at stake in women's performances of sex—particularly when thinking about and talking to women directly—and where does this lead, politically, socially, and sexually? Does performance have the potential to liberate? If so, what kinds of resistance do women imagine, and what can people learn from this? If empowerment discourses keep getting co-opted, how should people respond to this? How might people move toward a more liberatory sexual politics for women, and can performance inform these politics? Finally, how can people cultivate hope in the face of such pervasive power imbalances and conflicting messages about empowerment?

This book is both an indictment and a plea, though probably more of the former than the latter. I draw upon the richness of qualitative narratives in order to illuminate some of the conditions of women's contemporary sexual lives, particularly in relation to women feeling entrenched in contradiction and beholden to various kinds of performances. These stories reveal the *spoils of revolution*, that is, the confusing outcomes of fighting for sexual liberation during the women's movement of the 1960s and 1970s, yet nevertheless wrestling with newer, savvier, and more aggressive forms of disempowerment for women that manifest in different modes of performance. That said, embedded within these chapters are stories of pain and exploitation as well as glimpses into what might be possible if people get better at recognizing when empowerment discourses have shifted into disempowerment discourses. By illuminating themes of degradation and resiliency, women's stories reveal that performance need not exclusively represent the tragedies of sexuality; it can also show how women *survive, strategize,* and *build skills* to negotiate power in a context that engenders power-lessness. Performance, because it represents *discourse*, may serve as a gauge for women's social and political status. As such, *sexual* perform-ances speak to these political predicaments, priorities, and problems. As Audre Lorde (1993) said,

> When we look away from the importance of the erotic in the development and sustenance of our power, or when we look away from ourselves as we satisfy our erotic needs in concert with others, we use each other as objects of satisfaction rather than share our joy in the satisfying, rather than make connec-tion with our similarities and our differences. To refuse to be conscious of what we are feeling at any time, however com-fortable that might seem, is to deny a large part of the experi-ence, and to allow ourselves to be reduced to the porno-graphic, the abused, and the absurd. (p. 342–43)

Perhaps the most troubling aspect of performance is that it so often goes unnoticed, particularly in conversations about sex. Sexuality, espe-cially in public discourse, hides in the realm of biology or "the natural." People make choices without awareness about the larger mechanisms dictating those choices. As a collective body, people can work to rectify this problem by asking difficult questions about women and their sexu-alities. In particular, how can sexual freedom for women be imagined given the tensions they face in their lives? Can liberation be a goal?

These are hard questions indeed, made even more difficult by the fact of asking them at a tricky moment in the history of American fem-inism. Yet, while I do not necessarily believe in "liberation" per se—particularly as a point of arrival—I do believe that people can move closer toward, and further away from, a liberatory politics. People can have liberatory impulses, and acting in response to those impulses, they can infect the bigger narratives and change their meaning. People can set goals and then reevaluate and set new goals, particularly as the con-text of sexuality shifts. People can strategize, converse, build relation-ships, change their minds, and rework problems while striving for sexual liberation and social justice. For example, helping women to feel *embodied*—to experience their bodies from within, to feel what their bodies can do and what their bodies are capable of, to expect that women should inhabit themselves rather than rely upon others for external validation—seems like one such goal. Reimagining relationships between partners—whether through asking different questions of each other, evaluating the interplay between empowerment and disempowerment, or finding different ways to *speak* and *feel*—must have a role in liberation politics. *Talking to women*, while also thinking collectively, broadens existing perspectives on the meanings people derive from sexuality. These coming chapters, even in their focus on the way women feel *stuck* and conflicted, offer a variety of potential ways to change and evolve with regard to women's sexuality. Most centrally, maintaining the *permanence of the question*, and the elusiveness of the answer, must always remain a goal. As such, this book presents conversations that illuminate the troubling and unsettling distance between sexuality and liberation, while also offering glimpses into a world where these conversations can make us smarter, more strategic, and more radical in responding to sexual oppression.

CHAPTER ONE

GETTING, GIVING, FAKING, HAVING

Orgasm and the Performance of Pleasure

> We remain poised between the body as that extraordinarily
> fragile, feeling, and transient mass of flesh with which we
> are all familiar—too familiar—and the body that is so hope-
> lessly bound to its cultural meanings as to elude unmediated
> access.
>
> —Laqueur, *Making Sex: Body and
> Gender from the Greeks to Freud*

THE PHENOMENON OF women's orgasms has long troubled schol-
ars, therapists, theorists, activists, and scientists. Constructed as a symbol
of sexual satisfaction by some, it has also taken on political meaning in
the age of Victorian repression, during the women's liberation movement, and as the Western world moves into new frontiers of medicating
women's sexual desire. Such historical shifts—from orgasm as a treatment for hysteria to a signal of patriarchal obedience, from a measure of
women's liberation to a medicalized performance—reveal its importance as a cultural marker of gender politics. Orgasm unveils ideologies
about the status of women, beliefs about gender and sexuality, and it
serves as a concise reminder of the age-old claim that "the personal is
political."

This chapter examines orgasm—and, specifically, faking orgasm and the pressures women face to orgasm—as it relates to the cultural mandate for sexual performance. I interrogate several aspects of orgasm within partnered relationships: the construction of orgasm as a "gift" from a partner, similarities and differences in heterosexual and lesbian relationships with regard to orgasm, women's descriptions of themselves as "on stage" during sex, pressures women face to please partners, and, finally, women's justification for faking orgasm during sex. Key exploratory questions include: What are the effects of orgasm being constructed as something a partner "gives" to a woman? How do women experience themselves when performing a "fake" orgasm (and can one definitively distinguish a fake orgasm from a real one)? How do women negotiate the complexities of a partnered relationship in their performance of orgasm? What significance does orgasm have for women's sexual satisfaction? How is orgasm both personal and political?

HISTORICAL CONTEXT

The best laid plans of mice and men often go awry.
—Burns, *To a mouse*, as cited by Hirsch, Kett, and Trefil,
The New Dictionary of Cultural Literacy

A transition from orgasm as a regular and healthy part of women's sexuality to orgasm as a sign of social deviance dominated the moral anxieties of the Victorian age. Rachel Maines (1999) outlined the historical connection between orgasm and mental health: "In the Western medical tradition genital massage to orgasm by a physician or midwife was a standard treatment for hysteria, an ailment considered common and chronic in women" (p. 1). Orgasm became associated with an androcentric view of cure, whereby a woman's sexuality, when properly exercised, could remove any ailments of which she complained. Thus, if the marriage bed (i.e., penetrative vaginal intercourse) did not cure hysteria, the male doctor as a proper substitute assumed responsibility. Maines further argued that descriptions of this treatment date back to the first century A.D., with continued references until the 19th century. Carroll Smith-Rosenberg (1985) more clearly articulated this timeline:

"Highly respected medical writers in the 1820s and 1830s had described women as naturally lusty and capable of multiple orgasms. They defined women's frigidity as pathological. By the 1860s and 1870s, however, their professional counterparts counseled husbands that frigidity was rooted in women's very nature. Women's only sexual desire, these doctors argued, was reproductive" (p. 23).

Nineteenth-century views of women's sexuality sidelined orgasm as a possible, but not necessarily important, event: "The female is expected to reach orgasm during coitus, but if she does not, the legitimacy of the act as 'real sex' is not thereby diminished" (Maines, 1999, p. 5). Thus, the Victorian era normalized lack of orgasm and women's distance from their sexuality. Laqueur (1990) stated, "When, in the late eighteenth century, it became a possibility that 'the majority of women are not much troubled with sexual feelings,' the presence or absence of orgasm became a biological signpost of sexual difference" (p. 4). So, as the difference between the sexes came to justify a variety of social inequalities, so too did these inequalities breed *sexual* difference (in behavior, attitude, and socialization). Women were no longer entitled to sexual pleasure, and as Angus McLaren wrote in the late 18th century, "the rights of women to sexual pleasure were not enhanced, but eroded as an unexpected consequence of the elaboration of more sophisticated models of reproduction" (Laqueur, 1990, p. 8). Central to this loss of rights to pleasure, the relegation of orgasm to the sphere of the "deviant" accompanied these changes. Laqueur stated,

> Orgasm, which had been the body's signal of successful generation, was banished to the borderlands of physiology, a signifier without a signified . . . The assertion that women were passionless; or alternatively the proposition that, as biologically defined beings, they possessed to an extraordinary degree, far more than men, the capacity to control the bestial, irrational, and potentially destructive fury of sexual pleasure; and indeed the novel inquiry into the nature and quality of women's pleasure and sexual allurement—were all part of a grand effort to discover the anatomical and physiological characteristics that distinguished men from women. (p. 150)

Women became the symbolic representation of restraint, a carefully constructed (and politically significant) shift. Such restraint, in which women denied their sexual impulses in order to fit into polite society, also helped to define male sexual aggression, appetite, and desires. As women's sexuality was silenced, male sexuality came to the forefront. Havelock Ellis wrote in 1903, "[I]t seems to have been reserved for the nineteenth century to state that women are apt to be congenitally incapable of experiencing complete sexual satisfaction, and peculiarly liable to sexual anesthesia" (Gallagher & Laqueur, 1987, p. 16). During this period, the very existence of women's pleasure, desire, and sexual appetite was questioned and ultimately refuted. Chastity became, for women, a symbol of status; lack of sexual desire linked womanliness with social mobility.

Such social dictates placed women in the position of maintaining a modest, chaste exterior image, even while (in all likelihood) experiencing a vast array of sexual urges, desires, and fantasies. In this model, women maintained their hold on a "pure" externally projected image regardless of the realities of their internal life.[1] Deviations from this Victorian exterior placed them as cultural outsiders: madwomen, criminals, and disordered beings. Maines (1999) further argued that the societal restrictions on women's sexuality in the 19th century resulted in women acting out their sexuality in one of the few acceptable outlets: "the symptoms of the hysteroneurasthenic disorders" (p. 5). While in pre-18th-century Europe the *lack* of orgasm constituted sexual deviance and mental instability, in the Victorian age (and in the Victorian legacy), the presence of sexual appetite was enough to cast women into the classification of "mentally ill."

The Victorian era, which enforced women's sexual repression and, at times, their physical confinement, also famously asserted the (medicalized, eroticized) correlation between women's bodies and mental illness. Such correlations reinscribed notions of women's sexual repression, as women's bodies were labeled as entities to be controlled and tamed. The threat of the untamed female body enshrouded such discourses. This was particularly true for hysteria which, as Gilbert and Gubar (1984) noted, came into being during the Victorian era as a "female disease" that took its name from the Greek word *hyster*, meaning "womb."[2] Doctors believed women's ailments resulted from the uterus becoming dislodged from its proper place, resulting in the womb wandering throughout the body. This "wandering womb" caused women's "hysterical" symptoms and ultimately resulted in madness (Bullough, 1999). This fact was not insignificant, as such correlations have laid the foundation for existing definitions of mental illness today. The relationship between women's reproductive systems and their mental illnesses constructed mental illness as fundamentally a woman's problem that required male control and repression.[3]

Psychoanalysis and the Rejection of Sexual Repression (Early 1900s–1970s)

> The psychoanalytic solution restores speech to woman, only the better to rob her of it, the better to subordinate it to that of the master.
>
> —Kofman, *The Enigma of Woman*

By the end of the nineteenth century, "What came under scrutiny was the sexuality of children, mad men and women, and criminals; the sensuality of those who did not like the opposite sex; reveries, obsessions, petty manias, or great transports of rage" (Foucault, 1978, p. 39). Repression reigned, and women's orgasms fell into the shadows. Foucault (1978) argued that this focus on repression created a cultural obsession about sex; ironically, in the public denial of sexual interests and desires, sexuality became a dominant and pervasive force:

> This is the essential thing: that Western man has been drawn for three centuries to the task of telling everything concerning his sex; that since the classical age there has been a constant optimization and an increasing valorization of the discourse on sex ... Not only were the boundaries of what one could say about sex enlarged, and men compelled to hear it said; but more important, discourse was connected to sex by a complex organization with varying effects, by a deployment that cannot be adequately explained merely by referring it to the law of prohibition. A censorship of sex? There was installed, rather, an apparatus for producing an ever greater quantity of discourse

about sex, capable of functioning and taking effect on its very economy. (Foucault, 1978, p. 23)

Arising out of the context of severe repression of sexuality, the work of Sigmund Freud sought to make visible the connections between repression of sexuality and obsession with sexuality, allowing psychoanalysis to take root, both in Europe and in the United States. Suddenly, ideas about sexuality as a driving force of human behavior made sense. Like the sex research that was to follow psychoanalysis, the premise of psychoanalysis was to rebel against the repression of sexuality and to instead speak about sexuality in the public sphere. At the same time, these efforts to rebel against repression served both to free women's sexuality from the constraints of repression and to simultaneously constrain it.

Several important paradoxes appear in the way psychoanalysis shaped women's sexuality: (a) Though psychoanalysis functioned as the first "revolt" against the repressive discourses of the Victorian era, it nevertheless reinstituted these repressive discourses by portraying women as naturally passive and domestic and as having relentless "penis envy"; (b) psychoanalysis succeeded in partially bringing women's sexuality into public discourse, but it nevertheless kept women's sexuality hidden and obscure by its overemphasis on male sexuality and masculinist ideas of intercourse and penetration (consequently, women's orgasms could only occur via the vagina rather than the clitoris); (c) psychoanalysis allowed for the existence of women's sexuality (i.e., women *did* have sexual subjectivity), while simultaneously maintaining essential differences between men (as active, dominant, phallic) and women (as passive, inferior, and envious). Psychoanalysis was both repressive and antirepressive.[4]

The successes of psychoanalysis and its influence on the advancement of feminist thought, particularly surrounding orgasm, are worth noting. Some feminist scholars and analysts believed that psychoanalysis did function as the first theoretical revolt against repression, and as Smith and Ferstman (1996) stated, "The fundamental contribution of psychoanalytic theory to feminist social theory lies in its capacity and potential for explaining the origins of sexuality, sexual difference, gender difference, male domination, rape, perversion, pathology, the structure of the family, and group or collective behavior" (p. 17). These feminists felt that psychoanalysis refused to keep sexuality hidden and pathologized and instead brought women's sexuality into public discourse. According to Buhle (1998), psychoanalysis supported feminism by arguing that both men and women had the same instincts and, therefore, that women had the potential to be as sexual, and as orgasmic, as men. Certain tenets of psychoanalysis minimized sex differences (e.g., in Freud's earlier work, he argued for a theory of infantile bisexuality, in which children begin their lives without a sense of gender differentiation). Some feminists believed that Freudian theory did not naturalize sex differences, but rather offered an alternative explanation leaning more toward social and cultural construction of gender as a category. As such, some argued that psychoanalysis allowed women's sexuality to exist, both in public and in private, and it rejected the repressive discourses of the Victorian era. As Buhle (1998) stated, "Feminist have acclaimed Freud as a leading authority on the 'repeal of reticence' so central to their own lives" (p. 27). Psychoanalysis also fought for an end to the sexual repression of women by showing human behavior as a negotiation between the conscious and unconscious. As Buhle (1998) stated,

> psychoanalysis and feminists together advanced the modernist project of selfhood . . . Freud issued a mandate for a sweeping denunciation of traditional sexual morality and provided a distinctive rhetoric to make the case . . . Feminists ultimately succeeded in making women's sexuality and femininity central to the entire psychoanalytic project. (pp. 16, 35)

Kinsey, Masters and Johnson, and Critiques of Psychoanalysis (1948–1975)

Paradoxically, and despite these advances, psychoanalysis also further reinforced the discourse of repression while simultaneously advocating a new performance standard. Similar conflicts were also notable in the emerging research of Alfred Kinsey (1948; 1953) and Masters and Johnson (1966), as these American researchers sought to study both men's and women's sexuality from an empirical perspective. While psychoanalysis argued that both men and women were driven by unconscious sexual wishes and desires, Kinsey and Masters and Johnson sought to empirically demonstrate that mainstream Americans were engaging in a wider variety of sexual behaviors and "nontraditional" lifestyles. As Laumann (1994) noted, Kinsey was one of the first to study sexuality in a concrete way (i.e., what people do sexually, how often, and in what ways), and he found that people engaged in masturbation, nocturnal sex dreams, intercourse with same-sex and opposite-sex partners, "petting," and, sometimes, animal contacts.[5]

While this research brought sexuality into the public sphere and thereby normalized sexual variety, it also perhaps sparked new perceptions of the *normal*.[6] Women suddenly faced a shift in public perception of women as asexual and pure to a new definition of women as sexually obsessed (Freud), driven toward vaginal orgasm, and sexually active in a diverse group of sexual behaviors (Kinsey, Pomeroy, Martin, & Gebhard, 1953; Masters & Johnson, 1966). Within this changing climate, feminists were quick to criticize many aspects of psychoanalysis but seemed more ambiguous in their assessment of the work of Kinsey and Masters and Johnson (sometimes using the work of Kinsey and Masters and Johnson to argue against Freud's assertions) (Buhle, 1998).

With regard to psychoanalysis, feminist analysts in the era between 1940 and 1975, including Juliet Mitchell (1975), Helene Deutsch (1944), and Karen Horney disagreed with the ways that psychoanalysis portrayed women as naturally passive and domestic, attached to penis envy, and in need of "superior" vaginal orgasms in order to achieve sexual maturity.[7] Sarah Kofman (1980) argued that men suffered from "womb envy," saying that, though Freud's positioning of women rendered them in a masculinist framework, it also "proclaims the purely speculative character of the masculine/feminine opposition" (p. 15). Though she directly confronted Freud's distaste for feminism,[8] she pointed out that Freud took pride in the "mythic roots" (p. 18) of his theories.

In addition to the criticisms posed by feminist analysts, other feminists (theorists, writers, scholars) also criticized psychoanalysis[9] both on the grounds that it bolstered repressive discourse and that it inscribed a new form of sexual performance. These criticisms reflected some early markers of a change in public opinion that would ultimately lead to the sexual revolution and the women's liberation movement. According to its harshest critics, psychoanalysis represented the distillation of misogyny, in that "[t]he conclusions that Freud reached about women and their sexuality are about women as they exist within the fantasy structures of male psychic reality . . . Freud was haunted by women, obsessed with women, and in the end failed to understand them" (Smith & Ferstman, 1996, pp. 18–19).

Criticisms of domesticity and penis envy arose long before the formal start of the second wave of the women's liberation movement, first with Horney (1942), then with Simone de Beauvoir's (1953) critique of penis envy in her chapter, "The Psychoanalytic Point of View," and later, most notably, in Betty Friedan's *The Feminine Mystique* (1963), in which Friedan argued that Freudian theory directly contributed to misogyny. She also argued that women have been "bludgeoned into the belief that they can find happiness only by confining themselves to their 'feminine' role as wives and mothers" (Janus & Janus, 1993, p. 14). She was concerned about the spread of psychoanalysis, likening it to volcanic ash, which settles everywhere (Buhle, 1998). She was later joined by Kate Millet's *Sexual Politics* (1970), which named Freud "the strongest individual counterrevolutionary force in the ideology of sexual politics" (p. 178), as well as Germaine Greer's *Female Eunuch* (1972), which dismissed psychoanalysis outright as "nonsense" (p. 93). Robinson stated, "Pride of place in this litany of abuse belongs to Freud's theory of penis envy: the notion that women's psychology is based on a feeling of genital inadequacy, from which follows their inclination to passivity, narcissism, and masochism" (p. 13).

Arguments about vaginal and clitoral orgasm in Freud's writings also inspired much feminist criticism. Freud's celebration of the vaginal orgasm (a stance that rejected earlier ideas that women should *never* orgasm) established a new performance standard for women (i.e., that vaginal orgasm is superior to clitoral orgasm). Freud asserted that puberty represented a crucial moment of sexual differentiation, because girls transferred their sexual focus from the clitoris to the vagina. Freud argued that girls must "hand over [the clitoris'] sensitivity, and at the same time its importance, to the vagina . . . With the abandonment of clitoral masturbation a certain amount of activity is renounced. Passivity now has the upper hand" (Laqueur, 2002, p. 393). According to Freud, the clitoris, once the reigning site of sexual pleasure, must render itself inferior in the name of "mature adult sexuality." As Jane Gerhard (2000) argued, by assigning the clitoris to the immature or girlhood site of pleasure, while the vagina became attached to mature or adult pleasure, this theory essentially positioned the little girl as a "little man" (p. 452) who eventually realized the inadequacy of her clitoris and thus eroticized her vagina to compete with the penis. She stated, "Freud wrote, the clitoris would now come to function like 'a pine shaving' to help 'set a log of harder wood on the fire'" (p. 453). Importantly, if such a transfer was not complete, "she ran the risk of suffering from such psychological problems as penis envy, hostility toward men, hysteria, and neurotic discomfort" (Gerhard, 2000, p. 453). Fisher (1973) explained that analysts presumed a woman could not orgasm unless she had resolved her major (Oedipal) conflicts and had passed through the appropriate sexual stages.[10] Further, psychoanalysts Edward Hitschmann and Edmund Bergler (both trained by Freud) held "the absence of vaginal orgasm" solely responsible for the condition of frigidity, insisting that vaginal orgasm correlated with a reduction in "neurotic" tendencies (Buhle, 1998). To perform as a real woman, they felt, one must orgasm vaginally. Feminists fought vehemently against these claims, arguing instead that clitoral stimulation should be recognized as itself a positive and relevant experience for women.

Thus, as the Victorian era of repression and silence around sexuality gave rise to psychoanalysis and empirical sex research as "revolts" against repression, so too did the 1950s era of domesticity and passivity give rise to the women's liberation movement and the sexual revolution. These changes in climate around sexuality were, in part, nurtured by increasingly fervent criticisms of psychoanalysis, which naturalized women's passivity, anger, and hostility about women's continued subjugation in the bedroom (brought to light by the work of de Beauvoir, Friedan, Kofman, and many others), and increasing empirical evidence that despite efforts to silence public discourse about sexuality, Americans were engaging in a wide variety of sexual behaviors previously characterized as "fringe," including homosexuality, oral sex, anal sex, group sex, masturbation, and so on. Increasing distaste for repressive ideologies, as well as the spread of more information about women's actual sexual lives, contributed to the momentum leading toward sexual revolution and women's liberation.

Sexual Liberation and the Rise of Second-wave Feminism
(Late 1960s–1990s)

> It is no longer a question simply of saying what was done—
> the sexual act—and how it was done; but of reconstructing,
> in and around the act, the thoughts that recapitulated it, the
> obsessions that accompanied it, the images, desires, modula-
> tions, and quality of the pleasure that animated it.
> —Foucault, *The History of Sexuality, Volume 1*

Sexual Revolution and Women's Liberation Movement

While debates about the meaning of vaginal versus clitoral orgasm
occupied much of the public discourse surrounding orgasm, particularly in light of Freud's claim that women would outgrow the clitoral
orgasm as they became mature women, it is also noteworthy that
women's orgasms came to stand in for liberation in its entirety—a
symbol of women's improved social and cultural status. If women could
embrace sexual pleasure via orgasm and reject their repressed upbringings, they had arrived at a moment when, supposedly, other inequalities
would also vanish. Activism surrounding women's orgasms represented
a central feature of the midcentury women's movement and the sexual
revolution. It was at this point in history that women collectively
fought against the legacies of repression that had so long denied
women's pleasure and contained it within the mandates of propriety,
decorum, modesty, and silence. As Jane Gerhard (2000) said, "The vaginal orgasm, attained exclusively through intercourse, had long been a
keynote in the clamor of expert ideas about women's sexual health and
normality . . . During these early years of women's liberation, when
feminists came of age in and through the rhetoric of sexual liberation,
the female orgasm came to signify the political power of women's
sexual self-determination" (p. 449).

   During the women's liberation movement, women lobbied publicly
for orgasms—the right to have them, the right to talk about them, and
the right to reject the false claim of the vaginal orgasm as superior to
the clitoral orgasm (Jeffreys, 1990). For example, Anne Koedt (1973)
cited the then-recent scientific work of Kinsey and colleagues (1953)

and Masters and Johnson (1966)—which found that women orgasmed more frequently and easily from clitoral stimulation than vaginal stimulation—as more factual than Freud, and less attached to proper ideals of womanhood. Koedt argued, "The worst damage was done to the mental health of women who either suffered silently with self blame, or flocked to psychiatrists looking desperately for the hidden and terrible repression that had kept them from their vaginal destiny" (p. 201).

Other feminists in the 1960s and 1970s echoed these views, arguing for clitoral supremacy and women's self-determination. For example, Ti-Grace Atkinson argued that if women did not prefer heterosexual intercourse (and did not orgasm via intercourse), this was due to the institutionalization of patriarchal control over women and to the fact that intercourse itself did not appropriately stimulate the clitoris (Gerhard, 2000). She argued,

> The construct of vaginal orgasm is most in vogue whenever and wherever the institution of sexual intercourse is threatened. As women become freer, more independent, more self-sufficient, their interest in (i.e., their need for) men decreases, and their desire for the construct of marriage which properly entails children (i.e., a family) decreases proportionate to the increase in their self-sufficiency. (Atkinson, 1974, pp. 13–14)

She also famously said, "Why *should* women learn to vaginal orgasm? Because that's what men want. How about a facial tic? What's the difference?" (p. 7).

Kate Millet (1970) similarly argued that the practice of sexual intercourse upheld men's power over women, while Martha Sherfey (1970) argued against the heterosexist implications of the vaginal orgasm. If women believed that vaginal orgasm represented the only "mature" form of orgasm, this inscribed heterosexuality as the only appropriate and mature way for women to achieve pleasure. Not only did this denigrate the uniquely pleasurable potential of the clitoris, but it essentially required a penis for women to feel satisfied. Understandably, feminists attacked psychoanalytic ideas that differentiated mature and immature orgasms, saying that vaginal orgasm inscribed heterosexuality as the norm, repressed women's pleasure, and made all other sexual interaction inferior (Gerhard, 2000). Koedt declared, "The recognition of clitoral orgasm as fact would threaten the heterosexual *institution*" (Buhle, 1998, p. 217).

Activism around women's orgasms during this time focused on reclaiming orgasm on women's own terms, rejecting vaginal orgasm as a symbol of maturity, and embracing other means to achieve pleasure, most notably via lesbian sexual expression.[11] Celebrating the clitoris and its potential for pleasure had important implications for championing lesbian identification and lesbian sexuality. The combination of widely publicized sex research findings arguing that women derived the most consistent and powerful pleasure from the clitoris—along with rapidly changing sexual norms surrounding monogamy, partnering, and the meaning of sexual expression—paved the way for wider acceptance of lesbian sexuality as both normative and desirable (Singer & Singer, 1972). At one point, a common slogan during the women's liberation movement claimed, "Feminism is the theory; lesbianism is the practice" (Johnston, 1973, p. 166). In essence, the politicization of orgasm led both to an increased acceptance of nonpenetrative pleasure but also to the increased recognition of lesbian sexual identity as more legitimate on the whole.

As an outgrowth of the sexual revolution and the women's liberation movement, radical feminism garnered momentum, particularly in its attacks on conventional sexuality and conventional orgasm. While many feminists celebrated their newfound public right to claim orgasm in their personal lives, other radical feminist groups faulted feminist claims of sexual liberation. In particular, some radical feminists argued against *both* the tyranny of the vaginal orgasm *and* the championing of clitoral orgasm. They argued that the celebration of the clitoral orgasm mandated sexual performance in troubling ways. For example, the 1970s radical feminist group based in Boston, Cell 16, argued that patriarchy placed women in the midst of an "orgasm frenzy" (Densmore, 1973, p. 110), obsessed with women's right to enjoy their bodies at the expense of a larger social critique. This argument was echoed by Sheila Jeffreys (1990), who claimed retrospectively that sexual liberation in the 1960s and 1970s merely substituted one form of oppression for another. Instead of repressing women's sexuality and teaching women not to enjoy sex, these new norms forced women to have sex and to orgasm on demand. As evidence, she cited the multiorgasmic (and unbelievable) narratives of pornography, *The Joy of Sex* books, and widespread antilesbian sentiment. Roxanne Dunbar (1969) similarly argued that sexual liberation became equated with "the 'freedom' to 'make it' with anyone anytime" (p. 49) and that this ignored women's experiences of sex as "brutalization, rape, submission [and] someone having power over them" (p. 56). Other feminists argued that the sexual freedom campaigns of the 1960s and 1970s merely functioned to allow men to have sexual access to greater numbers of women and did not represent freedom at all. Such criticisms garnered backlash: As Laqueur (2002) notes,

> The whole clitoral–orgasm brouhaha, a sustained and widely publicized attack on Freud's theories of female psychogenesis, was, [Morton Hunt, editor of *Playboy Press*] thought, the work of 'extremists of the women's liberation movement' . . . who resented their own femaleness . . . feared male domination . . . used masturbation to help keep their distance from men. (p. 398)

Such criticisms reveal the unevenness with which ideas of sexual liberation based on orgasm took hold during the women's movement.

Contemporary Orgasm Research

> [W]e have also constructed more extensive typologies of orgasms, especially for women, on whom we have turned our sexual attention like a bright, unforgiving spotlight: multiple orgasms, vaginal orgasms, clitoral orgasms, uterine orgasms, G-spot, Z-spot, female ejaculation, and orgasms during anal sex . . . It may be that women learn to be less orgasmic than they could be solely from a physiological standpoint, through socialized inhibitions, fears, and gender roles.
> —Plante, *Sexualities in Context: A Social Perspective*

Of course, nearly all subsequent sex research has supported the "radical" women's movement claim that the clitoris best facilitated women's orgasms. Darling and Davidson (1987) found that, for many women, the quest for a high consistency of vaginal orgasm with a partner has become more burdensome than enjoyable. The notorious Hite Report confirmed this, saying that intercourse is not particularly suited for women's orgasms (Hite, 1976). Repeated studies have found that stimulation of the clitoris leads to the most consistent orgasms for women. Still, other research showed that many women still conceptualized intercourse as the ultimate sexual experience and believed that orgasm should be achieved through intercourse above all other sexual acts (Davidson & Moore, 1994). Cognitive pressures to orgasm during sex represent a major part of women's sexual lives (Dove & Wiederman, 2000).

Empirical research on orgasm has found conflicting reports of the frequency of women's orgasms. Reports of how often women experience orgasm vary widely and are rarely consistent across populations. Some researchers suggest that women experience orgasm in a fundamentally different way than men (Mah, 2002; Mah & Binik, 2001), most often pointing to women's increased difficulty achieving orgasm compared to men. Hunt (1974) found that 53% of 1,044 women surveyed reported coital orgasm "all or almost all" of the time, while Raboch and Raboch (1992) found that 52.2% of the 2,423 married women surveyed had experienced orgasm in the course of 70%–100% of "coital encounters." Janus and Janus (1993) found that 56% of women ages 18–26, 67% of age 27–38, 66% of age 39–50, and 50% of age 65 or over reported frequent orgasm during sex. Other studies reported the percentage of women who frequently experience orgasm at 25–30% (Butler, 1976; Hurlbert, Apt, & Rabehl, 1993; Wallin, 1960). Notably, measures of orgasm frequency most often rely on self-report, suggesting that frequency of actual orgasm might be lower if women do not know if they have ever *had* an orgasm.

De Bruijn (1982) found that many women with masturbatory experience still did not orgasm regularly with their partner during intercourse. Similarly conflicting reports were noted in studies assessing women's sexual dysfunction, with some research showing that women had high rates of sexual dysfunction[12] (Berman et al., 2003; Ellison, 2001; Shifren, 2008), while other research showed that women were generally not sexually dysfunctional (Walker-Hill, 2000). Importantly, very little attention has been paid to attributions of sexual dysfunction, in other words, whether a woman's sexual dysfunction is due to her own limitations or to her partners' limitations. Research on sexual dysfunction typically focuses on frequency (or lack thereof) of orgasm and/or arousal without attending to the specific causes for these dysfunctions or whether sexual disfunction even exists at all.

Research has also yielded conflicting reports on women's feelings about orgasm and its significance in their sexual lives. Such research has shown that, at times, women tended to downplay the significance of orgasm when reporting on sexual satisfaction, while at other times, women emphasized orgasm as the most important feature of sexual satisfaction. By downplaying the significance of orgasm, women may reveal that they do not value their orgasmic pleasure, or it could reflect women's emphasis on alternative definitions of pleasure, as women may value emotional connectedness over orgasm. For example, Sprecher Barbee, and Schwartz (1995) and Pinney, Gerrard, and Denney (1987) found that women linked sexual satisfaction with intimacy and close relationships, and Pazak (1998) found that emotional consistency, warmth, and time together were the most important factors (more important than orgasm) for women when determining levels of sexual satisfaction. Similarly, Haavio-Mannila and Kontula (1997) found that reciprocal feelings of love and versatile sexual techniques were most highly correlated with sexual satisfaction, while Kimes (2002) found that experiencing orgasm was much less important to women when assessing their sexual satisfaction than it was to men.

Other research, however, has found that women prioritized orgasm when assessing sexual satisfaction. This could reflect women valuing their own pleasure, or it could reflect a social norm in which orgasm becomes a benchmark of "good sex." For example, Means (2001) found that women identified orgasm as a major feature of sexual satisfaction and that single women were particularly focused on identifying orgasm and sexual arousal as key defining features of sexual satisfaction.

FAKING ORGASM

Coupled with this emphasis on orgasm as one common definition of sexual satisfaction, pressure to orgasm and faking orgasm have started to emerge in sex research. Bryan (2002) asked women about their experiences with faking orgasm and found that women faked orgasm because of concern for their partner's feelings, desire for the sex acts to end, enhancement of sexual excitement for self and partner, experience of themselves as abnormal or inexperienced, avoidance of conflict, and importance of orgasm to the relationship. Women faked orgasm most frequently during penile-vaginal intercourse without additional clitoral stimulation, less frequently during foreplay and penile-vaginal intercourse with additional clitoral stimulation, and during oral sex. She found that, on average, women faked orgasm 1 in 5 times they had sex with a partner, and that women who rarely orgasmed reported higher amounts of faking orgasm. Wiederman (1997) also directly addressed the issue of faking orgasm and found that more than one-half of women faked orgasm during sexual intercourse. Those who faked were significantly older, viewed themselves as facially more attractive, reported having had first intercourse at a younger age, reported greater numbers of lifetime sexual partners, and scored higher on measures of sexual esteem. Interestingly, this study also found that those who faked orgasm tended to have moderate to high self-esteem, high desire to please their partner, and difficulty communicating with their partner. Roberts, Kippax, Waldby, and Crawford (1995) also found that there were vast perception gaps between men and women about the occurrence of orgasm and that, while most women in their sample reported faking orgasm, few men thought they had ever been with a partner who faked orgasm. These studies strongly suggest that women internalize the need to perform as "good sexual partners" in ways that may prioritize performance over experience.

Some researchers have criticized the cultural emphasis on the performance of orgasm, calling instead for a more complicated understanding of women's sexuality. Research has shown that heterosexual women care more about achieving orgasm for their *male partners' sake* than for their own sexual enjoyment (Nicolson & Burr, 2003). Hyde and DeLamater (1997) argued that placing orgasm as the centerpiece of sex results in problematic consequences: "Our discussions of sex tend to focus on orgasm rather than pleasure in general. Orgasm is that observable 'product,' and we are concerned with how many orgasms we have, much as a plant manager is concerned with how many cans of soup are produced on the assembly line each day" (p. 261). Similarly, Jackson and Scott

(2001) argued for a feminist approach to women's sexual embodiment, in that they "contest both pre-social, biological accounts of sexuality and supra-social accounts: those that fail to locate desire and pleasure in their social context" (p. 99). Further, these researchers argued that pressures placed upon women to orgasm reflect a patriarchal interest in forcing women to "ejaculate" through moaning and vocal sounds: "Men make a mess, women make a noise" (p. 107). Roberts and colleagues (1995) added, "The demand for noise . . . indicates that heterosexuality becomes an economy in which the woman's orgasm is exchanged for the man's work" (p. 528). Adding to this, Burch (1998) argued, "Because sexuality is more or less a male province in industrialized cultures, a woman's sexual subjectivity does not flower" (p. 349).

CONTEMPORARY NARRATIVES OF ORGASM

> Must this multiplicity of female desire and female language
> be understood as shards, scattered remnants of a violated
> sexuality? A sexuality denied? The question has no simple
> answer. The rejection, the exclusion of a female imaginary
> certainly puts woman in the position of experiencing her-
> self only fragmentarily, in the little-structured margins of a
> dominant ideology, as waste, or excess, what is left of a
> mirror invested by the (masculine) "subject" to reflect him-
> self, to copy himself. Moreover, the role of "femininity" is
> prescribed by this masculine specula(riz)tion and corre-
> sponds scarcely at all to woman's desire, which may be
> recovered only in secret, in hiding, with anxiety and guilt.
> —Luce Irigaray, This Sex Which Is Not One

Despite this history of fighting for orgasms—by rejecting the supremacy of the (heterosexist) vaginal orgasm and by arguing for the centrality of orgasm in women's definitions of sexual satisfaction—current ideologies about women's orgasms suggest that orgasms fall far short of defining a liberatory politics. Orgasms represent a synthesis of cultural performances women are expected to enact, for even those women who do not fake orgasms often claim that a great deal of performative effort goes into the production of them. As Goffman (1956) has suggested, the difference between the real and the fake becomes obscured by the production itself; women struggle to generate orgasms wholly within a structure that demands their performance, making these distinctions of authenticity less possible or even fully impossible. Women's orgasmic performances signify limitations in "sexual liberation," in that, as radical feminists claimed during the sexual revolution, orgasm is a *requirement* of sex, rather than a mere pleasure. This signals an emerging gender politics based on sexual inequality, and it raises several questions: If women must always perform, does this preclude authenticity in their sexual expression? What kind of performances are orgasms? Can one differentiate between "real" and "fake" in meaningful ways, and if so, how (Lloyd, 2005)? How do women personally feel when they reportedly *fake* orgasm? How does orgasm function as a kind of sexual currency in women's sexual relationships, and does this differ in heterosexual or lesbian contexts?

Assuming a Marxist framework, orgasm functions as a product of labor. Orgasm is *produced*, via investment into the female body, and that production requires maximum efficiency and regularity. There are two ways of considering the Marxist implications of orgasm.[13] First, women are the laborers, and orgasm becomes a moment in which women demand of their bodies the production of an efficient, pleasurable response that affirms the power of the "overseer" (the sexual partner). She *produces* the product that is in high demand and therefore affirms her worth as a laborer (and, of course, in heterosexual contexts, gets to keep her job when competing with other women who may be interested in "her man"). This occurs most often in response to a phallic investment; as Plante (2006a) argued, "Women have long been expected to be responsive to penetrative activities" (p. 280). In the other model, if one constructs woman's *sexual partner* as the laborer, the woman's orgasm is merely a product of the sexual partner's efforts and is stripped from the woman herself. The success of the orgasm is attributed to the sexual partner, much in the way that Emily Martin (2001) has constructed the baby in the context of "labor" involving a doctor and a mother: "If the doctor is a supervisor, the women might be a 'laborer' whose 'machine' (uterus) produces the 'product,' babies" (p. 57). Either way, the labor implications of women's orgasms reveal the way in which orgasm becomes a *product* rather than an experience, a fact not without consequence in women's narratives of their orgasmic expression.

The Gift Metaphor

> The central proposition of the "pseudo-reciprocal gift dis-
> course" is that men require heterosexual sex to satisfy their
> sexual urges . . . [I]n order to do so, *this* discourse relies
> upon men viewing women as passive receptacles who must
> relinquish all control over their bodies, in "giving" them-
> selves, or in "giving" sex to their male partners. In return,
> the man must try to please the woman, which entails, in
> most cases, trying to "give" the woman an orgasm.
>
> —Gilfoyle, Wilson, and Brown,
> "Sex, Organs, and Audiotape"

Notably, the women I interviewed often conceived of orgasm as a kind of *gift* they received from a partner. Linguistically, the gift paradigm sig-nifies that women constructed their partners as having the power to *provide* orgasm *to* them rather than attributing the action to themselves. For example, 33-year-old Lori said, "I feel really good about my body and our relationship when he gives me an orgasm, and I think it kind of affirms him too, like he's been able to accomplish this thing, my pleasure, I mean." Though 43-year-old Dawn mentioned some mutual-ity, she echoed Lori's sentiment: "A lot of sex is timing, and that means we need connection. We give each other orgasms, but actually having physical intercourse doesn't happen as often as I might want it to." Bonnie, age 51, added another statement that implied the gift metaphor, saying, "I think he likes it when I orgasm. I think it makes him feel like, 'Oh, I'm talented' or whatever."

Women also regularly referred to their partners as *giving* them orgasm or doing things *to* them rather than situating themselves as fully embodied in the actions. For example, Margaret, age 54, took a rela-tively passive posture about *getting* orgasm from her partner: "I don't always orgasm. I've never had an orgasm through penetrative sex. So, usually after my husband has had his orgasm, he has to masturbate me in order for me to get an orgasm." Similarly, 24-year-old Ciara con-structed her husband as the *giver* of orgasm: "When I met my husband, he was able to give me an orgasm in different ways no one else had, so ever since then I enjoy sex and wish I could have sex with him every day if I could because he's the one that like did it for me." When dis-cussing her reasons for engaging in sex exclusively with women, Diana, age 50, talked about how men did *not* give her orgasms: "With men I had to use a vibrator to orgasm. Never once did a man give me an orgasm, either vaginally or through oral, clitorally. And, not always with women either." This suggests that women are stripped of their bodily agency and instead portrayed and experienced as objects that receive various external manipulations.

Likewise, the fact that lesbian and bisexual women described *giving* their female partners orgasms indicated that this construction of the gift metaphor appeared both in heterosexual relationships and in same-sex relationships. For example, lesbian-identified Leigh, age 21, described giving her partner an orgasm:

> Everybody likes orgasms but I think in most occasions I think I'd rather have my partner have an orgasm than me, because then I feel like, if I don't but that person does, I feel a sense of accomplishment with myself, but then if I do too that's like an added bonus. That's like my number one thing, to give her an orgasm, like that satisfies me when that happens to my partner.

Similarly, lesbian-identified Janet, age 21, described giving her partner orgasms as well:

> I just feel in the moment, I just let my body do whatever it's going to do. If it's going to orgasm it's going to orgasm, and if it's not then oh well, but with my girl it's like, if she doesn't orgasm . . . maybe her body just don't [sic] work right, or maybe mine don't work right. But it's like other times, like I said I'll make my girl orgasm a couple of times, or five or six times, and there'll be a puddle in the bed.

In lesbian relationships, the gift metaphor was sometimes mutual, where each partner *gave,* and neither partner *had* an orgasm. This implies that the gift metaphor applies to lesbian sexual relationships; even women who chose not to have sex with men still retained ideas about women's (lack of) sexual agency. In other words, it appears that gender socialization from an early age—oriented toward pleasing men and "receiving" orgasm—sticks with women regardless of their sexual identity as an adult. For example, 25-year-old Brynn described urges to please her partner via orgasm: "I'm more of a pleaser than needing to be pleased . . . I would rather please my partner than me have to be pleased. That said, you have to orgasm at least once. You have to get that out of you at least once. Otherwise, I would have to say something has to be done there, and there has to be some kind of communication to know what your partner's obviously not doing for you."

The gift paradigm also arose even when women discussed their own orgasms, as they distanced themselves from their bodily action. Some women, like Janet, seemed to claim that their body acted as a separate agent from their mind:

> I don't always orgasm, and sometimes I think it makes my girl feel like she's not doing something right, but it's not like that. I mean, I can't help that nothing comes out, that's not my problem you know? That's just my body, and if I orgasm I orgasm, and if I don't I don't. That's something you can't really control, like there's no button that you can just push and be like, "Orgasm now." I can't help what my body physically does, like whether I come or not.

When I asked Anita, age 46, about her feelings during orgasm, she described a similarly detached and mechanical sensation: "Sometimes he can make me orgasm, and I appreciate that. He'll just go to work on me, and I'll suddenly feel like my body gives an orgasm to him."

Interestingly, the gift paradigm almost never appeared when women discussed their male partner's orgasms, in that women did not construct themselves as "givers" of orgasm when having sex with men. More often, men *had* orgasms, rather than received them. Language of action and agency conferred upon men appeared repeatedly when discussing male orgasm, even while women ascribed responsibility for their own orgasms onto their (male) partners. For example, 54-year-old Marilyn described sex with her husband by saying, "He would always come. Well, he would have problems holding his erection, so he always came first . . . If he would hit the right spots, it wouldn't take very long, but um, he didn't always hit the right spot." Women only claimed agency in the act of "giving" their partner an orgasm when women discussed "giving" an orgasm to another woman or "giving" an orgasm to their (separated) bodies. To *have* an orgasm is to *get* an orgasm from someone else.

The tangible ways in which women's orgasm becomes a commodity here are startling; women's orgasms become products that partners (for Irigaray, *men*) invest labor into. As Luce Irigaray (1985) argued:

> Woman is traditionally a use-value for man, an exchange value among men; in other words, a commodity. As such, she remains the guardian of material substance, whose price will be established, in terms of the standard of their work and of their need/desire, by "subjects": workers, merchants, consumers. Women are marked phallically by their fathers, husbands, procurers. And this branding determines their value in sexual commerce. (pp. 31–32)

The demand for orgasm is complicated by the fact that it is linguistically difficult to construct the role of the supplier. If the orgasm is a commodity, what does this mean for women's experiences of it? How does the model of commodification affect their consciousness? Further, if one constructs women as themselves commodities, then what is the relationship between women (commodity 1) and orgasm (commodity 2)?

Demand for Orgasm

The clearly articulated demand from orgasm—something women perceived both directly and indirectly—contributed to the commodification of orgasm. When talking with women directly about orgasm, a prominent theme of feeling pressure to orgasm emerged, as women struggled both to *feel* pleasure and to demonstrate their pleasure to sexual partners. Often, this pressure was self-generated, as women described their partner's perceptions of pleasure as overshadowing their actual experience of that pleasure. This was well-articulated by Kate, age 25, who experienced a great deal of self-induced pressure to orgasm:

Putting pressure on myself to orgasm feels strange. For something that's supposed to happen spontaneously, supposedly, it feels like there's a lot of thought put into this and a lot of anxiety around it, like this is some kind of benchmark of not only the sex, but who this person is as a lover, or how I am as a lover, or how I am as a woman. It just is supposed to be an index of how liberated you are, how in touch with your body or yourself you are.

She went on to comment directly about orgasm as a kind of sexual performance:

I think it's always a performance to some extent, so it's just different degrees of conscious performance . . . I don't think I've faked it that often. Maybe a handful of times. Often times I was in a situation where it *did* seem to matter to the person, that they were performing well, or that they needed some kind of encouragement or some kind of reinforcement of their own experience. As I mentioned before, sex feels sometimes to me like a service. It's like, okay, I can do that thing for you if it's this important to you.

Other women articulated similar experiences, in that internally generated pressure to orgasm overshadowed the intrinsic pleasure they felt in the context of sex. Esther, age 44, articulated this when she said,

[Pressure to orgasm] makes it even harder. There's more tension, trying to figure out the right combination or position, the right stimulation or whatever, so that adds more pressure which means mostly likely it's not going to happen . . . I think that's like a society thing, because that's what we've been taught, you know, that women are supposed to have multiple orgasms, and if I'm not doing that, then there's something seriously wrong with me.

Other women directly perceived this pressure as overtly coming *from* their partners, indicating that the commodification of women's orgasms—and the construction of women's orgasms as *something partners invest labor into*—can be directly demanded from partners, particularly in heterosexual contexts. For example, Niko, age 23, said, "From my partners, I feel a lot of pressure. I feel like if a partner really wants me to feel good, orgasm probably means more to him than myself, so if I don't have an orgasm, it's a problem. When I'm by myself, I don't feel any pressure." When asked how this made her feel, she responded that she felt *pressured*: "In a way I feel very touched, but I also want to communicate to him that it's really not the most important thing to me, but it's hard to change how people see orgasm . . . He really wants me to have one. He really cares about me. I think it feels good emotionally to him, but I feel a lot of pressure." Jill, age 32, who described herself as completely nonorgasmic, communicated a similar sentiment of partner-induced pressure: "I have in the past felt as though my partner was trying to pressure me . . . I kind of got the impression that he was very invested in whether or not I had an orgasm and was somewhat annoyed or upset or distressed that he wasn't performing up to spec or something." Dorothy, age 19, communicated some of the hazards of being pressured into both sex *and* orgasm, saying, "I didn't even want to have sex in the first place! He'd say to me, 'I can't be done unless you're happy,' and it felt like so much pressure."

This feeling of partnered pressure appeared primarily in descriptions of heterosexual exchanges but also in the context of same-sex relationships. Bisexual women described that *both* men and women demanded the performance of orgasm, though the experience had different implications depending on the partner's gender. For example, Nora, age 23, said:

> Mostly I feel like it's a partner that pressures me to orgasm. There are a lot of men, again, that really expect you to, and it's been awkward with women even sometimes too. I guess with women I feel more pressured to pleasure them in turn, and that sometimes makes me feel uncomfortable. Whereas with men, I'm never really that worried because I like them to get off, but I know one way or another they can do it and that's not a big deal. Men will ask you, "Is it great?" You'll be like "Yeah, yeah." But usually it's more *them* that wants to get you off. I don't

enjoy it when a guy wants to get me off or is like looking for something to happen. I'm like, no man, you just need to do your thing, and it'll be fine. Don't waste 15 minutes trying to do whatever you're trying to do that's not really working.

This description reveals that eroticism remained laden with commodified overtones, particularly as the pressure to *give* orgasm overlapped with the pressure to *have* orgasm.

This does not suggest that all male partners were preoccupied with women's orgasms, though most women said that their male partners felt invested in ensuring that they had at least one orgasm. Some women, however, expressed ambivalence about how much their partner cared about their orgasms, at times citing length of the relationship as the predictor of increased pressure they felt to orgasm. This may reflect a pattern where length of relationship correlated with men's interest in women's orgasm, and as such, one-night stands or new relationships involved less concern for women's orgasms. For example, 23-year-old Courtney felt that short-term sexual encounters involved less pressure to orgasm:

I would say mostly guys don't really seem to care, but I think they enjoy it, and they like you to orgasm because that makes them feel better about themselves. It's just the ones that have really cared have been the ones that have had sex with me repeatedly for a while, and they're the guys that are more attentive to like, "Did you come?" Other guys, I felt like they didn't really care, like I'm sure they'd like me to, but it's not a must have.

Carol, age 38, also felt like her male partners did not always care about her orgasm, expressing both frustration and relief about this fact: "I've slept with men who don't seem to give a shit about whether I come. That makes me a little angry, but I also feel like I don't have to bother with faking." Clearly, these statements reveal the delicate balancing act that occurs about orgasm for those women currently in relationships, as partners *not* caring can feel as troubling as partners caring in a way that *demands* orgasm.

Self-blame about Orgasm

Many sex researchers have noted the profound psychological impact of differential experiences of orgasm for men and women (Tiefer, 2004). Because men more often say that they always or almost always orgasm in the context of sex, while women report a much wider range of orgasmic expression (e.g., many women report that, despite lifelong sexual activity, they have *never* had an orgasm), this difference can promote a complicated relationship between women and their orgasms (Laumann, Paik, & Rosen, 1999). Among the women I talked to, many struggled to achieve orgasm regularly during intercourse, and nearly all women commented that they did not *always* orgasm during intercourse without clitoral stimulation. This was occasionally framed as a response to their partner's inadequacies (e.g., Susan, age 45, said, "He just didn't do it for me. He wasn't skilled at oral sex at all"), though most often it was discussed as a failure of one's own ability to orgasm. Self-blame about not experiencing enough pleasure represented a major theme in my conversations with women. For example, 51-year-old Geena articulated the tension between not meeting other's expectations and not meeting her own:

> I've definitely felt pressured with a partner . . . I feel like if I didn't orgasm, the other person would think they were less, or they didn't do something well enough or right enough or good enough. That it would be somehow their fault. I don't believe that's true, because it's really up to me to have the orgasm. It lies with me, with my body; my body ultimately decides. Sometimes everything can be right with me, but my body doesn't want to have one . . . I'm either having too much internal dialogue, or I feel like I can't get into that moment. I'm more imagining what this looks like or some external view of this, and it's like I'm actually on stage as opposed to being in the moment with somebody. If I get stuck in that, I'm not going to be able to have an orgasm with somebody.

Ruth, age 46, echoed this sentiment even more forcefully, saying that she felt self-blame for not having an orgasm: "During times where I have not been able to orgasm, I felt worthless and angry at myself, like why would my body deny itself. It didn't make sense to me. I've never had an orgasm from intercourse though. It's always just been manually." Diana added that she felt distressed by a partner's impatience with her orgasm:

> When you have arousal and you're experiencing pleasure and being aroused and having an orgasm, that's letting your partner know that she's pleasuring you and that adds to her arousal and her complete experience, so yes, I feel pressure sometimes, because it helps her to feel more aroused . . . I've had a partner that gets impatient. I can feel her getting impatient . . . Ultimately, that's what you want, to please your partner. I certainly know how to pleasure a woman, but I want her to have an orgasm, definitely. If she's not, and I'm feeling inadequate, maybe she doesn't desire me, and there is no arousal, so maybe a little shame too.

Women who regularly experienced orgasm also mentioned self-blame surrounding orgasm as an important issue for them. Notably, orgasm as a *form of labor* inscribed as something (male) partners *invest into women* appeared frequently during the interviews. For example, Aya, age 25, described this context of labor directly: "I feel pressure from myself to orgasm, because I just feel like there's all that energy, like *work* that's being done that doesn't go anywhere. I'm really a very efficient person, so whenever that happens, it's like a waste. He wants to know that he can bring this about for me, and I want to show him that." Fiona, age 24, expressed similar feelings of wasted labor when discussing both male and female partners:

> I put pressure on myself to kind of coordinate an orgasm. For instance, if he was fingering me in my vagina and using his tongue, and/or I was using a toy, and it was just not progressing to a higher state of self-pleasure or pleasure in general, I think about how tired he's getting. I'm just kind of pressuring myself and saying that he's not interested anymore, that he's putting so much work into this. I do a lot of that kind of thinking, like thinking about how he's probably not enjoying himself rather

than focusing on how good it feels to for me. I used to feel that way with lesbians too, but at least lesbians could appreciate that feeling and had probably been in that position of having someone work on them for a long time and nothing was happening. With men, it can be really strenuous.

Self-blame about this lack of validation for (male) sexual labor was also communicated in women's frustrations at their sometimes inconsistent orgasmic ability. Priya, age 23, said, "It's just sort of frustrating when you want something to happen, and it's not happening, so you try and make it happen a little bit more. It's frustrating sometimes if you're trying to orgasm, and someone's trying to help you do that, and you just can't get there."

Thus, the self-blame women experience, and the blame they internalize from the outside world, maps directly onto other narratives that blame women for their perceived inadequacies, whether via rape myths that blame women for their own sexual victimization, mother blaming discourses that blame mothers (and *not* fathers) for all of children's shortcomings or delinquencies, or cultural tendencies to blame women for not being able to "keep their man." Each of these fits into women's *internalization of blame* as a key component of women's contemporary self-understanding.

Faking Orgasm

Given the amount of self-blame that surrounds inconsistent orgasmic expression, faking orgasm also represented a common technique to avoid the blame and pressure women felt to climax. This theme of faking orgasm appeared frequently in my discussions with women, as they invested sexual labor into the sexual exchange regardless of their actual physical experiences of orgasm. Questions of authenticity arose repeatedly when discussing sexual pleasure, as many women reported that they had successfully faked orgasm either occasionally or regularly, a finding consistent with recent research that suggests that over half of women have faked orgasm (Wiederman, 1997). Connected to discussions of performing well as a sexual partner, a majority of women reported that they had, with variable frequency, faked orgasm during sex with some of their partners in order to give the appearance that they enjoyed sex more than they actually did. Faking orgasm occurred not only in heterosexual couplings, but also in same-sex partnerships, though mention of faking orgasm in heterosexual couplings occurred far more often.

When asked about the reasons for faking orgasm, women reported that they faked for three primary reasons: First, to spare the partner's feelings; second, to end the sexual encounter and/or to encourage the partner to orgasm; third, to respond to the partner's pressure for them to orgasm. In many cases, women reported faking orgasm for all three reasons. For example, 29-year-old Mitra said:

> I fake often because, you know, he's going to feel bad about himself, or he's going to feel like I haven't enjoyed myself, so I just feel like I need to have one to make him happy, or sometimes you're tired and that's the signifier to be done. . . . I feel like orgasm is what sex is for men, and they think that that's what it is for women too. So, I feel like I could never really tell him that I'm faking, because men like to think, oh no one's ever faking with me. He's a good lover. It's not like he doesn't care about his partner's sexual satisfaction, and I think that makes me all the more compelled to fake. To me, it's much better to just fake it. Everyone's ego is intact, and you can just move on.

Courtney also claimed multiple reasons for faking orgasm, notably arguing that faking orgasm was a sign of her commitment or care for her partner:

> Usually if I fake an orgasm, it'll be just so I can go to bed because I'm tired, and I can see that that's what the guy is waiting for. I'll just fake it so that it can be over or because I really care about them and I want them to not walk away feeling like they were a let-down to me. Sometimes they could have been fine, and I could have had a good time, but since that's such a big factor in how guys value themselves, if I care about the person, I'll do it. Just telling them it was great doesn't work. They'll walk away and be like, "Yeah right, whatever, you didn't

come." I fake it when I care about the person, cause I'm not going to fake it if I don't really care. That's almost as much energy as having one!

Many heterosexual women claimed that faking orgasm allowed them to spare a partner's feelings, a theme that directly reveals the way in which cultural scripts demand attention to, and concern for, *men's* pleasure above that of *women's* pleasure. Such concern for the feelings of women's partners indicated an expectation for women to nurture and care for others (particularly men) in their lives. For example, Marilyn felt urgent about pleasing her husband: "I faked just to make him happy, and I'd just say I did to make him happy. We go back to the same thing. It was about pleasing him and keeping him happy. It was always, 'Was it as good for you as it was for me?' Oh yeah honey, oh yeah. So, you know, you just make the sounds that you did when you really didn't." Women spoke, at least implicitly, about the way in which their sexual partnerships demanded that they serve as a mirror for their partner's egos, such as Bonnie, who said, "I have faked it sometimes. I did it just to make [my] partner feel good or think that they've done a good job. I don't think it makes me feel bad or anything. It's just sort of something you do." When I asked Margaret why she faked orgasm, she responded by noting that she wanted to protect her husband's feelings: "Faking orgasm is strange, a bit theatrical really, and you're doing it for your partner, not for you. I did it probably because the other person was obviously into their own orgasm and seemed to expect that you were going to join in with whatever was going on for him at the time. I didn't want him to feel inadequate."

One can interpret these statements, perhaps, as a gesture of love and affection toward partners, as orgasms symbolize a kind of unique affirmation that *both* partners typically perceive as important. For example, when asked why she faked orgasm, Janet added that she wanted her partner to feel like a competent lover: "Because I felt like if I wasn't responding in any way, she'd really feel like she wasn't doing her job, or doing what she was supposed to be doing or she might feel like she was doing something wrong you know? I wanted to make her feel all right." Esther, who said she faked orgasm 80 to 90% of the time, echoed these sentiments, claiming that sparing the partner's feelings mattered more than her experience:

I don't want the person I am with to feel like they're not able to do what they think they should be able to do. If they think that they're good in bed, they wanna please a woman, and if I don't fake it, then there's something wrong with them, and they're not pleasing me, so that's part of my giving. Okay, I'll let you think that's what you did, but you actually didn't.

When asked how that made her feel, she responded, "A little bit guilty because it's a lie, but at the same time I feel like I'm building their ego, helping them feel okay as a man." Such statements suggest that, while, superficially, faking orgasm may symbolize deeply internalized oppression (e.g., one's own pleasure as frankly less significant than one's partner's pleasure), faking orgasm may also represent, for women, a gesture of care, affection, love, and nurturance.

On the more practical side—and perhaps indicative of women's busy, hectic lives that often demand caretaking of others—faking orgasm also resulted from fatigue and exhaustion. Indeed, most women reported working outside the home *and* doing a majority of the housework. Women sometimes said that they faked orgasm because they were physically and psychologically drained and wanted to stop the sexual interaction and rest. For example, Dorothy faked in order to end sex and go to sleep:

Sometimes with the "pressure guy" I'd be tired, and he just wanted to have sex, so I was like fine, let's have sex, but then he'd be like, "We can't finish until you have an orgasm." I'm like, "I'm tired, why can't you just let me be?" So to him, it wouldn't be complete unless I was fully satisfied . . . I faked it because I just wanted to be done with it, I guess, like it's 2:00 a.m., and I'm tired and want to put an end to it.

At times, this physical exhaustion was connected to emotional weariness or boredom with sex. For example, Susan said, "I've faked orgasms to get it over with. I wanted to go to sleep, or it was just kinda getting boring. It's like, all right already! Maybe this will help you. I'll scream a little bit and writhe about and then you can come, and I can go to sleep and you can go home."

Many women faked orgasm as a direct result of their partner's pressure to orgasm, revealing the way that sexual performance is at times *demanded* and *expected* both explicitly and implicitly. For example, Brynn faked in order to avoid conflict:

> I have faked an orgasm in order to just be able to have that person be like, "Oh okay, finally, they climaxed" or whatever. I don't have to worry about anything, and I can just let them have their ego trip. It just kind of got them off my back . . . If I didn't fake an orgasm, or if I didn't fake being pleased, then it was like he's obviously not done, and he's going to just keep pounding the hell outta ya until he hears something. I faked it all the time with him.

Charlotte, age 34, also faked to avoid conflict: "I've faked it because I knew he was wanting to do it, and I didn't want to turn him away and say nah I don't feel like it, or be mean or nothing [sic]. I wasn't really all the way into it, and he would be angry if he knew that."

Sometimes, partners communicated pressure to orgasm directly and intensely, often by using emotional manipulation, as in 44-year-old Charlene's description of her ex-husband:

> I've faked it because there were times where if I didn't seem to have one quick enough for him, then he would like start with the whole guilt thing, like, "You don't really love me do you?" kind of thing. If I was honest about not coming, he would say that it was a symbol of me not loving him . . . Once someone says you're not having an orgasm because you don't love me, it's pretty hard to have an orgasm then. I'd just fake it and that made him happy, so the pressure's gone now. So far as he's concerned, I always had one! He'd get off my back, excuse the pun!

Faking orgasm represents a complex emotional response to the intensely patriarchal culture in which women have sex and to the emotional dynamics of particular relationships. Among those I interviewed, faking orgasm allowed women to avoid guilt and shame about not experiencing orgasm as often as (or in the way that) they or their partners would like. Many women felt that their partners put a significant amount of emotional energy into their orgasms. As seen with the previous examples, the question remains open as to whether this pressure to orgasm represents a genuine indicator of generosity or affection; certainly, it seems clear that women's orgasms matter less than their *performances* of those orgasms.

Faking orgasm did not seem to correlate with women's level of sexual experience, orgasmic ability, or number of partners, though sex with men predicted faking orgasm. For example, highly-experienced and highly orgasmic Nora told me, matter-of-factly, "Generally all those situations where you're coerced into it by men or give into it or are pushed into having sex, you end up faking the orgasm and faking the pleasure. No doubt about it—just because you're like, 'Okay fine, let's just do this,' and you totally fake it. That's the easiest way to get rid of a situation sometimes." Maria, age 21, echoed this sentiment, saying, "I always faked orgasm with men, just to make it stop. I couldn't have been less interested in it, and I felt like if I didn't orgasm, they'd get angry and maybe violent."

Women who had never experienced orgasm also described frequent instances of faking orgasm. For example, Jill reprimanded herself for her lack of orgasmic ability:

> I am not entirely certain that I have ever in my life had an orgasm . . . My body does not seem to necessarily respond properly to things, so it's mostly my brain that's getting off . . . It would be nice [to orgasm]. I would like to know what all the fuss is about . . . I exaggerate the degree of pleasure I receive from something that I either think my partner enjoys or wish to encourage as it's headed in at least the right direction.

Similarly, Pam, age 42, who admitted to irregular orgasms, said that she often participated in various kinds of theatrics with her husband to encourage him to ejaculate: "You scream a little, deeper or whatever. You exaggerate. You use words, and you just hope."

Interestingly, one woman who claimed that she had never faked an orgasm said that she may consider doing so if the need arose, indicating the degree of acceptance and complicity women have in normalizing faking orgasm as an acceptable part of life. Newlywed Lucy, age 25, said,

I haven't [faked orgasm] yet. As silly as this sounds, at a girl-friend's house, they were trying to teach us how to fake orgasm, and I fully got into it because I haven't had to fake, so I'm kind of nervous. If at some point, if I didn't come repeat-edly . . . I don't know what I would do, because honestly, I don't know if I would fake it or not. As of right now, I've been honest with him, but I might fake it!

When asked why she would feel the need to fake it, she responded that faking orgasm represents being a "good wife":

Just that if my husband was trying to get me off, and I wasn't able to come, especially if it happened when he was trying to put forth effort, taking his time, and doing everything right, and he's still not able to, and if I didn't have a good reason, like I was not feeling sick or something, then I would probably feel bad. More than anything I wouldn't want him to feel bad . . . I hear so many women do, and she was trying to teach us, and she was like, "You need to be good to your husband! Be good to him!"

These statements indicate the intensity of the normative pressures women (particularly heterosexual women) face to put their partner's sexual needs, satisfaction, and desires above their own.

Even women who consciously resisted this often admitted difficulty with full honesty about orgasm with their partners. Julie, age 23, described a history of faking orgasm and vowed never to again return to faking orgasm rather than communicating authentic pleasure:

I hate faking orgasm and the pressure I feel, partly because I simply *refuse* to fake it. I used to fake it sometimes and then I realized that's a horrible thing to do. In the past, particularly my male partners have been like, "Are you coming? Are you coming?" I want to say, "Yeah," because, you know, for their little egos, but I sometimes do feel pressured. Most of the time, though, I just sort of insist on orgasms with my partners. Sometimes I really want one, and it's just not happening because the stars haven't aligned!

Thus, orgasm, in its many manifestations, reflects a number of dynamics in women's relationships: perceptions that they must please (male) partners at their own expense, concern for feeling sexually normal, and avoidance of negative consequences, whether emotional, physical, psychological, or literal.

CONCLUSION

This chapter provides a nuanced picture of the role of orgasm in women's lives, as despite the fact that women typically construct orgasm as an essential part of good sex, women often reported feeling a great deal of pressure to orgasm in order to *confirm* the "goodness" of the sex or the partnership. This pressure in part stems from the history of orgasm laid out in the first half of the chapter, as orgasm routinely symbolized a battleground about oppression, liberation, and sexual freedom. If orgasm once seemed like a distant dream to many women suffering within marriages and partnerships devoid of mutual pleasure, their newfound freedom to embrace orgasm (particularly clitoral orgasm) may have signified a major sign of progress. From the Victorian days to the advent of psychoanalysis, from the early empiricists to the sexual revolution, orgasm has stood in for much more than a mere physiological process. It harbors a great history of gender relations, power struggles, and political symbolism. This makes it all the more imperative to examine its meaning today, particularly as women experience this new *mandate* to orgasm as a defining feature of their status as "good sexual partners."

Part of the reason that faking orgasm, responding to pressure to orgasm, and constructing orgasm as a "gift" have such prominence in women's lives may be the way women learn to internalize ideas about orgasm as the primary reason for sex (itself a common cultural script) *and* because they constantly receive messages (from partners, from the media, from schools, from the culture at large) that women's pleasure matters less than men's pleasure. If women and men learn about sex from *families*, who often communicate that women should "not give it up" (Dilorio, Pluhar, & Belcher, 2003; Fingerson, 2005; Raffaelli & Ontai, 2001); from the *media*, which communicates that women are pieces of meat that others can consume and mold into the cultural whims of the day (Adams, 2003); from *pornography*, which normalizes not only extreme sexual power differentials but also flattens out women's orgasmic pleasure into constant moaning and thrashing devoid of any real climax; from *schools*, which routinely teach women that male ejaculation and ejaculate plays a central role in sex while their orgasms are rarely mentioned; and from *early partners*, who often bumble through premature ejaculation, distorted sexual socialization, and poorly socialized ways of treating women, women clearly face disadvantages with regard to their orgasms.

An important contradiction is also communicated to women as they negotiate their orgasms, in that women perceive that their partners value their pleasure, yet women still feel pressured not to fluctuate in their orgasmic ability. Most women experience their orgasms as somewhat scattered, fluid, inconsistent, flexible, and *highly* contingent upon the circumstances of the encounter. Again and again, women felt that their partners indicated that it was *unacceptable* for women not to orgasm during every sexual encounter. (To know whether men perceive this as true, more studies about men's subjective experiences with sex are needed). For women, the range of negativity that arose from this fact—from shame about their body's "failures," feelings of resentment toward partners for their lack of support, conflict about how to manage their need to support their partners' egos while sacrificing their own pleasure, and inability to explore different means of achieving orgasm— speaks to the conflicts and contradictions at hand when women negotiate sexual pleasure. Even if, hypothetically, women could orgasm 100% of the time, these narratives reveal that women would likely face *new* performance pressures, such as pressures to experience multiple orgasms during every sexual encounter. As it stands now, women, their bodies, their desire, and their orgasms are too often constructed as *commodities*, as *mirrors* to an investment of labor, and as beholden to cultural scripts that deprioritize them. Signs of real mutuality—where orgasm is seen as a complex and sometimes inconsistent bodily reaction to a variety of mental, emotional, physical, and psychological stimuli—remain sorely lacking in women's narratives of their sexual relationships. Women expressed concern about the *demand* they felt surrounding orgasm, which led them to feel inadequate and, at times, disappointed.

Indeed, one painful dimension of this chapter's findings is that faking orgasm may itself signify a gesture of *love* more than anything else. Not only did women discuss orgasm as something a partner *gave* to them, but they, in turn, frequently made attempts to sacrifice their own orgasmic pleasure in the name of affirming a partner's abilities or not hurting a partner's feelings. This presents a real dilemma: If women prone to faking orgasm fully disclose when they do or do not orgasm, this may emotionally wound some of their sexual partners. Is there a space where women can feel liberated enough *not* to orgasm and *not* to fake orgasm, if they choose? If women and their orgasms are constructed as *commodities*, how can women meaningfully resist the demands of those who construct them as objects? If women's orgasms symbolize (male) sexual prowess, how does this affect women's sexual consciousness? What does this dilemma reveal about sexual relationships, gender, orgasm, and power?

In moving toward a more up-to-date liberatory politics of orgasm, several possibilities become apparent. First, if people deconstruct and dismantle the existing definitions of pleasure and satisfaction, such that orgasm is one of *many* forms of pleasure women can experience, this opens up space to value other forms of pleasure that women enjoy. By not overvaluing orgasm at the exclusion of other acts (e.g., physical tenderness, extended arousal, power play, kissing, helping a partner to feel pleasure, flirting, deep intimacy, etc.), this lessening of urgency might facilitate better communication between partners about orgasm and increased pleasure more broadly. If orgasm remains the quintessentially authentic sexual act, this denies the fact that even the so-called *real* orgasm carries dimensions of performance within it. (Even among biologists, there is considerable debate about how to determine when a "real" orgasm has occurred, let alone what women's orgasms actually *do* in an evolutionary or social sense [Lloyd, 2005]). To avoid this double bind, people should expand definitions of pleasure such that orgasm is rendered one of many ways to enjoy the body and sexuality.

A second possibility when addressing the findings of this chapter is to recognize and value the enormous compassion that is *possible*, but not always present, in women's efforts to support their partner's egos *and* in their partner's desires to satisfy them. Evidence of this compassion is fundamental to discussions of how women relate to their part-

ners sexually and holistically. Women want to reflect back to their partners the affirmation that their partners long for; this is not itself problematic. The troubling elements here are the *terms* within which this
affirmation is demanded or extracted, particularly if these terms
demand performances that reproduce gender inequalities. How might
women and their partners differently negotiate affirmation, sexual
pleasure, and the mutual rewards of sex? Can orgasm become a *means*
toward something rather than an *end* goal? If women *have* orgasms
rather than *get* them as a "gift," will this facilitate a greater sense of
embodiment and empowerment? Might better communication about
orgasm facilitate more equitable relationships in general? Among these
interview participants, highly orgasmic women not inclined to fake
orgasm also were the women who had the most equitable relationships
with their partners, a fact that speaks to the symbiosis among sexual,
interpersonal, and cultural scripts. As this chapter shows, by examining
orgasm as a literal and symbolic marker of equality and inequality, one
can better explore the interplay among gender, power, sexuality, and
culture. As Elizabeth Grosz (1995a) has argued, such inquiries about
orgasm can help with "establishing new alliances, new connections
between and among bodies, desires, pleasures, powers, cruising the borders of the obscene, the pleasurable, the desirable, the mundane and the
hitherto unspoken" (p. xi) even while the study of orgasm may feel like
"a great disloyalty—speaking the (philosophically) unsayable, spilling
the beans on a vast historical 'secret,' about which many men and
women have developed prurient interests" (Grosz, 1995b, p. 279).

CHAPTER TWO

COMPULSORY BISEXUALITY?

The Challenges of Modern Sexual Fluidity

> So there is, *for women*, no possible law for their pleasure. No
> more than there is any possible discourse . . . If there is such
> a thing—still—as feminine pleasure, then, it is because men
> need it in order to maintain themselves in their own exis-
> tence. It is *useful* to them: it helps them bear what is intol-
> erable in their world as speaking beings, to have a soul for-
> eign to that world: a fantasmatic one . . . But it does not
> suffice, of course, for this soul to remain simply external to
> their universe. It must also be rearticulated with the 'body'
> of the speaking subject. It is *necessary* that the fusion of the
> soul—fantasmatic—and the body—transcribed from lan-
> guage—be accomplished with the help of their 'instru-
> ments': in feminine sexual pleasure.
> —Luce Irigaray, *This Sex Which Is Not One*

ADRIENNE RICH, in her classic and highly-influential 1980 essay,
"Compulsory Heterosexuality and the Lesbian Existence," argued,

[E]nforced submission and the use of cruelty, if played out in
the heterosexual pairing, is "normal," while sensuality between
women, including erotic mutuality and respect, is "queer,"
"sick," and either pornographic in itself or not very exciting
compared with the sexuality of whips and bondage. Pornography does not simply create a climate in which sex and violence

are interchangeable; *it widens the range of behavior considered acceptable from men in heterosexual intercourse*—behavior which reiteratively strips women of their autonomy, dignity, and sexual potential, including the potential of loving and being loved by women in mutuality and integrity. (p. 234)

Extending Rich's argument about the ways in which heterosexuality is not a choice, but rather, something enforced as the "normal," "natural," and socially acceptable necessity, this chapter considers the relatively new and rapidly proliferating phenomenon of heterosexual-identified women reporting that they engage in "performative bisexuality" in an effort to conform to what they perceive as sexually normal. Unlike other forms of bisexual erotic behavior, performative bisexuality is defined primarily as engaging in homoerotic acts with other women, usually *in front of* men and in the context of *social* settings. For example, heterosexual women increasingly report that, if they engage in homoerotic behavior, it occurs *exclusively* in settings like fraternity parties, bars, clubs, and other crowded, sexualized spaces. In my sample, while this was more common among younger women (18–38), older women (39–59) also reported an increase in pressures from their partners to engage in homoerotic acts. Further, 69% of heterosexual-identified women in the sample reported some form of same-sex behavior or attraction, and many of these women engaged in same-sex erotic behavior in front of men. These pieces of information raise questions about how these performances of bisexuality—where women literally act out bisexual behavior in front of men—imply that women's sexuality is often shaped to fit new manifestations of compulsory heterosexuality. Like all performances, the distinction between individual choice (e.g., "I choose to kiss women in front of my boyfriend") and cultural scripts (e.g., "Women are sexy if they kiss women in front of their boyfriends but do not identify as bisexual") is again blurred. This chapter explores the implications of this conundrum and the way in which many young heterosexual women report that performances of bisexual behavior feel compulsory or required in order to be sexually-validated within their heterosexual relationships or the heteronormative culture at large. Further, this behavior may challenge the conventional precepts of compulsory heterosexuality while also serving as an extension of compulsory heterosexuality, a paradox explored throughout this chapter.

Notably, what I term "compulsory bisexuality" arises out of "compulsory heterosexuality" and does not carry the same literal implications of compulsory heterosexuality. For example, the term *compulsory heterosexuality* functions as an *absolute mandate* for women to comply with, and it has dire consequences for those who violate it (e.g., hate crimes, job loss, discrimination, moral condemnations, etc.). Compulsory bisexuality—if there is such a thing—has far fewer severe consequences, in that women may suffer from social and economic consequences for not participating in these new sexual norms, but they will not likely experience them with nearly the same severity or penalties as they would with compulsory heterosexuality. Women performing as bisexual might arouse men precisely because it *violates* compulsory heterosexuality while still referencing it. Women do not stray far from the compulsory demands of *including men as their objects of desire* even while they technically choose women to "hook up" with. As such, the compulsory qualities of this behavior may be a reflection of how, for women, social norms take on qualities of *pressure, co-optation of power*, and, in some cases, *coercion*. Further, the compulsory qualities of bisexuality likely have drastically different meanings for those who identify as heterosexual compared with those who identify as lesbian or bisexual.

Building on chapter 1's analysis of women performing orgasm to please partners, chapter 2 closely considers the complexities of performative bisexuality as it relates to women's modern sexual lives and political attitudes. This chapter includes an exploration of women feeling pressured to perform sexual acts with women while having a male audience, their feelings about witnessing other women engaging in this behavior, and their reactions to *Girls Gone Wild* videos (i.e., performative bisexuality on camera). Further, the chapter explores women's experiences with same-sex attraction and/or activity and their sometimes conflicting political attitudes about homosexuality in light of these new trends of performative bisexuality for women. Key questions include: Does performative bisexuality represent a progressive trend of increasing acceptance toward bisexuality for women? Or is performative bisexuality a reactionary manifestation of ever-increasing efforts to control and manipulate women's sexuality for the purpose of serving

men's pleasure? What does it mean if it represents *both* of these positions
or even a middle position where *elements* of exploitation and empowerment inform this bisexual behavior? Is performative bisexuality indeed
(as Adrienne Rich suggested about heterosexuality) "compulsory," and
if so, how does that translate into women's sexual consciousness? How
does performative bisexuality *violate* compulsory heterosexuality while
also referencing it?

RESEARCH ON BISEXUALITY

> In a sex obsessed world, it appeared that no one wanted to
> know about bisexual sex. Why? Well, because it's not a
> "real" sexual orientation somehow. Reading about it is con-
> fusing because bisexuals themselves are just confused.
> Besides it's just a phase. Did I mention that bi is code for
> gay? And, you know, it's just a trendy way for straight girls
> to fit in with other radical and oppressed folks.
> —Baumgardner (2007), *Look Both Ways*

Research on bisexuality has revealed its contentious and often ambiguous qualities. Interpretations of what "counts" as bisexual vary widely
across groups, as some identify bisexuals as those who have *ever* had
sexual encounters with the same-sex, while others point to bisexuality
as a chosen political and social identity that does not require sexual
contact with the same sex. Others argue that bisexuality is a vehicle
through which women decide whether to be gay or heterosexual,
while still others claim that bisexuality is a legitimate and permanent
identity category. Some point to the chic and hip qualities of bisexual
identity, while others question whether the gay rights movement
should include bisexuals at all. Still others claim that bisexuality is a
transitory phase and not a real identity per se; constructs like "lesbian
until graduation" and "bisexual until graduation" speak to this assumption (Baumgardner, 2007). The popular *New York Times* article
"Straight, Gay, or Lying? Bisexuality Revisited" (Carey, 2005) touched
upon the reluctance on the part of mainstream media to accept bisexuality as a *real or fixed* sexual identity. This confusion is of course com-
pounded by the increasing emergence of performative bisexuality,

where women often deny the significance of same-sex encounters even while engaging in them, thus further challenging the meaning of bisexuality as an identity.

Examining the research, these tensions become increasingly clear. Bisexual experiences for women are relatively common. A recent study found that 11% of women ages 15–44 reported having had some form of sexual experience with women, and women were three times more likely than men to have had both men and women as partners in the last year. Younger women more often had same-sex encounters (Mosher, Chandra, & Jones, 2005). Thoughts or proclivities toward bisexuality are also common among women who call themselves heterosexual. After studying heterosexual-identified women from three geographic regions in the United States, 30% reported same-sex feelings (Hoburg et al., 2004). This number represents the considerable variability and sexual fluidity among women as compared to men, who are much less likely to report same-sex attractions and feelings (Laumann et al., 1994). Further, women's same-sex encounters occur often in the context of pleasing male partners' desires for threesomes, as research has shown that men tend to fantasize about group sex, particularly with multiple women (Wilson, 1987). Other research has found that significant numbers of women have had sexual encounters with other women outside of the context of men (Baumgardner, 2007), which presents a challenge *both* to compulsory heterosexuality and compulsory bisexuality.

Lisa Diamond (2003), in her longitudinal work on women's sexuality, found that those women who identified as bisexual or lesbian during their late teens and early 20s mostly did not lose their feelings of attraction to other women when surveyed five years later; in fact, 75% of them still identified as bisexual or lesbian five years later, and of the 25% who no longer identified as bisexual or lesbian, half adopted the label "heterosexual," and half abandoned labels altogether. This research points to bisexuality not simply as a phase but rather as a stable social identity. In Diamond's 2008 study, she found that women conceptualized bisexuality not as a transitional stage that they outgrew as they got older, but rather, as a label that *more* women adopted over time. Few women in her longitudinal sample relinquished bisexual and lesbian identities, indicating that sexual fluidity constitutes a central part of bisexual women's lives. These studies do *not*, however, account for women who engage in same-sex eroticism but still claim heterosexuality, as in the case of performative bisexuality.

Conflict about bisexual identity represents a common theme in research that addresses the topic. Moore (2005) found that bisexuals spoke in more conflicted ways about their sexuality than did heterosexuals or gay/lesbian individuals. Women have increasingly adopted the labels *bisexual* and *unlabeled* for their sexual identities rather than lesbian/gay identities, both as a descriptor and as a philosophical statement about being noncategorical (Savin-Williams, 2005). Bisexuality has also been adopted more and more by those who want to deconstruct traditional models of sexual identity, as bisexual takes on a more fluid and malleable quality than heterosexual or lesbian identity (Blumstein & Schwartz, 1990; Rust, 1992). This is further complicated by the idea that women's sexual desires "are even more situation dependent and less 'category specific' than those of men" (Diamond, 2008, p. 6). Ultimately, bisexual identity challenges people not to imagine a "third" sexual identity but rather to destabilize sexual identity itself (Garber, 1995). This raises the question: If women choose to *label* themselves a certain way, does this also reflect what they *want* sexually? How can performative bisexuality be differentiated from authentic bisexuality, or can it?

Historical Context

The historical context of bisexuality also reveals a fluidity of both definition and meaning, as scholars, sexologists, and theorists have struggled to situate bisexuality in relationship to heterosexuality and homosexuality for quite some time. As Jeffrey Weeks (1990) has argued, one must distinguish "between homosexual behaviour, which is universal, and a homosexual identity, which is historically specific" (p. 3). Thus, while bisexual *behavior* has existed as a persistent fact of human life, bisexual *'identity'* as a fixed concept represents a cultural invention that shifts in meaning as concepts like 'heterosexuality' and 'homosexuality' arise as opposites. As Angelides (2001) said, "[T]he elision of bisexuality from the present tense has been one of the primary discursive strategies employed in an effort to avoid a collapse of sexual boundaries—*a crisis of sexual identity*" (p. 17).

While much evidence suggests that male bisexuality was considered normative even as early as antiquity (though often labeled "homosexuality" by historians today despite the inaccuracy of the label), the history of women's bisexuality is much vaguer. While coming of age rituals sometimes involved men going through a homosexual stage during adolescence, women's bisexuality has rarely been constructed as ritualistic or a "normal" part of history (Ryan, 2007). The poet Sappho represents one notable exception to the dearth of female bisexual figures, as she was widely celebrated for her bisexual romantic and physical connections with others (Greene, 1999). Notably, however, the words *bisexual*, *homosexual*, and *heterosexual* did not appear until the 19th century, before which people did not acquire labels based upon *who* they felt erotically attracted to.

The nineteenth century ushered in a reconfiguration of thinking about bisexuality in the Western world. As heterosexuality and homosexuality gained momentum as opposite social identities, bisexuality emerged as a third possibility. In response to the changing sexual mores of the Victorian period, women's bisexual behavior led to attributions of them as "mad" and "unstable," as any expression of sexual interest was met with disdain during the age of propriety and modesty. Foucault (1978) said, "[O]ne had to speak of [sex] as of a thing to be not simply condemned or tolerated but managed, inserted into systems of utility, regulated for the greater good of all, made to function according to an optimum. Sex was not something that one simply judged; it was a thing one administered" (p. 24). Sigmund Freud (2000) proposed that bisexuality was an innate condition toward which every child had a predisposition. He argued that, via the process of sexual development, monosexuality (interest in only one gender) took hold and drove bisexuality into latency.

Later in the 20th century, Alfred Kinsey (1948; 1953) also famously found that 37% of men had had orgasm via contact with another man, thus asserting that sexual orientation should occur along a scale from zero (exclusively heterosexual) to six (exclusively homosexual). For women, Kinsey rated at least 10% of them as being a 3, 4, 5, or 6 on the Kinsey scale. He repeatedly argued that a large percentage of the overall population occupied the bisexual categories 1 through 5. These findings laid the foundation for the suggestion that sexual identity could *not* be described as exclusively heterosexual or exclusively homosexual, but rather that bisexuality may in fact be more normative than heterosexuality and homosexuality when the range of sexual behavior practices are fully accounted for.

Acceptance or Exploitation?

When examining popular culture today, increased visibility for bisexuality is apparent, perhaps because, as recent studies have shown, women's bisexual behavior typically turns heterosexual men on (Kimmel & Plante, 2002) and because women engage in experimental bisexual behavior, particularly with female friends, at an increasing rate (Thompson, 2007). Several television shows have begun to explore women's bisexuality, often involving a story arc in which the characters explore their bisexual feelings and then ultimately revert back to identifying as mostly heterosexual. Such characters as Claire on *Six Feet Under*, Samantha on *Sex in the City*, Buffy on *Buffy the Vampire Slayer*, Julia on *Nip/Tuck*, and Marissa on *The O.C.* serve as examples of mainstream television shows testing public acceptance of such sexual identity exploration. Notably, however, none of these women remained bisexual or lesbian for the remainder of the season. The only shows that have depicted heterosexual women choosing bisexuality or lesbian identity in a more permanent way include those shows like *The L Word* (notably on premium cable) that specifically promote themselves as lesbian shows. Films that depict bisexual and lesbian characters most often earn reputations as non-mainstream Indie films. Some examples include: *But I'm a Cheerleader, Election, High Art, Imagine Me and You, My Summer of Love, Puccini for Beginners, Gia, If These Walls Could Talk 1 and 2, Fire,* and *Kissing Jessica Stein*.

In contrast to the relatively thoughtful portrayals of women exploring different interpretations of sexual identity, the past several years have also ushered in a dramatic increase in the number of television shows that rely upon bisexuality as a form of crass entertainment. Howard Stern, with his taunting and objectification of "bisexual" women, has long encouraged women to behave as bisexual while on his show. In line with the highly publicized kiss between Britney Spears and Madonna at the 2003 Video Music Awards, shows like *A Shot at Love with Tila Tequila, Double Shot at Love, Flavor of Love, Next, The Real World, Parental Control, Rock of Love*, and *Elimidate* represent the exploitation of women's same-sex eroticism, as women kiss, engage in sexual banter, and sometimes compete for each other, typically in front of men either literally or virtually. Movies like *American Pie 2* and *Cruel Intentions* also follow these trends.

The proliferation of *Girls Gone Wild* videos—in which women show their breasts, hook up with other women on camera, and sometimes show their genitals or masturbate on camera—reveals the changing landscape of bisexual acceptance, particularly forms of bisexuality that can be appropriated into the male gaze. Ariel Levy (2005) wrote of this trend: "It sounds like a fantasy world dreamed up by teenage boys. A world of sun and sand where frozen daiquiris flow from faucets and any hot girl you see will peel off her bikini top, lift up her skirt . . . all you have to do is ask. It's no surprise that there's a male audience for this, but what's strange is that the women who populate this alternate reality are not strippers or paid performers, they are middle-class college kids on vacation—they are mainstream. And really, their reality is not all that unusual" (p. 17). Central to every *Girls Gone Wild* video is also the display of "friends" who kiss, fondle, and sometimes perform oral sex on each other. Levy recounts one scene from a recent *Girls Gone Wild* event (such events have notably included contests like "girl-on-girl box eating"): "'Girls! This is not a wet T-shirt contest' the MC bellowed over the sound system. 'Pretend you are fucking. Let me emphasize, pretend you are *really* fucking! I want you to pretend like you're fucking the shit out of her doggy style.' The women were too inebriated to achieve sufficient verisimilitude" (p. 14). The texture of these incidents reveals the challenges of deciding how to label these events—does this represent more acceptance of bisexuality in the mainstream culture? Or does it represent something else?

Hand in hand with such feigned acceptance is the potential for exploitation and manipulation of women's sexual identity fluctuations. For example, Baumeister (2000) found that women's sexualities tend to respond more readily to sociocultural and situational factors, regardless of sexual orientation. While this fact does not *justify* exploitation, it can help to explain why bisexuality as a *trend* has taken hold. Women's sexuality shifts in response to changing social trends and pressures more readily than men's sexuality, which can be particularly dangerous in a patriarchal climate that often exploits women and their bodies. On the positive side, such plasticity may make women more tolerant toward sexual variations as they "adapt to changing *cultural* scripts and expectations, along with making adaptations in the context of particular partners. Women may benefit by being more open to trying new things that partners suggest, seeking and taking advice about sex, and developing their sexual selves. But the detriment is that women may be more susceptible to pressure and coercion and more prone to confusion and discontinuity in their sexual lives" (Plante, 2006a, p. 223). Such plasticity may make temporary or transient bisexual identification possible, as women internalize messages that it is okay for them to experiment sexually with other women. At the same time, such plasticity may only be contextual and may not indicate any type of real attitudinal change. Moreover, if the behavior change only occurs in order to impress men, this constructs women as having the potential to be easily manipulated by the changing whims of the culture.

In the case of *Girls Gone Wild*, Jerry Springer, and "shock jocks," the films and shows exploit for profit the normative pressures women experience that tell them to behave as bisexual in front of men. Notably, women do not receive payment for their participation in *GGW* films (though they sometimes, ironically, receive t-shirts), and viewers are led to believe that women voluntarily want to engage in these behaviors both on and off camera. As Plante (2006a) argued:

> The video company markets their products by highlighting "young girls" subject to "no rules, no parents." They are "sweet innocent Daddy's girls" whose "corruption" occurs for your viewing pleasure. The women who engage in "girl on girl" sex are constructed as simultaneously sexually wild and innocent, coaxed into performing for the cameras "for the first time," outside the bounds of social conventions like heterosexuality, sex with men, and Daddy's implicit expectations that a girl like

his daughter would never do such a thing! We are led to believe that these innocent, white, "blond," college i.e., middle-class or upper middle-class girls are reluctantly showing the camera things they do anyway, but normally in the privacy of their own fantasies and (dorm) rooms. (p. 222)

Levy (2005) raises questions about the liberatory potential of this behavior: "And how is imitating a stripper or a porn star—a woman whose *job* is to imitate arousal in the first place—going to render us sexually liberated?" (p. 5). This implies that *real* acceptance of bisexuality is not inherent to its proliferation in the mainstream media. Just because women perform as bisexual, it does not suggest that they necessarily *want* to do these things; rather, it may indicate that this represents the newest form of selling women empowerment via exploitation. In essence, this hearkens back to the common strategies in advertisement, in which advertisers turn an apparently liberating practice into a commodity, much like Virginia Slims used women's newfound entry into the workplace as a way to sell cigarettes (Toll & Ling, 2005). With regard to performative bisexuality, Levy goes on to argue, "A tawdry, tarty, cartoonlike version of female sexuality has become so ubiquitous, it no longer seems particular. What we once regarded as a *kind* of female sexual expression we now view *as* sexuality . . . 'Raunchy' and 'liberated' are not synonyms. It is worth asking ourselves if this bawdy world of boobs and gams we have resurrected reflects how far we've come, or how far we have left to go" (p. 5).

Levy's analysis of *Girls Gone Wild* included a variety of interviews with women who performed sexual acts with other women on camera. Time and time again, women reported that their bisexual performances did not indicate lesbian or bisexual identity. One woman she interviewed said, "'I'm not at all bisexual . . . not that I have anything against that. But when you think about it, I'd never do that *really*. It's more for show. A polite way of putting it is it's like a reflex'" (p. 11). Such comments raise questions that this chapter addresses: Would women "do that *really*" outside of these circumstances? How is women's desire for other women co-opted in the name of empowerment and exploited as something "hot" to do for the men watching?

NARRATIVES OF PERFORMATIVE BISEXUALITY

> The theatrical imperatives that normally prevail in situations
> of domination produce a public transcript in close con-
> formity with how the dominant group would wish to have
> things appear. The dominant never control the stage
> absolutely, but their wishes normally prevail. In the short
> run, it is in the interest of the subordinate to produce a
> more or less credible performance, speaking the lines and
> making the gestures he knows are expected of him . . . Sub-
> ordinate groups endorse the terms of their subordination
> and are willing, even enthusiastic, partners in that subordi-
> nation.
>
> —Scott, *Behind the Official Story*

The diverse group of women I interviewed concretely represented a
wide range of sexual identities made possible by embracing and challenging conventional labels. Of the 40 women, 10 identified primarily
as bisexual, and 7 identified as lesbian, while 16 of the 23 heterosexual-
identified women reported same-sex experiences or same-sex attraction, often with brief stints of same-sex eroticism. In fact, only 7 of the
heterosexual-identified women reported *no* same-sex experiences or
attraction, indicating that same-sex experimentation, interest, experiences, and relationships were more the norm than the exception. This
allowed for a diversity of narratives from women who differently
defined themselves in relation to bisexuality, heterosexuality, and homosexuality. Most expressed awareness of, and had strong feelings about,
the increasing trend toward performative bisexuality.

This chapter considers several themes related to performative bisexuality, starting first with women who described engaging in this behavior directly, primarily at parties and clubs. I then consider women who
have observed this behavior, followed by an analysis of *Girls Gone Wild*
and women's opinions and feelings about *GGW*. I conclude the chapter by talking about women's resistance to labeling their same-sex experiences as "lesbian" or "bisexual" experiences, followed by an analysis of
the political implications of performative bisexuality for advancing (or
stalling) LGBT rights.

While some may argue that the motives for same-sex eroticism
may come from internal desire or earlier familial practices, my data sug-

gests that women often feel nudged into performative bisexuality by men, particularly male partners. When speaking directly with women, many of them—particularly the younger women—reported feeling the specific pressure to perform as bisexual in front of male partners or groups of men, often in order to accommodate men's sexual fantasies. (Again, in order to determine whether men themselves would agree, research on groups of men is needed.) This was true both for hetero-sexual-identified women and for bisexual and lesbian-identified women, but heterosexual-identified women reported that their bisexual behavior served to sexually satisfy or arouse their male partners, while bisexual and lesbian-identified women felt pressured more by men who were strangers or nonpartners. For example, Sally, age 20, described experiences "hooking up" with friends at parties, all while minimizing the authenticity of the sexual desire she had for her friends:

> I have kissed girls before. I made out with girls before, but it was mostly because I was drunk at a party, and they're my very close friends . . . The one girl, she's my best friend, and I felt like, well we both felt like kissing each other was completely a platonic thing, mostly because of attention you know. [My boyfriend] would say, "Oh look, let me see you guys make out," but I didn't feel, we didn't feel anything towards the other person other than you're my best friend, and that's how it's going to be . . . You know, you're at a party, and you're drinking a lot, and here's all these guys, and you know, "Oh you guys should kiss," and you know, we do . . . It was just because I was drunk. I would not make out with any of my friends if I was sober. It was like a mutual agreement, I guess, between me and the other girl, and we felt perfectly fine about it . . . We laughed about it, we had a good time. It was just a fun experience.

When I later asked Sally about whether she witnessed this happening for her friends and others she knew, she affirmed that women sought attention or the arousal of nearby men:

> *Oh yeah.* Oh, I'm sure, absolutely. I think that every time that I do go to a club, you know, there are always some girls kissing.

The girls are dancing close together, things like that, then there's the men behind them like, "Yeah, Yeah," drinking their beers and things like that. I think it's just a way to know you're turning someone else on, knowing that you're getting attention from it. I think it sometimes can feel good to a woman, knowing that you're the cause of their arousal.

Other women reported similar experiences with performing as bisexual, including Ciara, age 24, who described complying with a friend's demands for bisexual behavior:

I've done things with women in front of men, and I didn't have a problem with it. She was kind of crazy, and she had a friend of ours take pictures, and she took my skirt off and performed oral sex on me and then she had me do the same to her. It was a brief thing, but she was trying to have her friend take pictures in front of him. We were drinking, and she kind of came onto me and was having me try on outfits, and she said, "Hey, do you want to take some pictures without our clothes on?" and it just progressed from there. I was a little uncomfortable, and he was watching and taking pictures the whole time.

In addition to the obvious way in which alcohol played a role in these situations—perhaps by lowering inhibitions, giving women permission to be sexual, and encouraging women to engage in behavior they would not normally do—such scenarios also speak to the blurred lines between women doing things for *others'* pleasure versus their own pleasure.

Bisexual and lesbian women also reported feeling pressured to engage in performative bisexuality, as men recognized these women's sexual identity as something they could exploit for their own sexual arousal. For example, 23-year-old Julie talked about feeling exploited by heterosexual men:

I get asked to make out with women a lot because when people hear that you're bisexual, they automatically assume that you do it for men's pleasure, but really, a lot of my sex with women has not even included men at all, but some of it has.

I've definitely felt pressure to indulge in fantasies about men watching women together . . . I just don't want to be pegged as just for men's pleasure because I'm bisexual, because that can happen sometimes.

Lucy, age 25, reported having similar experiences of men pressuring her to perform as bisexual:

There's [sic] times you know when I was in college and I was with girls, and maybe I would be dating a guy that didn't mind if I was with a girl. I had two friends that we'd go out dancing, and we'd bump and grind and kiss each other, so I have done little things like that in front of guys. Most of the time we were out drinking and you kind of forget, "Oh, I came with that guy."

Lesbian-identified Leigh, age 21, talked at length about feeling like men exploited her sexuality. Notably, she and several other women defied and resisted their appropriation into male fantasy scenarios. Leigh described the following reaction to men pressuring her:

I have these guys, these neighbors down the hall that like, the other night they kind of know that me and my roommate are more than just friends. They keep saying to us, "Come on, make out," like that kind of thing. I've had people do that to me before, and I'm just always like, there are two guys here and two girls here, so if you want us to make out, you go first. Then they won't of course. I'm like, if I want to, I will, and if I don't want to, I won't.

Nora, age 23, expressed resistance to men's efforts to control her as well, talking about the ways in which performative bisexuality speaks to the commodification of women's bodies and the lack of space women have to express their sexuality without patriarchal control and influence:

I've been asked to [perform] on multiple occasions, even by guys who are totally homophobic toward gay men. It's so ego-centered and male-centered. It's like dude, if you're going to

celebrate sexuality, celebrate everyone's sexuality, not just these
two women. Of course we know that women turn you on, but
I find that most men can't handle two women because they
want to get, well they want to have their big penis waving
around somewhere to affirm themselves . . . I think they recognize that if women were self-sufficient like that, men would be
totally useless. I think they have secret fears about it that they're
not letting on. So I think if it's like only specifically for them,
and for their pleasure, they can accept that. I think it's a huge
hoax.

The notable differences between women reading performative
bisexuality as acceptable, normative, and even empowering compared
with those who read it as troubling and coercive also marks a key tension in the cultural framing of this phenomenon. At what point does
this kind of pressure translate into an expansion of women's sexual
repertoire and/or a change in their traditionally heterosexual worldview? Does it indicate that they are more open to same-sex experiences
or simply more coerced?

While many women noted some pressure to engage in bisexual
acts, the context in which this occurred followed some unique patterns.
One striking difference was between the older and younger women
(divided roughly at age 35 in my group), in that younger women
reported much more performative bisexuality that occurred in public
social settings, while older women reported more pressure in their private lives to engage in group sex and other bisexual behavior with their
sexual partners. The demand for conformity to performative bisexuality
was striking, in that even those women who did not engage in this
behavior in public (i.e., at a party, etc.) often experienced it in private
(e.g., partner's request for threesome). Women's own descriptions of
how it felt to have group sex, or same-sex encounters with men watching, revealed a deep ambivalence about these experiences. Many
women, particularly the older women, felt pressure to engage in homoerotic behavior in front of their sexual partners, indicating that this
behavior was both arousing to the partners and demanded as a part of
"normal" sexual life. About half of the women found it arousing, both
because it pleased them personally and because they found pleasure in
pleasing their partners, while the others felt turned off by the context

of coercion and pressure involved. This points to conflicts about the degree of *intrinsic* pleasure women have when being sexual with other women in these contexts.

Many of the older women, as compared with the younger women, discussed their partners' requests for group sex in a critical manner, often saying that they outright rejected, or at least questioned, these demands for them to perform as bisexual. For example, Dawn, age 43, said,

> I have been asked to have sex with another woman in front of men, and I've declined. You know, there's a situation where the guys or the husbands or the partners are like, "Wow, this is my fantasy to see my girlfriend getting it on with another girl." You know, sorry buddy, and there've been times where I have engaged in sexual situations with another woman where the husband has been there. It was more like an ego thing for him, or a notch on his belt or whatever. It didn't feel like I was being honored as a person.

Similarly, Esther, age 44, reacted to the pressure she felt in a critical and uneasy way. She said, "I've been asked to [perform as bisexual], yes. As a matter of fact, this one guy asked me to join he and his girlfriend, and it ended the relationship . . . I think that is again for the man's benefit, and it is not necessarily for the women's benefit. It is coercion. They basically want it for their own pleasure." When I asked her how it felt to hear such a request, she expressed fear and unhappiness about the arrangement:

> I felt pressured and embarrassed because we did not talk about it. That was not something that was agreed upon. I was afraid that I would go to his house, and he would have someone there waiting for me, and I would have to figure out how to get out of that situation because I'm not going to do that, and it's not what I want. In my younger life, I may have been that, but not now. That's not what I need.

In our later discussions about ideal sexual partners, she mentioned discussing this with her partner: "He said, 'Any man that would ask you to [have sex with another woman in front of him] doesn't love you,' and that's a powerful statement for me."

The deep ambivalence about group sex that involved other women came across both in response to a partner's pressures and when considering their own viewpoints about it. For example, Charlotte, age 34, expressed ambivalence about agreeing to a threesome: "He asked me one time, after we had done something, had I ever thought about it . . . I told him yes because that would get that out of his head, and it wouldn't happen again, but then it would also be like the satisfaction of a bi-curiousness in my head at the time. But then I gave him the no. I said once she does it, there may be times that we're not around each other, and you can be with her . . . That would make me mad."

Similarly, Fiona, age 24, articulated serious caution about threesome sex:

> I think my current boyfriend would like to have a threesome, and I guess that's a very common male fantasy in general. He likes the fact that I was a self-described lesbian in my past years, and I tried to explain that when I was a lesbian, I had a shaved head and piercings and that I didn't necessarily look like the kind of lesbian that he fantasized about. I don't think that the female that I would be attracted to would be somebody that he would want to have sex with.

In general, older women more often experimented with bisexuality in private compared with younger women, who experimented in public, indicating a generational or cohort divide about how women responded to performative bisexuality pressures.

Witnessing Performative Bisexuality

The consequences of performative bisexuality were not confined to personal requests by men that the women knew. After speaking with these women and confronting my students' ideas about this topic, it became increasingly clear that even those women who did not engage in this behavior did *witness* some form of performative bisexuality, either in person or on television. As such, most women had plenty to say about their interpretations of watching other women engage in performative bisexuality both in public and in private. Reflecting the tension women felt about moral relativism and judging other women's sexual behavior—in that an overly harsh or judgmental stance can oppress others and reinforce discourses of women as "sluts" while, at the same time, having no judgment can imply condoning or accepting such behavior—women's responses fell along a spectrum between nonjudgmental and judgmental (or, more precisely, a continuum of seeing the behavior as liberating or *recognizing* exploitation of women).

When asked what they thought about women engaging in bisexual behavior in front of men, a few women approved of this based on the idea that it was consensual and noncoerced. For example, Edie, age 19, imagined performative bisexuality as a way to "feel something":

> Upon the premise that they're pressured to and don't want to, I think it's terrible. If they want to just be freaky for perform-ance['s] sake and reaction['s] sake, I think it's good when people want to do something abnormal to feel something. But, how-ever, it's becoming normal to do that, and if it makes them feel horrible, or if the result is feeling bad about themselves, then I'm against it. If the result is feeling empowered, then I suppose I'm for it though I'd never encourage it in an actual situation. If they do it to please men, then it doesn't seem right to me.

Analyzing this scenario from a generational perspective, 56-year-old Ophelia noted how common performative bisexuality had become and how her generation also behaved in "unpopular" ways: "It's popular, and both people are consenting and having fun. I'm sure there were things that we did in my generation that were popular at the time too but I can't remember."

In addition to the issue of consent, some women—from a range of sexual identities and political orientations—raised questions about the implications for gay rights and/or actual lesbian identification. For example, queer-identified Dawn, age 43, urged other women not to insult real queer identity by playing around with queerness:

If you're not wholly into [same-sex behavior], then please don't do it, or please don't do it again. Maybe you can learn from that and set a bigger boundary . . . The other thing too is that it shows there's a little more freedom in our society. It's interesting how it's okay for two women to make out at a party, but it wouldn't be okay for two men to make out at a party. These are the same groups of people. That makes me sad, very sad, 'cause we're in a hetero-male dominated situation, and it's a lot of hetero males, hetero acting, hetero males' fantasy.

Niko, age 23 and heterosexual, also felt that it exploited queer sexuality: "I feel that it's disrespect to real lesbians, 'cause if you're doing it for other people to watch, it's bad, but I find it arousing if they really love each other, if they really like each other or find each other attractive. But if it's just a pure act, I find it kind of disgusting." Charlene, age 44 and bisexual, argued that homophobia is at the root of performative bisexuality:

I think it's a double standard because men think it's sexy when women are together but they have no real concept of real lesbians or who lesbians are. It's a double standard because if it was two men kissing they'd be totally grossed out, because whether you're lesbian or gay or transgender or whoever you are, it doesn't have a lot to do with sex. It has to do with who you are, so to just have two women on stage kissing, I guess it's degrading to true lesbians. It's homophobic.

Lesbian-identified Maria, age 21, expressed similar sentiments, saying that she felt mistreated by men exploiting her identity: "I feel constantly made into a fetish by men. They think it's hot that I'm a lesbian. I tell them to get the fuck away from me. It's insulting and painful."

Other women expressed conflicts about performative bisexuality, recognizing it as potentially liberating but ultimately concluding that it exploits or coerces women into accommodating patriarchal fantasies about women. For example, Susan, age 45, described it as solely a male fantasy: "I think that the bisexual woman fantasy is very much in reaction to a man's fantasy, and my desire is to respond to a man's fantasy.

Whether I would have thought of that on my own, I don't know . . . I think it goes back to this cultural norm where that's part of what heterosexual men have defined as interesting." Many women described self-awareness about the way they responded to men's fantasies, noting that in the case of performative bisexuality, these problems were heightened. For example, Mitra, age 29, argued that it reflected men's fantasies at the expense of women:

> I think [performative bisexuality] is exploitative too because it's not really about them. It's about pleasing some male fantasy. It's like our culture has become so oversexed, but I still feel like it's the male version of what sex is. I don't feel like there's a female voice in defining what's sexy in our culture.

Sonja, age 24, also felt that performative bisexuality exploits women into accommodating male fantasies, saying, "If they're just making out at a party, but in front of other men, I just find that irritating. It's just doing it to kind of make a spectacle for men . . . I can also see that in some ways it is sexually liberating, but for some reason it seems to irritate me because I feel like it's again related to the male-dominated world. Again, it's another instance of female sexuality dominated by men." Lesbian-identified Brynn, age 25, agreed, saying that men use threesomes to satisfy their egos: "I mean, if that's what gets you off, more power to ya, but I think that's more of a male ego trip. You know, they can walk around and be like, 'Oh yeah, I had two women, what'd you have? One?!'"

Other women spoke more strongly against performative bisexuality, such as 25-year-old Aya who, using direct language of commodification, said, "I think it's just catering to market demand for things like that. I assume that people that do that need large amounts of approval from men in order to feel some sense of value, or to feel like they've achieved this standard of sexiness." Nora, age 23, expressed objections to performative bisexuality based on its relationship to treating women and their bodies as commodities: "I just wish that we could stop the commodification again. I wish we had topless beaches. I wish we had more affirming natural body things. It's just so silly. It's this 'sorostitute,' a sorority-prostitute concept." Outraged by the implications for young

women in particular, Lori, age 33, commented on the damaging power
imbalances in these performances:

> I hate that women learn how to be women only by imagining
> themselves as objects. I mean, we don't even know what they
> actually want here. We only know that they pretend to want to
> be bisexual, that they'll do whatever they've been brainwashed
> to do that makes their boyfriend happy. Women are not objects,
> and I wish they'd stop acting like that and actually value what
> they really want. Maybe they do want to hook up with
> women, and if so, go and do it alone. Don't do it for your
> boyfriend's pleasure.

Some women took a more critically distant approach to analyzing
performative bisexuality, arguing that it did not make sense given that
men were partly excluded from the physical aspects of the sexual
exchange. For example, 32-year-old Jill said,

> It has always somewhat baffled me, this heterosexual male fasci-
> nation with actual or mock lesbians. It['s] just, like, okay, that is
> an act that you have absolutely no part in, so why does it fasci-
> nate you so much? I think that anyone playing that kind of
> game had better be damn well sure that the other people
> involved are at least aware of what level they're playing at,
> because I don't think it's fair to engage in any sexual activity
> without reasonably in one way or another letting your partner
> know to what extent you mean it.

Pam, age 42, also expressed bafflement about men's interest in women's
same-sex experiences:

> It's offensive that men are going to find some pleasure in that. I
> don't know why they do though! I can't figure that out
> because you're not in it. I could understand if it's two women
> on a man, but for me, watching two men, that would do noth-
> ing for me. It would actually disturb me. But you watching two
> women? Now if it was me, and it was two men on me, and not

touching each other, I'd probably still be disturbed, but it just seems better. It's all about me.

Thus, most women reacted directly to performative bisexuality, either by approving of it based on consent and "having fun" or by directly opposing it based on its implications for queer identity or its exploitation of women's desires.

Girls Gone Wild

Some women encountered performative bisexuality purely through mediated forms. Given the proliferation of shows and films that depict performative bisexuality—most notably the *Girls Gone Wild* films and reality shows such as *Next*, *A Shot at Love with Tila Tequila*, and *The Real World*—even those women with no personal experience with performative bisexuality still felt affected by the mediated exposure of these images and scripts. When asked about their feelings about *Girls Gone Wild* and its meaning for women's sexuality, particularly in light of the fact that women agree to appear in these films without receiving any monetary compensation, responses ranged from identification with the women in the films to emotional responses of rejection to outrage about its implications for "real lesbians." Again, ambivalence about what it means to *have* desire versus *perform* desire informed these responses.

Identification and sympathy for the participants in these *GGW* films, while not the most common response, did appear in my conversations with women. This indicates that performative bisexuality appears as a part of women's (private?) sexual lives but also as a form of entertainment en masse. Predictably, the women who identified with (or at least condoned the behavior of) the women in the films tended to also engage in public acts of performative bisexuality. For example, Ciara, age 24, said, "I mean, that's a choice, and I can't say that if I was there, I probably wouldn't do it, 'cause I'm fun like that . . . I mean, personally I don't think there's anything wrong with it, but it does have an effect on what people think about women. If I had a few drinks, and I was in that situation, I probably would do it. I was in New Orleans on Bourbon Street, and I did the flashing for beads. I'm comfortable with myself." Leigh, age 21, argued that it might be fun, saying, "I guess it's kind of funny, but probably four years ago I would have loved to have been on it. Now I might even still consider it because it would be fun. I think it's funny to think about those girls that are in it and their parents are watching TV and saying, 'Oh, there's Amber, our daughter.'"

Along these lines, a small number of women minimized the significance of the potentially exploitative qualities of GGW by stating that flashing on camera represents sexual fun and acceptance of women's sexuality. For example, Sally said she would consider flashing in certain circumstances: "If I was ever in that kind of situation on *Girls Gone Wild,* and I was just really drunk, I would probably show my boobs off too. I think that's just showing that sex is more accepted in our society. We want to see young women taking off their clothes and showing off their boobs and things like that." When I asked her whose pleasure mattered here, she responded,

> It's for men's pleasure. Well I'm sure that it's for women's pleasure too, but I think that for the women actually on *Girls Gone Wild*, I think that it's just an exciting experience for them. Who knows, someone might recognize them or something . . . Women actually want men to pay attention to them and feel more accepted I guess. It's empowering.

This idea of participating in *GGW* as a possibly liberating act again reflects the conflicted and confusing messages women receive about their sexuality. Can certain behaviors both exploit and liberate at the same time? Does it matter whose pleasure is valued, and if so, does it make it acceptable if women claim that it *feels* empowering?

Edie perfectly articulated the resulting confusion and ambivalence around the liberatory potential of *GGW*, saying:

> Who are they flashing their tits for? Men's masturbation. I'm not against men's masturbation. But I think for women's sexuality, it may do two things . . . I think it lets a younger, more vulnerable, less-developed woman at 13 years-old think that that's okay. I also think it's kind of for self-respect. I don't know if it's self-respecting or not to flash your tits. You have them so

why is it different than your ear? You know what I mean? Why? It's been made that way. Out of ease, we're punished in that way because it's covered. I know that it confuses me.

Here, she raises a central problem in the deconstruction of women's sexuality: Just because something is socially constructed (in this case, the construction of breasts as sexual and something to be revealed in the context of "going wild"), does *knowing that* change the impact that it has on people? In this way, Edie touches upon a central problem of feminist theory: Despite defining sex as an "unnatural act" (Tiefer, 2004), women still respond physically, emotionally, and culturally to the dominant narratives of sex. The frames and scripts people inherit from their socially constructed world often organize and justify prevailing power structures. The impulse to construct *GGW* as fun and empowering fits with cultural expectations for women to comply with cultural demands for performative bisexuality (and compulsory heterosexuality).

Even so, while some women read a possible liberatory impulse to *GGW*, most saw the exact opposite. In part as a response to seeing the social consequences and implications of *GGW*, most women described outrage at seeing *GGW* boom in fame and publicity. For example, Brynn expressed disgust at the way women condone their exploitation:

> That is very demeaning, seriously. So here's this guy who walks around with this camera and who wants young women who are very much under-the-influence of whatever it may be, whether it be alcohol or drugs or whatever. The whole *Girls Gone Wild* thing is just not my cup of tea. I don't see where you can actually provide yourself with any kind of self-worth like that if you're just gonna walk around and say, "Here, let me show you what's underneath my top or here, I'll pull my pants down for you, no big deal. Sure, you want a scene of me in the shower with my best friend, and neither of us has any clothes on, no problem!" I don't see where they would actually find that appealing, or even believe that for themselves.

Ruth, age 46, argued that the blame lies not with the women themselves but with the exploitative director:

I think that the women in it are being duped and used. I feel anger at the director. Unfortunately, I fear that a lot of these women don't go into it with their eyes open because they're looking for that idealization. Personally I don't think that is going to bring them the attention, respect, and the fame and fortune that they're looking for. I think that they're just being used and discarded like an old Kleenex.

Though Ruth disliked the director, her statement that he uses the women "like an old Kleenex" hearkens back to ideas about women as polluted, contaminated vessels (as "sluts," perhaps), again situating *women* as the ones tarnished and ruined by the exposure of their breasts.

Comparisons between men and women also appeared when discussing *GGW*, in that women recognized the lopsidedness of the representation. Lucy, age 25, argued that men should be exploited in similar ways:

Maybe it wouldn't bother me if there was a *Guys Gone Wild* out there too, you know. Not that I think men and women should ever be completely objectified only at the physical and sexual level, but I think that women should not ever have to get to that level to where it's sheer entertainment for guys just to watch them be drunk and show their boobs. But at the same time, if women were open with their sexuality, does that mean that there would be a *Guys Gone Wild* too? . . . I'm all about equality and fairness, and if there's going to be one, there's got to be the other."

Shonda, age 44, recognized the lopsided representations as they exist now: "We don't have men on TV exploiting their private parts, so I don't think it's proper. I don't think it's right." Notably, *Guys Gone Wild* does exist now, marketed mostly to other men. This suggests that, even if the gender imbalances are rectified for representations of those "going wild," the videos still target *men* as their primary audience. Heterosexual, bisexual, and lesbian women do not *consume* this imagery; rather, they *are consumed*.

Similar to some women's responses to public displays of performative bisexuality, some women raised concerns about the implications of

GGW for actual lesbian sexuality, constructing *GGW* as a setback for lesbian rights. Janet, age 21, felt insulted by *GGW* because of its antiqueer politics:

> As far as the whole *Girls Gone Wild*, the whole girls kissing girls and things like that, it portrays real bad things for the real gay people, the real lesbians, because I don't see me or any of my friends acting like that! It just makes us look bad. Don't flash your tits and kiss whoever just because that's your friend, and you're on Spring Break. If you're not lesbians, then don't do things like that. If you're not gay, don't be gay, just be yourself. If you're straight, be straight, and don't play around."

This concern about what *GGW* means for "real lesbians" brings up the central tension about the heterosexist ramifications of performative bisexuality: Does it represent *greater acceptance* of queer sexuality, or does it represent *greater exploitation* of women and their bodies? Can a nuanced argument account for both of these positions? It seems troubling that women increasingly report self-objectifying feelings about their bodies and their sexuality, always imagining, for example, that others watch and judge their actions. Performative bisexuality evokes the male gaze as a profound and always-present aspect of women's sexual lives. *Who is watching* matters as much as *what I'm doing*, giving power to the (imagined) observer even while the actor might be subverting some sexual norms. For example, heterosexual women engaging in performative bisexuality assume some degree of personal agency in exploring different sexual partners and in breaking out of the heteronormative paradigm of finding pleasure only with men. At the same time, the *presence* of men begs the question of whether a meaningful distinction exists between men's physical and visual participation. Do *participating* men and the *observing* men have different abilities to enact power and exploitation?

In thinking about this more deeply, the question of pornography, a medium in which men's physical *and* visual participation are paramount, arises. While strides have been made to increase the production of feminist pornography that potentially subverts dominant paradigms and narratives of mainstream porn, pornography as a whole (particularly the top-selling pornography) nevertheless remains painfully consistent in its portrayal of women, most often treating them as objects used for men's pleasure. Women's same-sex experiences in pornography again embody the partnership between mainstreaming (faux?) lesbian eroticism and exploiting women's same-sex interactions for the purposes of (men's) pleasure. When considering how such pornography has begun to sneak into media depictions of mainstream sexuality more prominently, as explored in Levy (2005), performative bisexuality may signify the integration between media and life, between the artificial and the real. The mainstreaming of "girl-on-girl" action, the rapid increase in sales of thong underwear, reports of more and more women undergoing plastic surgery procedures, and the changing culture of fraternities and sororities all reveal this integration (Levy, 2005). Perhaps performative bisexuality exists *because* of pornography, rather than merely in tandem with more same-sex eroticism in pornography. If this is the case, then women are taking cues about sexual liberation from a medium widely known for mass exploitation of women, reckless disregard for women's sexual health (e.g., there are still few regulations about condom usage in the industry, let alone regular and mandatory STD testing and sexual health screenings), and archaic and repetitive ideas about what is "sexy" (Jensen, 2007).

Questions about the role of sexual fantasy in people's lives abound when addressing pornography, a theme that I take a closer look at in chapter 6. To illustrate this more concretely, the common pornography technique of "facials," where men ejaculate onto women's faces, may actually symbolize a backlash reaction to the perception of women's increased social power and may itself constitute a form of sexual violence (Franklin, 2004; Haugh, 2005). Also, most women's bodies do not conform to the narrow conventions of pornography (e.g., massive breasts, thin body, completely shaved/waxed, etc.), and most women *do* enjoy extended oral sex to orgasm (Barrett, 2004; Pinkerton et al., 2003), something often distorted in pornography by women's endless, vague, and nonspecific "orgasm." Yet the fantasy world of pornography has come to influence women's lives in important ways. Increasing numbers of women report mimicking behavior they see in pornography, and new industries for labiaplasty and genital cosmetic surgeries have arisen throughout the country, particularly in wealthy areas (discussed more in chapter 6). Levy (2005) argued that women imitate porn stars more and more, evidenced in part by booming sales of porn star memoirs. The reality show industry has as its staples the construction and reconstruction of women's bodies, women's temporary stints into bisexual identification, and competitions between women to best accommodate patriarchal fantasy (e.g., *America's Next Top Model* dressing women in beef bikinis, making them up as high-fashion dead girls, and doing photo shoots comparing women to garbage). Plastic surgery shows—where women shape their faces to look like celebrities—permeate the airwaves. In short, distinctions between the "real" and the "artificial" are becoming more and more narrow. Such a breakdown of these distinctions, while being useful in helping people to further envision a postmodern or cyborg sexuality (i.e., deconstructing human from machine, challenging what is *real* versus *fake*), may also have damaging and lasting effects on the ability to imagine sexual relationships *outside* of this context.

Performative bisexuality represents one version of the way that the artificial world of pornography collides with women's real sexual lives. Cultural scripts about in-vogue bisexuality may stem from these media representations. Performative bisexuality may also represent the co-optation of women's sexual desires into discursive fantasies about the "plasticity" of women's sexualities. Such shows define women's empowerment by their degree of *adherence* to cultural scripts about bisexuality and heterosexuality. And yet performative bisexuality may signify a shift in sexual consciousness whereby, even *despite* such mandated adherence, new possibilities emerge for women to explore same-sex desire and attraction. Perhaps the most interesting paradox occurs when women *experience* same-sex eroticism while minimizing its significance. In the face of girls going wild, *real* same-sex desires forge ahead quite timidly.

"I'M NOT A LESBIAN BUT . . ."

Though 23 of the 40 women I interviewed claimed "heterosexuality" in the prescreening questions, more than 69% described some version of same-sex eroticism in their lives, either through same-sex attraction, occasional same-sex sexual behavior, or same-sex relationships. Heterosexual-identified women described strong feelings of attraction toward women's bodies, childhood kissing, sexual experimentation with women, one-night stands with women, and repeated sexual encounters with women, often *not* involving men.

This expansive repertoire of same-sex eroticism reported by "heterosexual" women calls forth multiple interpretations. First, it may indicate a strong cultural pressure to repress one's sexual identity and/or desire for women, in that many women identified as heterosexual when their behavior suggested a label of "bisexual" or "lesbian." Women's willingness to acquiesce to heteronormative pressures (indeed, "compulsory heterosexuality" in its classic form) appeared in their statements when they claimed, "I'm not a lesbian but . . ." or "I'm not really bisexual but . . ." even while describing meaningful same-sex experiences. For example, Mitra said, "I don't really think any of these feelings make me a lesbian or even bi. I think they're just something that's there for me."

Alarmingly, women described much of their same-sex attraction and behavior by minimizing its significance, primarily by claiming that the actions were girlish and a product of youth. For example, Susan remembered an experience practicing kissing with a friend:

I remember the summer when I was 13, I practiced kissing with one of my girlfriends. I don't remember that being sexual so much as that we needed to practice. I don't remember being turned on necessarily, but it was fun. So I guess I was turned on, in a roundabout way.

Geena, age 51, also minimized the significance of her early experimentation with other girls:

I remember I experimented sexually with a female friend, but we were pretending like we were a boy and a girl. I can't really explain it. It didn't feel like we were being sexual with each other. We were just acting out what we thought it would feel like to be with a guy. We were fantasizing about boy/girl relationships with each other.

Bonnie, age 51, also described a same-sex encounter where she practiced kissing, saying that it only facilitated better encounters with men later on:

I do remember two times practicing kissing. I was like I think around twelve or thirteen. We wanted to make sure we knew how before we actually kissed a boy in real life . . . I mean we knew we weren't attracted to each other. We were just practicing so that we could get good for our future boyfriends.

Heterosexual women's reluctance to identify their early same-sex experiences as significant contrasted sharply with the early sexual experiences of the lesbian and bisexual women. For lesbian and bisexual women, they remembered their early same-sex eroticism as exciting, rewarding, and developmentally important for them, even despite negative social feedback from their parents. For example, Dawn recalled looking at *Playboy* with a girlfriend:

I was probably nine years old with another girlfriend. We looked at my dad's *Playboy* together and then we kind of we simulated what we thought might be going on, but we weren't quite sure. It was a playful thing in a lot of positive ways. My parents didn't provide any education or availability to talk about sexuality, so this was how we learned . . . When I was a young teenager, I came to the realization that I was attracted to women and had a conversation with my mother about it, which was really kind of a bad choice on my part, and she pretty much was shocked and shut me down and then let me know that that was not okay. It probably affected me a little bit more than I would like to admit.

Janet also had no qualms describing early sexual attractions to women and the solidification of her gay identity:

I always was attracted to women . . . My mom always said, "Well, this is just a phase, this is just a phase, you're going to get over it." I'm like, "Mom, I'm 21 now. This is not a phase" . . . When I was younger, I would date guys or whatever, but it was more just to make my mom happy, like my mom would think I'm normal if I had this dude that I was hanging out with, and I'd kiss him, and it'd be totally disgusting because I knew what they had under their clothes, and I didn't like that . . . I've known I was gay since I was really small. I think I was like maybe 9 when I started kissing girls . . . It's not a phase. It's something that's a part of me, since before I knew it was a part of me.

Fiona also felt proud and joyous about her childhood sexual experimentation with neighborhood girls:

As a kid, I had a couple of girlfriends that I would sneak around and do that kind of stuff with. I was a very naughty little girl. I'm happy to go on and on about it. I remember making out with female friends at camp at ages 7, 8, 9. I remember convincing other little girls to make out with me, and I found a lot of satisfaction doing that . . . I did a lot of making out through my middle school years.

Such contrasts—between heterosexual-identified women's reluctance to disclose same-sex experiences compared with the often bold ways in which lesbian and bisexual women reported their experiences—reflects the way in which "compulsory heterosexuality" predictably has more strongly aversive effects on women who identified as heterosexual yet experienced some same-sex desire. However reluctant they are about it, women's reporting of same-sex desire outside of the context of men may represent a shift away from compulsory heterosexuality.

In addition to reflecting a small subversion of compulsory heterosexuality, other narratives also explain why heterosexual-identified women reported same-sex behavior: Particularly for those trying out bisexuality *now*, they may respond to a cultural push toward mainstreaming and performing same-sex behavior with other women. Many women, particularly younger women, felt *pressured* to engage in sex with other women (typically in front of men), or to express attraction to other women, as they perceived this as a predominant cultural expectation for *good femininity*. These responses raise an important question: *Is bisexuality compulsory?* Is there something about same-sex expression that feels mandatory to women? If so, what does this mean?

The narratives previously described in this chapter represent the push toward bisexuality as an emerging social norm for many women.

In those stories, performative bisexuality reflects a desire to please (male) partners and accommodate in-vogue cultural fantasies about women and their bodies. Here, same-sex behavior seems less authentic or internally driven, as women report engaging in it, or watching other women engaging in it, for the primary purpose of pleasing or sexually arousing a male partner or audience. They respond to normative pressure to perform as bisexual even when they say it does not excite them personally; even those who merely observed performative bisexuality often noted its power over women. Yet, however powerful these normative pressures were, women still reacted in ways that communicated their *resistance to compulsory heterosexuality*. In this way, these narratives show that same-sex behavior, *even that behavior that occurs in front of men*, can resist the culturally demanded strict adherence to heterosexuality. This raises the even more difficult question: *Can (compulsory) bisexuality function as a resistance narrative against compulsory heterosexuality, even while compulsory bisexuality references compulsory heterosexuality?*

If the cultural push toward normalizing women's bisexuality (despite competing pressures to pathologize bisexuality, as evidenced by the Defense of Marriage Act and other such political efforts) can be interpreted in an expansive, emancipatory way, one of its obvious benefits is that women now describe an increasing acceptance or openness toward same-sex sexuality, even if they do not directly act on that attraction. In other words, perhaps performative bisexuality—in *making visible* women's same-sex eroticism, regardless of the exploitative context—allows women to internally explore the *possibilities* of same-sex attraction. For example, Priya said, "I usually am just mostly attracted to men. But I have lots of female friends where I'm like, if you were only a guy. But, I think I have been curious about what it would be like to have just a sexual encounter with a female, but I've never really acted on it, and I'm not sure that I would." Such assertions—both in what she believes and in terms of what she feels comfortable saying out loud—may be consequences of the "chic" qualities of bisexuality today. Dorothy expressed similar feelings about her openness toward same-sex attraction:

> I'm definitely attracted to women a lot but I've never had an experience with a woman. I know I'm definitely heterosexual

if anything. I've thought a lot about female contact, but it's
never really come up in my life. I'm definitely really aroused by
female bodies though. I think they're beautiful. I think even as
a teen going through adolescence and puberty, I think I was
more aroused by women than men . . . I don't know if that's
something that everyone feels, or if it means anything. I've
never had an experience with a woman, so I really wouldn't
know about that. I mean, I'm open to it, so I'll see . . . In general, I don't think there are any absolutes, and also I think sexuality is very defined by culture. Like in the Indian culture,
men have sex with men, but they're not gay. They have wives.
It's just an act. People should realize that sexual preferences are
very much defined by culture, if you're going to make it your
identity or not.

Perhaps the new norms around bisexuality make these feelings possible.
Furthermore, perhaps Marjorie Garber (1995, cited in Kermode, 1995)
was right when she said that bisexuality would be universal except for
"repression, religion, repugnance, denial, laziness, shyness, lack of opportunity, premature specialization, a failure of the imagination or a life
already full to the brim with erotic experiences, albeit with only one
person, or only one gender." This suggests that repressive institutions are
still fairly strong, but may be losing their grip slightly.

Many of the older heterosexual women described a newfound
openness toward same-sex attraction that they had not acknowledged
in their younger lives, though traces of the performative qualities often
still arose. Same-sex eroticism became a possibility, as Susan, age 45,
said:

I definitely prefer men, but I have fantasies about other
women. I think that if it wasn't so awkward to negotiate, I
think I would have tried it. I think that part of my interest in
other women is that it would entertain men. Even if a man says
he's gay, he thinks it'd be hot to watch a woman with another
woman. It's something hard-wired in their little American
brains or something . . . I have friends who told me I just have
to meet the right woman, so yeah, I think that I'm much more

open to the idea than I used to be. I didn't give myself the freedom to fantasize about that until the last 10 years or so.

As most sex-positive theorists and scholars have argued, openness to new sexual experiences can help women to develop a stronger sense of their own internal erotic life (Queen, 1997). The possibilities of transitioning a platonic friendship between women into something erotic opens up possibilities for women to explore new and different ways that they can relate to each other. While this evolution from friendship to love is not a new phenomenon (Smith-Rosenberg, 1985), it was notable how often women comfortably relayed stories about their "crushes" on friends or fantasies about having "more than a friendship" with women in their lives. For example, Charlene described erotic feelings for a close friend, a phenomenon that many women mentioned about their own lives. She said, "I have one friend now, and I've told her that she's the only woman that I've ever been attracted to. It's not that I want to have a physical relationship with her, but I find her extremely attractive, and she's just a wonderful person, and she's just the only woman that I've thought about in any other way than just being my friend."

Such openness to same-sex attraction, particularly with friends, was not limited to women with socially liberal views. Several conservative women also expressed interest in same-sex attractions, even when such attractions did not resonate with their political sentiments. Ruth, a self-described Evangelical Christian and lifelong Republican, described her interest as present but still repressed by the restrictions of her lifestyle choices:

> Every once in a while I'll have a conversation with a lesbian friend, and it's not like she's trying to talk me into it, but I ask her a lot of questions about it because women are so much more nurturing than men. She doesn't blame women going into lesbian relationships because after a certain point you're tired of the men and game-playing and stuff. I don't know if I totally agree with that, but I could see myself thinking about having a relationship with a woman, but I don't think my beliefs would ever let me do it.

When I asked her what she meant by that, she responded by citing biblical principles as the key deterrent to initiating a sexual relationship with a woman:

> It would be against the biblical principles that I believe in and hold dear. I'm not really a strong proponent of gay rights . . . but every once in a while with some of these women, even my friend, I have actually thought about what it would be like to have a sexual experience with them. I've never told her that though. I'm attracted to women, but I just don't think I would act on it because of my religion . . . You know, the books and stuff like that—*I have two mommies, I have two daddies*—to me it's still a breakdown of the American society of the family, and I'm not a real proponent for gay rights. It's just not a world I want to be in. Maybe if something happened once with one woman, but I don't think I could ever completely turn myself into becoming a lesbian. It just doesn't appeal to me.

Esther, also a self-described conservative and religious woman, reported both same-sex attraction and same-sex behavior, saying,

> I do find myself attracted to women, and I have had one sexual experience with a woman in my life, and even though I can look at a woman and say, "That's a nice looking woman," that's about as far as it goes, even if there is a physical attraction. It's not something I would probably initiate, though attraction to women is something I experience in my life. It took me a long time to realize that because I grew up with those magazines that my dad had—*Hustlers* and all of those—so that was my first experience, seeing women with great big boobs. I kind of just learned, whether I wanted to or not.

Notably, she minimized the importance or significance of such attraction and behavior, constructing her feelings as based on the images she viewed in pornography.

Similar attitudes were described Courtney, age 23, a self-described conservative who more directly referred to her same-sex attraction and behavior in the context of performative bisexuality with her female friends. Minimizing the significance of these events, she said,

> I grew up always thinking that it's guy/girl, and to this date that's never really been a conflict in myself. I've never questioned or thought that I was attracted to a female. I've always been attracted to guys, and that's pretty much just been that. Well, sometimes me and my girlfriends will like give each other a kiss or something when we've been really drunk, but we've never taken it farther. That was more like teasing the guys that we were dating, just teasing them because they were like, "Oh my God, they kissed." It's not that big of a deal. I like to tease them. They thought it was funny.

Given the apparent conflicts between conservative political views and women having same-sex experiences, a key question emerges: Does performative bisexuality translate into a shift in women's political consciousness, particularly about LGBT rights?

Political Perspectives

The demographic groups of women reporting a newfound openness to same-sex eroticism reveal both the enormous potential of, and the enormous perils of, mainstreaming bisexuality for women. If women's sexual identities and practices are actually more flexible and "plastic" compared to men's—that is, more subject to the changing social norms of the time—openness to same-sex attraction may be just another way in which women's sexuality accommodates changing social norms. The rebellious or subversive potential of such eroticism is perhaps destroyed and diminished by its allegiance to male, patriarchal constructions of pleasure. The central problem becomes whether such same-sex eroticism signifies *a shift in consciousness* or not. While arguments can be made for its subversive potential, particularly in the way that performative bisexuality at least presents different options for women, the seeming lack of shift in *political* sensibilities presents a more frighteningly conservative picture. If women's feelings toward the *political context* of same-sex eroticism do not consistently change as a result of participating in performative bisexuality, this suggests that it fails to politicize women about the perils of heterosexism. In other words, if bisexuality is compulsory or merely a performance, it loses some of its capacity to provoke progressive social change and enact social justice. Moreover, if heterosexual women do not see the sexist aspects of performative bisexuality, they may never become involved in social movements that directly challenge the institutional practices that discriminate against sexual minorities.

In tandem with the dissonance that conservative and/or Evangelical women experienced with regard to same-sex sexuality, many women described political views that did not match up with their behaviors, attitudes, and beliefs about same-sex sexuality. While the vast majority of women I interviewed supported LGBT rights, including gay marriage and antidiscrimination laws, several women did not support gay rights despite reporting same-sex erotic attractions or behaviors in their histories. For example, when asked about her political beliefs about homosexuality, Ruth, who reported same-sex attraction, also articulated homophobic views:

> Religiously, I'd rather see families of heterosexual couples, though I see that they are just as much of a person and should be as loved as anybody . . . I pretty much take things on a case-by-case basis, but I do not like the political agendas and the strength the groups have. It's almost like they have a chip on their shoulder of "because I'm gay, because I'm this, you should, we should this." I am not against rights, but I don't like the idea of marriage, of it being called "marriage," 'cause to me that's between a man and a woman.

Esther, who reported both same-sex attraction and same-sex behavior, also voiced homophobic views when asked about her political beliefs on homosexuality, drawing notable distinctions between lesbian and gay sexuality:

> I really don't like the idea of two men being together, and that's mostly because of what I've been taught. My best friend in

high school was gay. I knew that he was, and I accepted him for who he was, but I didn't necessarily like the fact that he did it. It goes back to the Old Testament in the Bible, you know, that's something that God says. Men should not lay with men, and women should not lay with women, and men should not lay with beast, and man should not be with his daughter, so that kind of makes it hard. I feel the same way about women, but for some reason society has made that a little bit more acceptable than having two men together. So to me, and I know that's kind of weird in my mind, it feels more wrong for two men than for two women.

When I later asked her about her beliefs about gay rights, she reverted to common beliefs promoted within some conservative communities, including the idea that heterosexuality does not promote itself and that homosexuality is on par with bestiality:

I don't dislike gay people. I really just don't see the need to promote sexual preference as a group of people. If that's what somebody wants to do then that's fine. You go home to your partner, and that's it. I don't see heterosexuals having parades. There's no reason to go out and promote that fact. I don't need to wear a t-shirt that says, "I like men" . . . If people need to go have sex with animals, I don't agree with that either, but there's no reason to go advertising it on the street.

When I asked her about whether she supports gay marriage, she sharply voiced her opposition:

No! I go back to the Bible and when God said that's just not something we should do. I think we need to acknowledge all the groups. I think pedophiles should be able to marry children. I think people should be able to marry their horse, or their dog, or their cat, or their sheep, or whatever it is that is their sexual preference. I don't think it's right to acknowledge one group and say that this is okay without acknowledging the other groups that are different from mainstream society.

Self-described conservative Courtney, who had experiences with performative bisexuality, also expressed a variety of homophobic views:

> [Homosexuality] must be so sad for the person. I mean, I don't want to marry a gay guy and then find out five years later, because that would make life horrible for me. People should choose what they are and stick with that. I have real problems with people who lie . . . It's a religious issue, and I think it's okay to ban them from your church so God can't bless them, but I'm not sure that this is the role of the United States government to uphold these sacred ideas. I'm okay with the church doing that though. Maybe it's better if we didn't have gay people there.

These passages collectively reveal the disconnect that can occur between behavior and attitudes, as openness toward same-sex attraction or behavior did not always translate into an antihomophobic worldview.

Performative Bisexuality as Commodification?

Returning to a Marxist paradigm of women's sexuality, women's same-sex experiences may represent a way for women to increase their value as sexual commodities. The way in which performative bisexuality enhances women's status as commodities (e.g., they are *looked at, evaluated, consumed*) indicates that this sexual culture demands that women participate in patriarchal fantasies to determine their worth. Perhaps this talk of "spicing things up" in the bedroom indicates women's investment in bettering their commodity status; in other words, by hooking up with women at parties, engaging in sexual acts they do not necessarily always find appealing (e.g., anal sex, "facials," etc.), and serving as a willing partner in group sex, women solidify and enhance their role as sexual laborers *and recipients of men's sexual labor.* Further, their desire becomes itself a commodity.

Along these lines, feminist theorists have consistently argued that women shape their sexual desires to please others' fantasies about women, both directly, as they assume their male partner's fantasies, and indirectly, as they assume cultural fantasies about women more broadly. This makes it increasingly difficult to determine what women really *want*, particularly if they become internally oppressed. If men's fantasies dominate the landscape of sexuality, and men's fantasies become normative and widespread, women may more often internalize men's fantasies in order to feel accepted, loved, and, perhaps, objectified and sexualized. In this way, women may assume men's desires and abandon any alternatives. French feminist Luce Irigaray (1985) explained this by stating:

> Woman, in this sexual imaginary, is only a more or less obliging prop for the enactment of male fantasies. That she may find pleasure there in that role, by proxy, is possible, even certain. But such pleasure is above all a masochistic prostitution of her body to a desire that is not her own, and it leaves her in a familiar state of dependency upon man. Not knowing what she wants, ready for anything, even asking for more, so long as he will "take" her as his "object" when he seeks his own pleasure. Thus she will not say what she herself wants; moreover, she does not know, or no longer knows, what she wants. (p. 25)

As such, women's assertions of whether they *want* to engage in performative bisexuality are less relevant than the demand they perceive from their heterosexist contexts. Because performances of bisexuality result in much contradiction and conflict for women, can they resist these? Can they perform something else or generate something else? Such questions point to the complexities of studying and analyzing women's descriptions of their bisexual encounters, particularly in performative spaces where women feel that men literally watch, analyze, and, in many cases, get turned on. What is at stake in such an arrangement?

CONCLUSION

The narratives in this chapter offer several cultural and discursive readings of performative bisexuality: First, compulsory heterosexuality, regardless of the growing prevalence of compulsory bisexuality, still holds great power in women's lives. This fact is notable in heterosexual women minimizing the significance of their same-sex feelings, attractions, behavior, and experiences. Compulsory heterosexuality also appears when women feel that the *literal* and *figurative* presence of men is required during same-sex encounters. Women, particularly heterosexual-identified women (whose sexual experiences constitute the central analyses of this chapter), reported that they engaged in same-sex eroticism in order to arouse men. Women therefore reveal a cruel contradiction, as some women enhance their standing *as heterosexuals* by pretending to embrace bisexuality for male partners. Women are *heterosexual even while performing as bisexual.*

Second, the potential for exploitation of women's same-sex desires and behaviors becomes evident when examining the interface between popular culture and women's behavior. Women kissing women or having sex with women becomes a form of *entertainment* most prominently, while private or self-generated expressions of same-sex eroticism are discouraged and driven further underground. *Girls Gone Wild* features girl-on-girl action but tightly regulates the kind of women who appear in the films (e.g., young, thin, blond, "feminine" in appearance, etc.) and always imposes the male gaze onto the action. Television shows such as *Elimidate, Next, The Real World, Howard Stern, Double Shot at Love*, and *A Shot at Love with Tila Tequila* require women's same-sex eroticism to boost the show's ratings and prove women's openness to male-dominated, male-controlled, male-observed group sex encounters. Mainstream pornography, similarly, has mandated "lesbian" sex only within the narrow confines of *particular* bodies, *particular* actions, and *particular* audiences. Butch women, fat women, and older women, for example, rarely appear in mainstream pornography.

Women said that this exploitation of women's same-sex eroticism led to negative consequences, particularly for women forging sustained bisexual and lesbian identities. When their genuine attraction for each other was transformed into a spectacle for men's viewing pleasure, bisexual and lesbian women felt that their genuine feelings, desires, and sexualities were exploited. When same-sex eroticism became fetishized, this narrowed or diminished other kinds of potential explorations of same-sex desire. The blurring of lines between "real life" and pornography became evident in this construction, as women struggled to define sexuality on their own terms, particularly in light of unflattering "entertainment" representations of their bodies and sexualities.

Yet, as in everything that potentially exploits and manipulates women, perhaps some subversion of compulsory heterosexuality can arise from performative bisexuality. If jaunts into bisexuality are becoming more common, this may open up more opportunities for women who traditionally *never* discussed or explored same-sex desire to think about, talk about, or even experiment with this desire. This seemed particularly true for traditionally conservative women or older women, where married heterosexual encounters were expected. Conversations about attractions to female friends indicated some degree of openness to bisexual and lesbian sexuality. However exploited or taken advantage of, perhaps it is never a bad thing when women explore new avenues of desire, particularly with each other.

One would hope, ideally, that women's mutual eroticism would lay a foundation of mutual respect for each other and, more importantly, social justice for women of *all sexual identities.* As evidenced in these descriptions of women's political beliefs, this hope is only partially realized. While most women argued for full civil rights for bisexual and lesbian women—perhaps as a result of their same-sex experiences— many women still felt justified in retaining homophobic worldviews *despite* their same-sex attractions, actions, or experiences. This suggests that *women's same-sex eroticism does not always translate into a shift in political consciousness,* a finding that should concern those who read performative bisexuality as subversive or as having the potential of expanding women's sociopolitical consciousness. Perhaps this unevenness in political views can be attributed directly to the sexist and homophobic context in which women's same-sex eroticism often currently exists. Gender hierarchies often breed exploitation and power imbalances in order to maintain and reproduce themselves. Cultural scripts often demand only the narrowest vision for how both men and women must behave sexually. *Anything* that does not accommodate mainstream scripts must be demeaned and diminished; *anything* that does not support the status quo must be rendered insignificant. The near-extreme denial of, and cultural contempt for, *men's* same-sex desire, for example, reveals the limitations of acceptance for anything other than (compulsory) heterosexuality. And yet something of the increasing trendiness of bisexuality speaks to a cultural flirtation with rejecting compulsory heterosexuality or embracing same-sex desire, all the while remaining just enough inside of those boundaries to garner social acceptance. This

makes it difficult to fully see the ways that the performance of bisexuality may reinforce the status quo even while it plays with the boundaries
of compulsory heterosexuality and feigns rule violation. What other
visions are possible? What other options exist besides choosing a man
for a sexual partner or choosing a woman with a man's approval? Surely
one need not "go wild" to experience the power of same-sex eroticism;
the more American culture encourages such displays, the further away
we become from truly subverting the compulsory demands placed
upon women's sexuality today.

CHAPTER THREE

THE RISE OF VIAGRA FOR WOMEN

How Sexual Pharmaceuticals Medi(c)ate Desire

Women's bodies—through their use, consumption, and circulation—provide for the condition making social life and culture
possible, although they remain an unknown "infrastructure" of the
elaboration of that social life and culture. The exploitation of the
matter that has been sexualized female is so integral a part of our
sociocultural horizon that there is no way to interpret it except
within this horizon.

> —Irigaray, *This Sex Which Is Not One*

What a lot of people may not know is that for some time now,
pharmaceutical company marketing strategies have focused on
promoting illness, rather than simply promoting drugs. Underpinning many of the marketing strategies of big drug companies is a
very sophisticated and comprehensive plan to widen the boundaries of illness, and create an environment in which more and
more formerly healthy people are defined as "sick." The strategies
have many components—the most visible being TV and newspaper ads that make us think that our ailments and inconveniences
are the signs and symptoms of genuine medical conditions. A sore
stomach is "Irritable Bowel Syndrome," a mild sexual difficulty is
"Female Sexual Dysfunction," and overactive grown-ups now
have "Adult Attention Deficit Disorder."

> —Moynihan, as cited in Stephen J. Dubner,
> "What Don't We Know about the Pharmaceutical
> Industry? A Freakonomics Quorum"

THE RELATIONSHIP BETWEEN the pharmaceutical industry and
the feminist movement has been rife with conflict, as drug companies
square off with groups advocating a more natural approach to physical
and mental health. While many have lauded the pharmaceutical industry for improving people's lives in myriad ways (e.g., inventing medications to lower blood pressure, reduce symptoms of arthritis, assist with
childhood hyperactivity, etc.), others have criticized its tendencies to
medicate aspects of people's lives that could potentially benefit far
more from other approaches such as psychotherapy, better diet, vigor-
ous exercise, less toxic chemicals in foods, stress-reduction techniques,
communication with partners, and so on. While feminism exists as a
progressive force that tries to counter, circumvent, or smash the sexist
practices that damage women in numerous ways, the pharmaceutical
industry pushes a for-profit agenda that follows traditional ideas about
gender norms by medicating women into compliance with "appropriate femininity." These competing priorities often do not gel. The interplay among feminism, the pharmaceutical industry, and women's lives
represents a key battle between social change and social stagnancy. For
example, what does it mean when doctors (or even employers, spouses,
parents, teachers, jailers) medicate behavior in order to enforce conformity to gender norms?[1] Why do corporations market antidepressants as a way for women to be "better mothers" and men to be
"better workers"? Why have corporations repackaged Prozac in a pink
container and labeled it as the cure for "Premenstrual Dysphoric
Disorder"?

   These questions clarify the context in which Viagra for men (the
"little blue pill" that "changed sex in America" [Loe, 2004a] by inducing erections in men) has taken hold of today's cultural consciousness, as
masculinity becomes equated with potency, power with sexuality. Viagra
(and its equivalents) has transformed the landscape of "lifestyle drugs,"
taken over television commercial spots, and sold record numbers of
drugs to men all over the world. Sales of male Viagra have exceeded
$48 billion, with 35 million men worldwide taking Viagra; notably,
Viagra accounts for an enormous percentage of pharmaceutical sales
worldwide (Arndt, 2008; Strong Viagra, 2008). Given this profitability,
and the patterns of pharmaceutical companies always expanding into
new markets in order to increase profits, it makes sense that researchers

have started to hone in on the potential for *women* to take such drugs. Increasing numbers of studies are (conveniently?) finding that women report sexual dysfunction at high rates, a fact that feminists have criticized. For example, recent studies claim that *over 40%* (!!) of women suffer from sexual dysfunction (Kohn, 2008; Shifren et al., 2008), a finding that has left feminists suspicious, nervous, and worried about both the methods of such studies and the potential ways that drug companies can capitalize on pathologizing women's sexual health.

The obvious money-making potential in medicating sex has predictably led to a slew of attempts to create, in essence, Viagra for women, sparking a battle among frenzied pharmaceutical companies to recreate the successes of Viagra for men. These efforts make sense: given the findings of chapter 1—where women describe incredible pressure to orgasm when in sexual relationships—Viagra for women could tap into women's anxieties about being "good enough" sexual partners. Further, if male Viagra draws upon men's anxieties about potency and power, Viagra for women could draw upon women's desire to please their (male) partners by increasing the frequency and intensity of sex. After all, women as a group report less interest in sex, less frequent orgasm, less physical arousal, and, for the most part, less sexual satisfaction than men as a group (Haavio-Mannila & Kontula, 1997). Viagra for women could fit into this trend by both providing women with heightened physiological arousal and better chances to perform as "good enough" partners and by providing men with another tool with which to pressure women into sex.

In light of recent pharmaceutical attempts to develop Viagra for women (and other pharmaceutical drugs that medicate sexual arousal for women), this chapter explores the symbolic and literal meanings of such medicated sexuality: What would a medi(c)ated sexuality look like? *Why is gender medicated?* Unlike the other chapters in this book, chapter 3 is a *prospective* chapter; rather than interrogating what is currently happening in women's lives, it raises questions, by talking directly with women, about the *future* of women's sexual performances. What kinds of performances will be demanded in the future, and how might women respond to them? How do women feel about the new frontiers of women's sexual performance, particularly as they align with medicalization?

Specifically, this chapter draws upon a variety of sources that have a multitude of different agendas. I first consider mainstream newspaper articles on the development of Viagra for women (particularly the *New York Times*), as well as psychological studies about female sexual enhancement drugs. While the newspaper articles underlie the mainstreaming of the pharmaceutical industry in women's sexual lives, the psychological studies highlight women's conflicted feelings about such drugs. Most centrally, this chapter considers women's narratives about their *anticipatory* feelings on this subject in order to highlight the relationship between sexual performance and medication. These narratives reveal the conflicts women face when weighing their (often inconsistent) bodily responses, cultural expectations for sexual performance, and their partner's sexual demands. I also examine the evolution of Female Sexual Dysfunction (FSD) as a series of clinical diagnoses (widely used in *The Diagnostic and Statistical Manual of Mental Disorders-IV*), paying special attention to the discourse of sex therapy as it mandates certain kinds of (heterosexual) female sexual behaviors. To frame this discussion, I draw from *The New View* campaign—a group of feminist sexologists who have rejected efforts to medicate women's desire—while more directly situating these issues in the framework of women's stories about anticipating the release of Viagra for women and other sexual pharmaceuticals.

In short, this chapter adds to the existing literature on the subject by contextualizing women's *imagined* need for female sexual enhancement drugs within the larger framework of mandated sexual performance, particularly performances encouraged by drug companies and by women's sexual partners. By looking closely at the way drug companies invent and use women's sexual worries to further their corporate interests, women's own conflicts about these drugs reveal the extent to which sexual performance permeates not only their cultural surroundings (e.g., media, advertising, doctor's offices) but also their personal ideologies about sexual normality and pharmaceutical intrusiveness. Key questions in this chapter include the following: How do pharmaceutical companies manufacture women's need for a sexual enhancement drug, and how do women speak about this manufactured need? What might it mean in women's lives if drug companies successfully develop Viagra for women? Would women resist these drugs or comply with cultural expectations that they need them? How would the introduction of women's Viagra onto the marketplace change women's experiences of sex and/or complicate expectations of sexual performance? What do women's feelings about sexual pharmaceuticals say about the norms of sexual performance?

RESEARCH ON VIAGRA FOR WOMEN

A man knows he has a problem. But in the case of a woman, she can perform. She doesn't necessarily think of herself as having a problem.
—Mazer, vice president for clinical research at Theratech, Inc., as quoted in *New York Times*, April 25, 1998

Studies continue to overwhelmingly argue that more and more women report diagnosable sexual dysfunction, with some studies reporting that nearly half of all women are sexually dysfunctional, based on self-reported sexual problems (Shifren et al., 2008). While these studies have received harsh criticisms based on the wording of the survey items (e.g., most studies, aside from Shifren's study, that interrogated sexual dysfunction, asked women only about the problems themselves and not about the subjective distress about those problems), cross-cultural comparison data (e.g., British women report numbers hovering around 10% rather than 50%), and who sponsored the research, these studies have been used by pharmaceutical companies to justify the apparent need for the development and marketing of Viagra for women and other sexual pharmaceuticals designed for women (WebMD, 2007). Shifren's research found that 43.1% described some kind of sexual problem, while 39% reported diminished desire, 26% had problems with arousal, and 21% acknowledged problems with achieving orgasm (Gardner, 2008). These kinds of data open up opportunities for the pharmaceutical industry to attempt to profit enormously from women's so-called sexual dysfunction.

Mainstream media discussions about the development of, and failure to acquire FDA approval for, Viagra for women have permeated newspapers and websites for the past several years. This mainstream newspaper coverage of Viagra for women, along with feminist criticisms of the emerging market for female sexual enhancement drugs, reveals the cultural investment in women's *performances* of sexual interest and activity; after all, Viagra is a quintessential device of enforced sexual arousal, supposedly overriding the body's "natural" functions and inclinations in favor of artificial excitement. Drug companies' conflation of increased blood flow to the vagina (the physiological result of the drug) and subjective feelings of excitement (the unmet psychological goal of the drug) has yielded less than stellar results for fledgling Viagra for women. Research and reports on Viagra for women reveal the intense clashes between the feminist and medical model of constructing sexuality, particularly as it relates to women's bodies, desires, and behaviors.

The quest for Viagra for women started in 1998 following the blockbuster success of Viagra for men, as a variety of pharmaceutical companies became invested in the development of the female version of the drug. Scientists initially wanted Viagra for women to mimic the men's version, in that it would stimulate increased blood flow to the vagina, thus resulting in women finding it easier to become lubricated and to reach orgasm during penile-vaginal intercourse. *The New York Times* reported on Pfizer's attempt to develop Viagra for women by describing the various impediments that emerged throughout the development phase from 1998 through 2005. Often, reasons for Viagra's "failure" stemmed from two primary assertions: 1) Women and men are different, and therefore Viagra does not have the same effect on women; and 2) women do not connect physiological arousal and psychological desire in the same way as men (supposedly) do.

Consider this: a March 2004 *New York Times* article points out that scientists had given up on developing a female version of Viagra (Harris, 2004), citing its inability to ignite women's arousal patterns. The article stated, "[Female] Viagra's failure underscored the obvious: when it comes to sexuality, men and women to some extent are differently tuned. For men, arousal and desire are often intertwined, while for women, the two are frequently distinct" (O'Connor, 2004, p. F–5). Another *New York Times* article from the same month, also discussing the failure of Viagra for women, stated, "Although Viagra can indeed create the outward signs of arousal in many women, that seems to have little effect on a woman's willingness, or desire, to have sex" (Harris, 2004, p. C–1). Researchers were puzzled by Viagra's inability to convince women to have sex with their partners, citing that many women do not feel sexual arousal until they actually begin to have intercourse. The article concluded by saying, "Getting a woman to connect arousal and desire . . . requires exquisite timing on a man's part and a fair amount of coaxing. 'What we need to do is find a pill for engendering the perception of intimacy'" (Harris, 2004, p. C–1).

Thus, while it is difficult to fully determine the extent to which such a statement reflects the actual priorities of the pharmaceutical industry (i.e., do people really want to develop a pill that engenders *desire*?), these statements reflect a kind of orientation toward the creation of new diseases, whereby pharmaceutical companies—in an effort to generate profits and hook people on lifestyle drugs—literally *invent* disorders in order to convince people that they need treatment for them. While women *do* experience changes in their sexual health through the processes of aging, illness, childbirth, and the like, critics wonder whether drug companies have acted too hastily in identifying these changes as a potential new market. As one recent article asks, "*Is a new disorder being identified to meet unmet needs or to build markets for new medications?*" (Moynihan, 2003). Feminist critics of the pharmaceutical industry have long pointed out that disease mongering is a standard practice, particularly for "diseases" that require lifelong medications (e.g., antidepressants, antianxiety drugs, etc.) (Tiefer, 2006b). Further, it speaks to these drug companies' tendencies to reduce women's desire and women's sexuality to exclusively a physiological function (much in the same way that sexual identity has been figured prominently in the mainstream news media as a biological/physiological matter [Hegarty & Pratto, 2001]). Here, desire is not a function of, say, any social factors of a relationship but instead of the woman's malfunctioning brain chemistry. This characterization completely leaves out the role of social relationships, power struggles, partnered inequalities, lack of communication, major life changes, stress and health issues, and other related factors that have little to do with physiological brain chemistry issues.

The insistence upon the difference between men and women's physiological reactions to sex showcases the belief that, for men, sex represents "hydraulics," while for women, sex represents a mixture of desire and physiology. Biological essentialism forms the underpinning of these clinical trials. For example, Leonard Derogatis, president of

Clinical Psychometric Research, Inc., was quoted by the *New York Times* saying, "In men, erectile dysfunction is relatively dramatic and some-what catastrophic . . . In women, problems are more subtle. Arousal blends with desire, and problems can be medical or nonmedical. And whereas it's hard for a man with an erection not to think about sex, a woman with increased blood flow will say she feels nothing" (Duen-wald, 2003). The emphasis on women's pathology versus men's "natural decline in functioning" is evident in Julie Heiman's statement: "With-out having a good, clear physiological picture of how all the organ sys-tems work together, you can't know if a woman has a genital problem, something interfering in her brain processing, or, quite possibly, both" (Duenwald, 2003). Even the way scientists measure arousal reveals gen-dered problems; David Ferguson told *The New York Times*, "How do you prove lubrication? . . . Do you put tampons in their vaginas and weigh them when you take them out? Do you aspirate vaginal fluids?" (Kolata, 1998). The frustrations that women do not sync with men's sexual experiences as fully as scientists and doctors would like reveals the way that the *social* aspects of sexuality (including various interfer-ences with sexual desire) remain completely ignored.

Along these lines, some reports argue that men's failure to give Viagra a "real try" or men's resistance to using Viagra altogether stems from their female partners. The construction of men's resistance to Viagra as the fault of their partners situates men's sexual dysfunction as the fault of women (Vares & Braun, 2006). For example, a recent article (Arndt, 2008) posited:

> Many suspect the real problem lies in the fact that it takes two to tango. The major consumers for these products are older men . . . These mid-life men may be desperate to get back in the saddle again yet they are often partnered by women who would far prefer to spend their evenings with a good book . . . Women started writing to advice columns complaining that the drug companies were wrecking their marriages. "Please tell those smart-aleck scientists and those big drug companies to work on a cure for cancer instead and quit ruining the lives of millions of women who have earned a rest."

Such discourse situates women as resistant to sex, putting up with sex because they "must," and unable to generate their own desire, even though this is far from the whole truth (Loe, 2004b). Men's desire, by contrast, is situated as always active unless they do not have willing female partners. Such a contrast fails to locate the intensely gendered nature of these sexual dyads. Further, by blaming women for resisting sex—particularly without interrogating the pressures to perform that women face in this situation—people recklessly construct women as merely the gatekeepers to men's pleasure rather than sexual agents in their own lives.

Several more recent *New York Times* pieces reflect these priorities, as the social constructedness of sexuality takes a backseat to the idea that *desire* can be manufactured biologically or physiologically. Implications for the *enforced performance of women's sexual interest* are overwhelming here. An April 2007 piece argues:

> [Viagra for women] enhanced engorgement of vaginal tissue, just as it had of the penis, but that extra bit of pelvic swelling did nothing to amplify women's desire for or enjoyment of sex. What is needed for the treatment of so-called female hypoactive sexual desire disorder, researchers decided, is a reasonably safe and effective drug that acts on the central nervous system, on the pleasure centers of the brain or the sensory circuitry that serves them. (Angier, 2007)

In essence, the pharmaceutical companies seem to believe and hope that sexual desire arises from brain chemistry rather than a complex array of *social* practices. Thus, if biology governs sexual drives and sexual performance, seemingly nothing is out of bounds to pharmaceutical intervention, including women's desire for sex.

The overreliance upon biological essentialism as an explanation for the differences between men and women remains at the center of these controversies about Viagra for women. A July 2008 article reports that "[m]ost women with sexual problems suffer from a lack of desire, while men with sexual problems are more likely to suffer from lack of arousal, the physiological ability to become excited. In men, Viagra works on arousal by increasing blood flow to the penis . . . The most prevalent female sexual dysfunction is not arousal but desire. Viagra doesn't have a direct effect on that" (Kohn, 2008). Or, as *The Los Angeles Times* puts it, "In women, the drug increased engorgement of genital tissue but failed to enhance women's enjoyment of sex" (Gellene, 2008), as if enjoyment of sex related primarily to women's physiological arousal *outside the context of the social.*

RESEARCH ON OTHER SEXUAL PHARMACEUTICALS

> Not to discount psychological aspects, but at a certain point all sex is mechanical. The man needs a sufficient axial rigidity so his penis can penetrate through labia, and he has to sustain that in order to have sex. This is a mechanical structure, and mechanical structures follow scientific principles . . . The "typical resistance" posed by an average vagina is a measurable two pounds. The key is to create an erection that doesn't "deform" or collapse when engaging that resistance. I am an engineer . . . And I can apply the principles of hydraulics to these problems. I can utilize medical strategies to assess, diagnose, and manipulate things that are not so straightforward in psychiatry.
> —Goldstein, "The Second Sexual Revolution" 2000

The search for the female equivalent of Viagra has not ended simply because researchers cannot find a way to attach desire and physiological arousal; rather, researchers have begun testing, marketing, and selling drugs that cover new female "sexual pathologies" and attempt to increase the frequency of women having sex with their (male) partners. Interestingly, these efforts often attempt to *make women more like stereotypical men* (e.g., medicating a more aggressive desire for sex, physiological arousal, etc.), often while packaging the drugs in the conventional color of pink (or otherwise feminine colors).[2] For example, in recent years, doctors have begun to prescribe off-label testosterone prescriptions (i.e., prescriptions given without FDA approval for the use of that drug in that particular way) to women, despite lack of FDA approval and absence of long-term safety data (Cook, 2005). Procter and Gamble developed Intrinsa, a testosterone patch that "delivers small transdermal

pulses of the sex hormone thought to play a crucial if poorly understood role in male and female libido alike" (Angier, 2007). The FDA
declared it unsafe because the medical risks far outweighed the modest
benefits of the drug, yet the patch is now being picked up again by
P&G after they buy the rights from Noven Pharmaceuticals (Procter &
Gamble, 2008). A recent study found that women using the testosterone
patch increased their likelihood of developing breast cancer, yet
researchers still argued, "I think most women would be more than
happy with it" (Harding, 2008).

Nevertheless, off-label of testosterone continue to rise in numbers,
fueled in part by the coupling of men and sex drives along with pressures placed upon women to maintain their sex drive throughout their
lives. In 2006 alone, doctors wrote over a million prescriptions for off-
label testosterone (Kwan, 2008). As Ganahl (2006) recently said, "And
for a lot of women, losing one's sex drive feels equivalent to being
dead." Pfizer has begun sponsoring research on whether male Viagra
itself will help women, which has resulted in mixed findings. Two studies found that male Viagra helped some women with sexual problems,
including subjective feelings of arousal (Kohn, 2008; Nurnberg et al.,
2003). Leonard Derogatis noted, "It's not a blockbuster study, but it's
interesting. The large majority of women with sexual dysfunction do
not respond to Viagra" (Kohn, 2008).

Another recent study with a very small sample size found that male
Viagra may help women on antidepressants to have orgasms, though it
did *not* increase women's sex drive. Further, women who took Viagra
reported a host of negative side effects, including severe indigestion, hot
flashes, visual problems, nasal congestion, and the like (Szabo, 2008). *The
New York Times* reported that Viagra caused women to have headaches
and indigestion (Venkataraman, 2008). Still, some researchers continue
to believe that women's bodies simply need more testosterone in order
to feel better. Reichman (quoted in Cook, 2005) said, "Women need
estrogen for lubrication and comfort during sex. But they need testosterone to feel desire in the first place. With diminished testosterone . . .
women don't just lose desire for their partners, they lose desire for *any*
partner." A *New York Times* piece cited German researchers saying,
"Testosterone might have direct effects on cognitive behavior, e.g.,
influence the awareness of sexual cues, but it is also suggested that

testosterone may act peripherally to enhance sexual pleasure and thereby increase sexual desire and even sexual activity, circumstances and partner permitting" (Sweeney, 2005). This implicitly suggests that the only reason for women's lack of desire for sex is their lack of physical arousal, in essence, their lack of ability to *be like men*. The implications here suggest that women are less able to pick up on sexual cues or feel sexual pleasure. Such claims seem "patronizing, dismissive, and irresponsibly uninformed" (Rako, quoted in Cook, 2005) in their assertions that women's bodies should mimic men's bodies in order to be acceptable, desirable, and high-functioning.

Another attempt to medicate women's sexual desire, Bremelanotide, has also been the subject of much controversy over the past two years. The hormone, a synthetic version of a hormone that contributes to skin pigmentation, initially sought to prevent skin cancer by creating artificially tan skin. Once it was discovered that the drug created spontaneous erections in male college students, the drug was tested as a treatment for hypoactive desire problems for women. While the drug had some mild aphrodisiac properties, the unspecified "embarrassing side effects" and the fact that the drug only worked when women had "control over the mating game" (Angier, 2005) led to its ultimate demise. One of the lead researchers for this drug, Michael Perelman, was quoted saying, "I'm interested in helping people respond more to the right kind of stimulation from the right person when that's just not happening naturally for them, in the way that they would like, or that it used to" (WebMD, 2007). Again, the implications are overwhelming: it seems that scientists want to develop a drug that will, in essence, override a woman's own social feelings with regard to sex so that she wants sex even when she perceives a variety of social barriers or problems with her partner(s). Also, the idea of a "right kind of stimulation" comes awfully close to portraying any male effort to stimulate women as adequately skillful while women's *responses* to that male effort are labeled as "dysfunctional." Women *must perform if he "correctly" stimulates her*, they argue.

In recent years, doctors have prescribed a whole host of drugs to "cure" sexual dysfunction despite lack of FDA approval and lack of formal evidence for their effectiveness. The antianxiety drug Buspirone (marketed as BuSpar) has been prescribed to women off-label as an antidote to sexual dysfunction (Lyon, 2008), as have a variety of sexual creams and nasal sprays promising to increase women's enjoyment of sex (Palmer, 2007). For the drugs that act on the central nervous system, many doctors consider that kind of intervention to be something that should only be attempted as a last resort for a severe disorder; many doctors do not see women's sexual dysfunction as a "disorder" severe enough to warrant manipulations of this kind. Clearly, danger matters less than women's conformity to social norms about sex.

Given this intense pressure on women to perform their arousal, it comes as no surprise that sexual pharmaceuticals have become increasingly aggressive in their efforts to corner the market for informal treatments of female sexual dysfunction. As early as 1999, following the blockbuster success of male Viagra, a variety of companies patented creams, devices, and pills that claimed to enhance women's sexual drive or orgasmic abilities. Michael Wysor and Wanda Drinnon Wysor patented an ointment in 1999 that allegedly induced multiple orgasms in women when applied to the clitoris. They told the *New York Times*, "It increases blood flow tremendously and basically eliminates the need for foreplay. This is going to have an impact equal to that seen with the introduction of the Pill" (Riordan, 1999). In the past nine years, this ointment invention has not gained commercial success.

More recently, BioSante Pharmaceuticals has focused its efforts on developing LibiGel, a gel-based testosterone that women rub onto their upper arms in order to boost libido. Scottish scientist Liz Paul has invented a patch women wear on the inside of their wrist called "Scentuelle." Women are instructed to sniff the patch all day long, stimulating a better mood and sense of well-being associated with the brain's production of dopamine. Paul, who has yet to submit Scentuelle to a placebo test, was quoted saying, "It's aromacology. It works entirely on the smell. Nothing goes into the bloodstream, and it works on the limbic area of the brain, which controls our emotions and attitudes" (Ganahl, 2006). While the placebo effects for such a "drug" seem quite plausible, it also forces confrontation with another set of problems with regard to medicating desire and arousal for women: sometimes drug companies insist upon extreme secrecy about their products. Some pharmaceutical companies keep their products shrouded in mystery, such as Boehringher-Ingelheim Pharmaceuticals, who sponsored the drug flibanserin, rejected by the FDA in June 2010 for lack of clinical effectiveness (Wilson, 2010). This drug, allegedly an antidepressant, "hasn't been approved previously for any use." All people know is that "flibanserin is a molecule acting on the central nervous system and is not a hormone product" (WebMD, 2007). The drug has been purposefully kept enshrouded in secrecy about its chemical makeup and direct side effects, again showing the relative lack of demand for more information about what doctors prescribe or impose upon women in a pharmaceutical sense. Perhaps the lesson is clear: if they do not tell the public *how* the drug works, the public will accept the drug more readily.

In short, efforts to corner the market on female sexual dysfunction continue in earnest, as drug companies sense the enormous profits to be made not only by inventing disorders but by convincing women they need to treat those disorders with *their* drugs. The story *underneath* these many botched drug trials, failed attempts to medicate women's sexuality, and laughably bizarre techniques used to induce desire is clear: *women must perform desire even if they do not physiologically experience it.* The requirements for women to not only discipline their bodies to *produce* sexual responsiveness at the correct moments but also to perform their *desire* for their (male) sexual partners reveals the increasingly aggressive ways drug companies enforce women's mandatory compliance with proper gender roles. Women become, in essence, desiring machines.

FEMINIST CRITIQUES OF SEXUAL PHARMACEUTICALS

The common thread in most research on sexual pharmaceuticals posits the following assumption: *Most women are sexually dysfunctional* and *that is an important problem.* This carries with it the troubling implications that *not desiring sex is itself a fundamental problem.* This implies that the artificial inducement of sex matters more than women's inclinations toward sex, in other words, that women should *not* attend to their own internal processes about when (and how often) they want sex but should instead demand from themselves a constant level of interest in, and orientation toward, partnered sexual activity. These assertions sharply deny the reality that women's sexual desire fluctuates daily and throughout the lifespan. In sharp contrast to the medicalization of sexuality, some studies have shown that, even if women struggle with lack of sexual desire, most women do not report feeling distressed or bothered by that fact (Shifren, 2008). The study found that only 12% of women suffering from a low sex drive are bothered by the problem, though one would do well to interpret such distress findings with a bit of caution, particularly given the varied social norms that different age groups face. For instance, another study found that 24% of women reported distress about sex, with variable numbers for women of different ages (Bancroft, Loftus, & Long, 2004). From a feminist lens, perhaps low sexual desire throughout parts of women's lives is a normal occurrence, not something that deserves medical and psychological attention. Interestingly, women between ages 45 and 64 reported *more* distress about sexual problems than either 18–44 year-olds or those over age 64 (Collins, 2008), indicating that pressures to perform arousal may be especially strong for women during the menopausal years.

Leonore Tiefer, one of the most outspoken critics of female sexual enhancement drugs, argued that sexual desire cannot be separated from its object and that a host of problems can affect people's sexual experiences, including socialization as a child (e.g., sex guilt, sex negativity, etc.), body image difficulties, emotionally distant or hostile partners, distrust in relationships, other life events (e.g., grief, stress, work, etc.), and so on (Tiefer, 2004; Tiefer, 2006a). She lists a litany of outside forces that can disrupt good sex: "They don't have a partner, they just had a baby, they just lost their job, their husband is philandering, their marriage is on the fritz . . . Just because you don't have an orgasm doesn't mean you are unhappy about this" (Kirkey, 2008). Rosemary Basson agreed, arguing that women and men "'have multiple motivations to be sexual, and 'desire'—as in urging 'lust,' 'horniness,' or 'drive'—is only one of these reasons'" (WebMD, 2007). She also stated that it is too often assumed that all women have a constant amount of sexual desire or that there is a "normal" amount of desire; these claims are not supported by data about aging, menopause, pregnancy, and other *natural* hormonal fluctuations that occur across the lifespan and disrupt the constancy of women's sexual desire.

Feminist critics have also pointed out that fluctuations in sexual desire are common and that many other factors aside from physiological dysfunction may contribute to sexual impairments for women. One recent study argued that many cases of impaired sexual response or decreased interest in sex for women are psychologically understandable or even adaptive and hence not dysfunctions at all (e.g., postsexual trauma, postdivorce, etc.). Until people can distinguish between adaptive versus maladaptive inhibitions of sexual response, pharmaceutical treatments have the potential to exploit and abuse women (Bancroft, 2002). As sex researcher John Gagnon said, "People are not necessarily unhealthy or in need of medical treatment if they do not feel like having sex all the time. 'Many people find their hobbies more interesting . . . Sex is a modest pleasure'" (Grady, 1999).

As another related critique, feminists have expressed concern with the gender, sexual identity, and social justice implications of sexual pharmaceuticals, as drugs such as Viagra and Eros reinforce ideas about masculinity as "potent," femininity as "receptive," and sexual identity as "always heterosexual." The prescriptive implications of the drugs render "atypical" gender and sexual expressions, desires, and appearances invisible and marginal, also calling into question "what counts" as legitimate sex (Fishman & Mamo, 2001). Some have argued that the pharmaceutical industry serves male desires of women as constantly available for sex (Nicolson, 2004).

Because of the relative lack of attention to the social constructedness of sexuality, sex therapy has particularly suffered from the pressures to shift toward a more pharmaceutical understanding of women's sexuality. Tiefer (2006b) has argued, "The classification of women's sexual dysfunctions has been rewritten repeatedly over the last few years in an effort to provide diagnostic categories useful in clinical trials, and yet difficulties persist in producing a list of conditions that match the diversity of women's descriptions of their experience" (p. 367). As such, treatment of women's sexual problems has increasingly turned less to social methods like psychotherapy and social networking and has instead embraced more medical methods like medication and surgery (FDA, 2000). For example, women routinely hear that something is wrong with their bodies, that they need various kinds of medication, and that their partners are irrelevant to their "sexual dysfunction."

In response to these technologically patriarchal inventions, the New View campaign, started in 2000 by Tiefer and a group of other

sexuality scholars and practitioners, has argued against the medicalization of women's sexuality and instead focused on pleasure, satisfaction,
and the social aspects of sexuality. The front page of their website
declares, "The New View Campaign was formed in 2000 as a grass-
roots network to challenge the distorted and oversimplified messages
about sexuality that the pharmaceutical industry relies on to sell its
new drugs. The pharmaceutical industry wants people to think that
sexual problems are simple medical matters, and it offers drugs as
expensive magic fixes. But sexual problems are complicated, sexuality
is diverse, and no drug is without side effects." They go on to argue,
"The Campaign challenges all views that reduce sexual experience to
genital biology and thereby ignore the many dimensions of real life."
The New View campaign sees male Viagra as laying the groundwork
for an even more aggressive medicalization of women's sexuality in the
future, something they work against via activism, scholarship, and therapy (Tiefer, 2001). They also fight against direct-to-consumer pharmaceutical advertisements (Hartley & Coleman, 2008), sex therapy that
ignores the social aspects of sexuality (Tiefer, 2007), and the profitability of lifestyle drugs that keep people hooked on drugs for long peri-
ods of time rather than phasing them out over a set period of time
(Tiefer, 2003).

Members of The New View have provided a much-needed voice in
the debates about how to best treat female sexual dysfunction. In an
interview, Tiefer was asked, "If drugs for low desire aren't a good solution, what is?" to which she responded,

> The only thing you need a solution for is a problem. I hope
> some women who take a look at their sex lives won't need a
> solution. But if you do decide you need a solution, there are
> lots of them: Conversation and communication with a partner;
> sexual education with a partner; education for yourself about
> sexual realities and options . . . The mind leads and the body
> follows. (Lyon, 2008)

Rather than relying upon the pharmaceutical industry to solve
women's sexual problems, many feminist critics argue that women need
to reassess the mythology around "wanting" and "needing" sex all the

time throughout their lives; instead, women should reimagine their interest in sex as having normal fluctuations in response to life events, biological changes, and partnered relationships.

Other feminists have centered their critiques on the implications for sexual performance embedded in sexual pharmaceutical discourse. For example, if heterosexual women report lower sexual desire than their male partners, might these drugs open up new avenues for performance pressures? If a man has more desire than his partner and does not receive the kind of affirmation he wants about his desire or skills, might he badger her to medicate herself rather than face his own short-comings (as a sexual partner, as a communicator, etc.)? The pressure women describe about trying to experience multiple orgasms, for example, reveals these kinds of heteronormative pressures, as women face constant pressures to perform as *more* orgasmic, *more* efficient, *more* desiring, as established in chapter 1.

The medicalization of women's sexuality may actually represent, in addition to sexual *performance*, a form of sexual *repression*. Allina (2001) has argued that pharmaceutical treatments for sexual dysfunction come out of the lack of desire to *speak about* sexuality; market-driven research and medication, therefore, enter the sexual landscape precisely at the same time that there is an increase in abstinence-only education, con-servative political climates, and a dearth of conversations about healthy sexual relationships and sexual decision making. Thus, sexual pharma-ceuticals not only map onto cultural silences about sexuality, but they also *make a profit* off of the cultural reluctance to speak about sex.

Many scholars, particularly feminist sexuality scholars, have expressed extreme alarm at the infiltration of medicalized ideas about women's sexuality within academic, pharmaceutical, and medical cir-cles, often at the expense of any kind of social critique. Heather Hart-ley, one of the original authors of the New View manifesto, argued that drug companies have worked to medicalize women's sexuality via sexual pharmaceuticals by focusing on three main efforts: first, mass dis-semination of estimates of disease prevalence (often overestimating women's "sexual dysfunction" despite contradictory evidence); second, the institutionalization of Female Sexual Dysfunction in academic cir-cles, including the strategic revision of disease definitions as well as the creation of a legitimized infrastructure for dissemination of supporting research and education; and third, public relations stimulated main-stream media coverage (Hartley, 2006).

Some even argue that the pharmaceutical industry represents a vast conspiracy to invent disorders as a way to make a profit (Kingsberg, 2008), a claim supported by much of the evidence reviewed so far. While this chapter has until now addressed the corporate push for female sexual pharmaceuticals, the rest of this chapter examines how women themselves respond to such an agenda. What impact does Viagra for women have on women who are just beginning to grapple with the introduction of sexual pharmaceuticals into their sexual lives? If women struggle with many demands placed on their sexuality now, how do they feel about *new* demands placed upon them in the foreseeable future? When speaking with women about their willingness or reluctance to try Viagra for women, conflicts between sexual performance, partnered pleasure, and self-identified sexual "function" and "dysfunction" become apparent.

WOMEN'S NARRATIVES ABOUT VIAGRA FOR WOMEN

> A commodity—a woman—is divided into two irreconcilable "bodies": her "natural" body and her socially valued, exchangeable body, which is a particularly mimetic expression of masculine values.
>
> —Irigaray, *This Sex Which Is Not One*

Women's reactions to the emerging medicalization of their sexuality—and the potential for new social scripts about their sexual performances—reveal the conflicts of negotiating sexual empowerment. While most women experienced pressures to orgasm (chapter 1), and some women grappled with performative bisexuality pressures (chapter 2), Viagra for women represented a cutting edge way that women's sexuality may be shaped and molded in the future. When asking women for their opinions about the development of Viagra for women and other sexual pharmaceuticals,[3] and how they would decide whether to use such drugs, responses predictably ranged from positive and supportive to relatively ambivalent to intensely negative. Questions about Viagra for women allowed women to grapple with performance in an *imaginary* and prospective sense—that is, women typically reflected on whether they hypothetically would use such a drug, whether they felt a need for such a drug, and how they felt about medicating their sexual responses in general. These responses, in essence, reflect *anticipatory* aspects of performance.

Their stories reveal the way that women's attitudes about sexual pharmaceuticals could lead to positive, negative, or ambivalent outcomes, a range driven by a variety of factors: the degree to which women were open to trying pharmaceuticals and other drugs in general, their skepticism or trust (or both) in the medical field, their perceptions about their own need for such a drug, and their beliefs about gender and the construction of themselves as a "good partner." Embedded within these narratives were the relationships women have to ideologies of sexual performance and their constructions of *themselves* within a culture that demands women's sexual performance.

Positive Reactions

During the interviews, women were asked how they felt about the possibility of taking a female version of Viagra. In line with women responding to the medicalization of their bodies—and perhaps similar to the liberal feminist argument that women should seek full equality by being *similar to men* (Scott, 1988)—several women reported positive and supportive feelings about sexual pharmaceuticals such as Viagra for women, citing in particular the way that such drugs paralleled those available for men and opened up new avenues for sexual expression. Women who felt sexual dysfunction relative to their peer group expressed particular support for sexual pharmaceuticals. Such willingness to try Viagra for women indicated specific ideas about the distance between how women *do* feel sexually and how they think they *should* feel sexually. For example, Jill, age 32, expressed positive feelings about these drugs based on ideas of her body as not responding properly to sexual stimulation:

> Assuming it didn't have any side effects I was worried about, it
> might be nice to try female Viagra. I feel a lot like my brain

wants sex as much as possible, but my body doesn't always seem to be getting in on the program. It might be nice to have my body responding at least as much as my brain is rather than having to sort of coax and prod my body into getting interested.

Jill's response reveals the crux of the tension between sexual pharmaceuticals and the feminist movement; if women feel they *should* respond a certain way, but their bodies do not comply with their mental state, drugs seem like a viable option. Drug companies capitalize on this precise perception, knowing that women will *medicate* their bodies to comply with societal expectations. Diana, age 50, who sometimes struggled with feeling fully sexually functional, also expressed willingness to medicate her sexuality: "Yes, I would try it, absolutely! If it enhanced sex, I would enjoy it because if I go into menopause, and it affects my libido, I would try it."

Women also cited the fairness issue as a reason to support Viagra for women, in that if men had their own version of Viagra, why shouldn't women also have theirs? For example, Courtney, age 23, told me, "They have it for guys, so they should have it for girls too! We should have the option. As long as we're carrying their babies, we might as well have an orgasm." Pam, age 42, who also believed strongly in fairness with regard to medicalizing men's and women's bodies, said, "If they need it, more power to them. I think that that's one of the examples of these sexist practices in medicine. We know that insurance will pay for Viagra for the man but not for fertility treatments for the woman. It doesn't make any sense. Viagra for women might help that unfairness."

Women of all ages also expressed feelings of fear about their sex drives slowing down or their relationship to sexuality changing as they got older. Twenty-five-year-old Lucy talked frequently about her fears that her sexual relationship with her husband would shift once they finished their newlywed phase of marriage, particularly surrounding the dampening of their sex life (see Klusmann, 2002). Remember, too, that Lucy also anticipated *potentially needing to fake orgasm* if her desire waned later on in her marriage (see chapter 1), revealing that performance has a *strongly anticipatory quality* at times. She said of Viagra for women, "I think now I have a lot of sex, and I'm pretty much open to it even when I'm not exactly in the mood, but if my husband was trying repeatedly, and I wasn't able to do it, I think I'd be open to Viagra. I hear when you get older that your sex life slows down and so need things to help. I don't want that to happen." Lucy's anticipation of performance indicates the pervasive qualities of performance pressures that women often face in long-term relationships; though she has plenty of sex now, she worries about the inevitability of that slowing down and has prepared herself for getting various kinds of "boosts" to ensure that that does not happen.

Having experienced her sex drive slowing down, Bonnie, age 51, also expressed an interest in Viagra for women to help alleviate the sexual pressures she felt from her husband:

> I'd try it. I'm an experimental person. Right now, I think my lack of sexuality is caused by something external rather than something internal. I'm referring to the problems with my husband. He would say it was internal though. He just says it's the way I am. I have always been a very sexual person my whole, life so I say it's not the way I am.

The attribution differences here between women's own sense of why they lack desire for sex and their (male) partners' sense of why sex has waned speaks to false images of sexual desires for people in real relationships and the intensity of pressures to perform as sexually aroused in women's lives. In a paradigm where men's desires reign and their power is exercised and reinforced repeatedly, beliefs about women as dysfunctional, particularly in heterosexual contexts, seem far less threatening than a nonflattering assessment of men's sexual abilities. Women's *bodies* become the targeted problem, not men's *abilities*.

Ophelia, age 56, expressed positive feelings about Viagra, given her physiological experiences going through menopause: "After menopause, there is no lubrication, so I use lube to avoid tearing and things like that. Creams probably aren't much different from these drugs, and I think all drugs are good." Faced with the realities of aging and the inevitability of bodily changes, as well as the high likelihood of fluctuations in sexual desire, some women, particularly older women and women in partnered relationships, felt more open to pharmaceutical intervention than others, revealing again the ways that norms of sexual performance affect women's lives. Additionally, women's different kinds of relationships to drugs and altered states in general seemed to play into their responses to Viagra as an option, perhaps revealing another reason why women try off-label prescriptions of testosterone or other non-FDA-approved sexual enhancement drugs.

Ambivalent and Conditional Reactions

The requirements of sexual performance for women also appeared in women's ambivalent attitudes toward Viagra for women and sexual pharmaceuticals. These ambivalent women reported that, in certain circumstances, Viagra for women may help women to feel more sexual. That said, they expressed concern about the risks or social implications of such a drug, most often citing their own lack of need for the drug now, their concerns about side effects, and their reluctance to believe that pills can definitively solve sexual problems. For example, Mitra, age 29, described feelings about Viagra much in the same way that some women describe the anticipation of plastic surgery as a result of aging and "needing help":

> I might be interested in taking it, but I'd feel a little weird taking it too. To me, Viagra is for old men, and I have a real problem with what I think of as our overmedicated society right now. I just feel like there are emotional problems that people would be better off dealing with than taking a pill, but I'd be curious to see if it affected me. I would try it once, and my decision would be based on how it made me feel. Sometimes I wonder why my interest in sex feels like it has waned. Everyone always talks about 30 being your peak, but I don't see it.

Aya, age 25, also expressed some reluctance about the potential success of Viagra, yet expressed openness to it as well:

> I feel ambivalent about it. I assume that Viagra has a very visible goal. You can tell when a guy has an erection or when he doesn't, but then with Viagra for women, I guess you could

probably measure the blood flow, but I don't know if we're that defined. For myself, I wouldn't pay for it, but if it was free, I might try it, assuming that I have a partner and that we have intercourse and that he liked to have intercourse. I would want to take a pill that made it as pleasurable for him as it was for me, otherwise it's unfair.

Some women expressed openness to trying Viagra for women but were not fully comfortable with the gender and health implications. Twenty-five-year-old Brynn likened Viagra for women to other gestures of "spicing things up in the bedroom":

I see myself as losing my sex drive a lot of the time, so that would be an interesting thing to play with or experiment with to see how that plays out. There's something out there on the market for males, and males aren't the only ones who have a need. There are plenty of women that have a need as well. Sometimes I feel like I need something else besides, "Here, let's introduce new things into the bedroom and experiment with different stuff." That's not what heightens my sex drive. That said, there are a lot of things I would want to know, like side effects and what possible other things could come out of it aside from heightened sex drive.

Ciara, age 24, also said that she would try it but expressed some reluctance about the health implications: "I know that testosterone is supposed to help women increase their sexual desire. I saw them do this study on that, but I don't know much about the pill Viagra. I might use it after menopause or if I lost my sexual desire, but I don't know if it's good for women."

One of the more surprisingly ambivalent reactions I heard was from Janet, who jokingly expressed that she would like to give her lesbian partner some Viagra for women without her knowing about it, again affirming a particular kind of gendered relationship to the idea of sexual performance. Janet, age 21, said: "Me myself? I don't think I would need it. Maybe give my girl some, pop her some when she ain't looking! Then she'll be coming on to me, and I'll be like, 'All right! It worked!' (laughs). That would be cool, but maybe that's just in my fantasy."

Collectively, women's conflicted narratives of Viagra for women represented the extent to which they responded to the pressures of gendered social norms while also holding out some reluctant feelings about medicating their sexual desire or responses. When contrasting these perspectives with the women who supported Viagra for women and felt little or no reservations to taking the drug (mentioned earlier) and those who rejected Viagra for women (mentioned below), the range of responses women have both to the medicalization of sex and to the norm of sexual performance in general can be seen. Given the conflicted range of responses women had to thinking about Viagra for women, the question remains: How do these drugs medicate not only *sexual responses* but also *gender itself*?

Negative Reactions

About half of the women expressed intense negativity and distrust of the medicalization of sexuality, noting the overuse of drugs at the expense of other things such as communication or psychotherapy. Women's negative responses to Viagra for women included less content about their *imagined* physical experience of using the drugs; instead, women who rejected Viagra for women offered observations about the dangers of medicalizing sex. As such, self-identified feminists far more often expressed negative reactions to their imagined use of Viagra for women. Women expressed particular concern about the social implications of sexual pharmaceuticals, the gendered messages embedded within these drugs, the physical risks posed to women, and the clear financial gains drug companies have when medicating women's sexuality and desire. This reveals that, compared with women who articulated positive or ambivalent anticipatory reactions to sexual pharmaceuticals, those who reported negative responses focused more on critiquing sex research and drug developments in a more *abstracted* sense. Emily, age 22, expressed clear concern about the conflation of drugs and the emotional and social processing of sex for women:

> Taking drugs that are supposed to make you more horny? No. I think in general people just use drugs to replace dealing with their emotions and stuff. I don't think it would be any better

for a sex drive than it would be for any other thing that all the
psychiatric drugs are supposed to help. God, in my case I would
just be masturbating to death. I just think that there are so
many other issues in people's lives that are related to their sexuality, and they need to look at those and make sure that that's
all healthy instead of just trying to pop a pill for a quick fix.

Dawn, age 43, also expressed concern about the overreliance upon
drugs and the underreliance upon psychological and social processing
of sex, even while herself disclosing some recreational drug use. Interestingly, she, like Emily, also drew some parallels between Viagra for
women and vaginal plastic surgery:

There's probably something natural to take instead, and that
could be just as good. How many drugs do we take that mask
over some of the core issues and just kind of deal with a little
bit of the symptoms? With female Viagra, I can just see guys
slipping it into girls' drinks, can't you? It's not consensual then.
It's just like saying, "Hey, there's something wrong with you, so
take this pill," just like the vaginal plastic surgeries. Oh my God
it makes me sick! It makes me so mad.

Notably, women never mentioned concerns about *women* slipping
men Viagra or forcing them to use it nonconsensually In line with the
critiques of how Viagra for women intrudes upon women's lives at the
expense of dealing with their emotional and psychological issues with
sexuality, other women contested the intrusions of the pharmaceutical
industry in general. For example, Nora, age 23, saw Viagra for women
as standing in opposition to women learning to accept their bodies:

I have issues with the pharmaceutical industry in general. I feel
like there's not a pill for everything, and I'm really an advocate
of going back to holistic stuff, of getting back in touch with
your body. I think that we're just getting farther and farther
away from ever fixing anything and creating a real solvency . . .
I think we need to get back to women feeling and being in
their own bodies, and I think giving you another drug is only

going to move it farther away from that. It's not going to fix the larger problem. It's this artificial thing.

Priya, age 23, argued a similar reasoning, citing the manufactured need for such a drug:

> I could see women feeling a lot of pressure to take something like that. I think now our society jumps the gun. If anything is wrong, all of a sudden they'll look to medicine as a way to fix it. Personally, the way that I find stimulation is about the person I'm with, so if there's a problem, I need to work on the relationship and the way I am not feeling stimulated rather than jumping right to the medication.

Anger and resentment at the medical field and its priorities also arose when discussing women's reservations about Viagra for women, as the drug symbolized corporate and medical greed, the prioritization of medicines over other aspects of women's lives, and the recklessness of the medical profession with regard to women's bodies. For example, Kate, age 25, critiqued Viagra for women as a socioeconomic class problem:

> I think there are a lot of other things that medical research, time, and money could be spent on. I think it's interesting that this kind of thing is developed while we're still waiting for that male birth control pill. I just wonder why this is seen as a concern for either men or women. You only see this in the north, in wealthier countries. I don't mean to devalue sex, but if you're starving, or if your family is facing complete annihilation, then it's not like your sex drive is going to come first.

Fiona, age 24, articulated similar sentiments, paying particular attention to the messages Viagra for women sends about medical priorities for women:

> I'm very frustrated that pharmaceutical companies or health care companies won't pay for women's birth control or the

morning after pill, but they'll pay for Viagra. If there's a female Viagra, would that make it equal? I think there's a stigma in our society that women don't desire or want sex as much as men do, and I don't necessarily think that's true. This shows that they think women can't keep up with men's sexual desire.

Fiona's statements about the gendering of sex also show her resistance to constructing herself as a woman with deficient sexual desire in need of pharmaceuticals. Notably, Fiona said earlier in the interview that her antidepressants had made her desire sex less (something that concerned and upset her) yet still felt reluctant to support a drug that would potentially increase her sexual desire.

Concern about Viagra for women as a means to exploit women financially also appeared in these discussions. For example, Jasmine, age 37, likened drug companies to drug dealers: "I don't condone people pushing drugs on you. It is just the medical society being drug pushers, and that's not right. They don't care about the side effects. They just want to make a buck. I know that it's a man's world, and he is probably promoting it, and that's bullshit." Sonja, age 24, who used to work at a neurotherapy clinic, told me that she saw Viagra for women as an extension of the corporate greed she observed working at that clinic: "I feel like medications just kind of mask the issues sometimes, and they don't always target specific areas. They're just kind of general drugs."

Messages about gender also appeared at the center of women's resistance to Viagra for women, as women expressed reluctance to support ideas about women's sexuality as fundamentally different from men's sexuality. As Dorothy, age 19, said, "Are you having sex with a pill or a person? I'm a person, not an invention." Along these lines, Geena, age 51, told me, "My first thought is, we get second dibs again. The guys got theirs first. Red flags go up for me when it's in the pharmaceutical form, though, because I have questions about safety, and I'm worried that a lot of other things in women's lives are going to be ignored because this pill is going to be a fast fix." Similarly, Edie, age 19, talked about the way that Viagra for women constructs gender, noting that women's reluctance to have sex will not be solved in pill form:

It's just going to be a horrible tool in the hands of men to pressure their wives and such. I don't know if it's only in America, but there is this widespread social idea that women don't like to have sex, and men do, that men like to have significantly more amounts of sex. It's hard to consider what kind of women would take that. It seems like a lot of women just don't want to have sex, so why would they take a pill to make them want to have sex? If people were actually open with each other, they wouldn't need pills to force women into having sex. I think honesty is the essential platform for a good sex life.

Forty-five-year-old Susan's argument had an even stronger gendered analysis, in that she posed that women resist sex to garner more autonomy and independence from their male partners:

I think that female sexual response is so much more complicated than men's. The people I talk to socially about Viagra—the guys—they say they're not coming any better; they're just getting hard. I think with women it's a little easier because we can use lube if we're not that excited. I'd hate to see something come out that's thought to be like a panacea. Women aren't interested in sex with their partners because they're too busy taking care of the kids or doing this or doing that. Or perhaps some other kind of resentment. Or perhaps they don't have a good relationship. How are they going to feel when the pill doesn't help that?

Collectively, these negative responses to Viagra for women indicate a hopeful and heartening distance between these women's ideas about sexuality and the overarching social and cultural norms about sex that dictate a constant level of sexual arousal and sexual interest for women. Many women echoed feminist concerns put forth by The New View. Somehow, these women have both challenged and distanced themselves (however abstractly) from the cultural mandate for performed sexual arousal by instead arguing that genuine bodily feelings, positive and communicative relationships, healthy psychological and social processing of sex, and anticonsumerist, antimedicalization stances matter more than drug-induced desire.

CONCLUSION

When speaking with women about sexual pharmaceuticals, few women seemed particularly curious about how these drugs concretely affected women's bodies. Though women offered their ideas about their (lack of) willingness to try Viagra for women—or their resistance to it in theoretical and practical ways—they rarely asked questions about the effects it could have on their bodies or how the drug functioned. This seemed like a representation of the general willingness to accept the biological and medical interventions of the pharmaceutical industries without questioning the drugs themselves and how those drugs might connect directly with other priorities (e.g., greed, the invention of disorders, recklessness with women's health, etc.). The question remains: Why do women not ask more questions about their sexual health? And, consequently, how does this *facilitate* the pharmaceutical industry's efforts to medicalize women and their bodies?

The corporate and pharmaceutical quest for, marketing of, and selling of female sexual enhancement drugs represents most centrally the way that women's sexualities have become *vehicles of sexual performance* that must make themselves constantly sexually available to men, a finding that will be illustrated more clearly in chapter 5 when taking up questions about sexual violence and coercion. Women's sexual availability to their (male) partners matters more than their examination of the rewarding or unrewarding aspects of their sexuality. True assessments of the interplay among arousal, distress, and pleasure seem lacking in the discussion of sexual pharmaceuticals, in part because drug companies will not acknowledge that large numbers of women often feel completely fine with not having sex. If women express satisfaction despite lack of sexual activity, this represents a finding worthy of further exploration and analysis. Does this mean that women have "settled" or that sex has less salience for women's personal happiness than this culture has made people believe? Might some women have a low bar for sexual satisfaction such that sex and satisfaction don't always go together?

Given the mandates within American culture to equate (heterosexual) masculinity with sexual potency *and* eliciting women's sexual desire, it makes sense that women feeling peaceful and content with having less sex would possibly be threatening—to men (though researchers should ask men directly in order to say this with any certainty), to drug companies, and to cultural institutions. It is less clear, however, what this means for women themselves. How do changes in sexual desire or interest in sex affect them? If arousal becomes another culturally induced performance, do sexual frequency and subjective pleasure also fall in line as performances? Returning to Goffman's claim that there may be no "face behind the mask," what is "real arousal" and "real desire" anyway? Truly, women may find pleasure outside of arousal, and they may experience distress *despite* arousal. They may find pleasure when *medicating* arousal or in resisting medication. Pleasure and arousal may be deeply connected or entirely separate. These factors reveal a messy set of outcomes and subjective sensations for a pharmaceutical intervention (let alone women themselves!) to contend with.

Sexual pharmaceuticals bring up issues around the mediation and medication of sexuality, in that pharmaceutical industries communicate their clear priorities in the drug markets they create and respond to. The linkage between performance and sexual access is a consistent thread running through these discussions. Women learn, fairly early on, that their bodies *must* respond properly (e.g., orgasm, lubrication, etc.) and that they must make themselves available for sex, even when situational, attitudinal, or psychological factors present legitimate impediments to that availability. Women behaving as *responsive* (if not desirous) sexual beings is essential to the maintenance of traditional gender roles. As such, the ravenous qualities of drug company efforts to medicate women's desire, particularly as revealed in women's own narratives of willingness to try Viagra, are among the most troubling aspects of this chapter.

When examining women's responses to the corporate forays into Viagra for women, it seems relevant to ask: *Which* women will be more affected by the development of female sexual pharmaceuticals? While younger women tend to respond more willingly to performance pressures, older women may, as a function of their biology, be more susceptible to believing that they need these drugs because of natural life processes that slow down libido and arousal (e.g., menopause, aging, postchildbirth, etc.). The performative implications, then, affect *all* age groups; while older women may not fake orgasm (chapter 1) or hook up with other women at parties (chapter 2) as often as younger women do, they may feel more susceptible to pressures that they should continue having frequent sex despite their (potential) physiological and psychological lack of desire to do so. While women in newer relationships might feel pressure to engage in a wide repertoire of sexual acts, women in long-term relationships might feel pressure to *want* sex more often than they actually do. One can imagine that race, class, and size may also affect women's relationship to sexual pharmaceuticals—as cultural ideologies about *whose* sexual arousal is desired and *whose* bodies should be responsive—continue in earnest. The more important question here is too often ignored: If women do not want to have sex with their partners, might this reflect the gendered inequalities they face outside of the bedroom (e.g., lack of conversation, inequitable division of labor in the family, raising children without enough help, etc.)? No pill can resolve that issue.

The discourses of Viagra for women raise the question of what sexuality will look like once it is further medicalized. If American women continue to veer away from social constructionism as their primary way of understanding desire, attraction, satisfaction, and pleasure, and instead move into the medical realm, how will this change women's experiences of sex? If women conceive of low sexual desire as a *disorder* rather than a normal life event, how might that change their understandings of their bodies? One clear possibility is that, with the increasing stranglehold of medicalization, women will demand that their bodies perform in the same way throughout the lifespan. No longer will women accept or tolerate or embrace the cycles and highs/lows that their bodies experience sexually, but instead, they will demand a constant amount of sex (and orgasm?) throughout their lives. Similarly, women's partners may become less tolerant of these fluctuations and may intensify their demand that women *perform* sexually in the same way throughout their relationship. This could potentially further distance women from their bodily processes, much in the same way that birth control pills that eliminate menstruation create constant states (e.g., lack of menstrual blood) fundamentally unintuitive to the body. Women may feel less entitled to skip on sex when they feel low desire for it; the old biological rejoinder of "I have a headache" will no longer suffice.

With the loss of the social view of sex, a number of catastrophic results could ensue: first, women may stop looking to the dynamics within their relationships as something they should improve or think more deeply about. Instead of having communication or dialogue about sexual difficulties or mismatched sexual desire, they might instead blame their bodies and seek out medical treatment for their "sexual dysfunction" without considering the role of their partners in their sexual responsiveness. Second, sex therapy and medication therapy may become synonymous, as women with "sexual difficulties" may start to seek out pills rather than psychotherapy. This means that women may miss out on the deeper analyses of their sexual blocks, issues, concerns, or needs. Third, women may internalize the "realness" of the variety of new "disorders" the pharmaceutical industry creates, thus furthering a tendency to blame women for everything that goes wrong in families and relationships, thereby adding to the ahistorical and acontextual understanding of sexuality. Suddenly, "clitoral numbing" or "vaginal tiredness" might become conditions accepted as real medical conditions. Disorders are often portrayed as existing outside of their social and cultural contexts, something that has proven to be quite dangerous in other aspects of mental and physical health (e.g., depression as a "chemical imbalance" rather than a response to one's social environment, thus prompting women to avoid analyzing social inequalities or other contributors to their depressive states, etc.). Fourth, the medicalization of sex opens up the door to continued intrusions of the medical industry in people's lives; for example, the numbers of vaginal surgeries continues to rise, as people believe that they need plastic surgery to tighten, trim, or "rejuvenate" their genitals. Pfizer's comment that they need a pill to engender the sense of intimacy is not actually a joke but, rather, a priority. The mere fact that they would start a quest for such a drug represents the degree to which drug companies develop unnecessary interventions in order to satisfy profit margins.

When considering the potential impact of Viagra for women, the implications for enforced sexual performance overwhelm. Sexual pharmaceuticals essentially attempt to trick the body into responding in a way that it does not want to respond. These drug companies in turn can enforce certain kinds of social priorities that women need to: 1) be more like men (see chapter 1); 2) make themselves sexually available at all times to their partners (see chapter 5); 3) never wane in their sexual interest; 4) construct all sexual dysfunction as "their fault" or existing within their bodies alone; and 5) change their bodily chemistry in order to satisfy gender norms that dictate women's sexual availability. The demand for women's sexual performances of arousal and desire clearly serves the interests of existing discourses and institutions, though it is less clear whether men themselves, or corporations, are actually making these demands. The fact that Viagra for women may have disastrous health consequences, or encourage women to have sex when they do not want to, or construct conformity to the morals, ethics, and sexual standards of the day does not deter those in the pharmaceutical industry. They know they can make a vast amount of money via the invention of disorders, particularly those disorders that play on women's insecurities about being "good women" (or, as Irigaray would say, "good commodities").

As the tidal wave of sexual pharmaceuticals crashes down, it is imperative to reimagine people's relationships to sexuality, the medical field, and their bodies. Many women I spoke with expressed resistance, at least in an anticipatory sense, to the intrusions of the corporate and medical interest in their sex lives. Most women recognized that sexual pleasure and its accompanying manifestations, particularly orgasm, are finicky and sensitive elements of their lives, subject to being impacted by all kinds of different events: physiological changes in the body, sickness, aging, childbirth, stress, anxiety, trauma, relationship shifts, and so on. The whole of sexuality is much larger than one specific form of pleasure or one specific sexual behavior. Rather, a more interesting approach might ask women to imagine a nongenital sexuality altogether or a sexuality that valued intimacy or comfort over that which emphasizes particular goal-driven kinds of sexual performance such as erections and orgasm (ironically, doing so might actually generate more *frequent* erections and orgasms). Still more, women could focus on constructing sex as one of many ways to relate to partners and achieve intimacy. By removing the demand for consistent sexual performance and access—or at least by moving in that direction—women could potentially lead happier, healthier, less drug-induced lives, particularly if they can tap into the newfound wealth of erotic experiences available to them.

CHAPTER FOUR

ON THE MANY JOYS OF SEX

Pleasure, Love, and the Gendered Body

to save ourselves from the brittleness of being
"the-one-who" this one that one
we must be prepared to fall out of our own sky
and find
a friend or lover with brown hair and green eyes and
a presence we can curl up into and
save ourselves and fall away
appear and reappear
and no way I mean no way this is not terrifying
but there is eroticism in trust when
we have finally ploughed through all the fantasies
all the barbarism and criminal elegance of
our imposed sexuality there is nothing left but
yourself real in a real world
when the divesting process is nearing completion
is complete
and all the tableaux of pain and oppression
rape and necrophilia
coprophilia pederasty and prostitution
are destroyed
when
we are finally descended finally here and now
and found and present in time and space

—Fallon, "Sextec"

THIS CHAPTER REVISITS the classic question, What do women want? by adding the questions: Can women want? And, What do the things women want reveal about the ways they learn to perform their desires? The project of interrogating pleasure—what it means when women find sex pleasurable, whether scholars can (or should) judge what other women find pleasurable, whether pleasure translates into *words*—is one fraught with difficulty. What does it mean if women derive sexual pleasure from feelings of love? What if they derive sexual pleasure from painful experiences? If women *say* they take pleasure in recreating conditions of relative powerlessness, what does this suggest about gender?

As established in the previous three chapters, when numerous iterations of women's pleasure have taken on qualities of performances—whether via faking orgasms (chapter 1), performing bisexuality (chapter 2), or medicating desire (chapter 3)—imagining pleasure outside of *power* becomes convoluted and, at times, impossible. Pleasure does not represent uncomplicated, inexplicable, simple joy; rather, it arises out of a context rife with contradiction. And yet the sexuality literatures have relatively little to say about women's sexual pleasure. Some evolutionary perspectives even argue that women's sexual pleasure means relatively little, and scientists should not investigate it at all because it does not directly facilitate reproduction (Lloyd, 2005). Still, as pleasure often reflects women's social and political status—particularly *how* and under what conditions they negotiate their needs—interrogating the positive aspects of sex can prove fruitful. Sexual joy might fuel better connections between women and their partners, women and their bodies, and women and the culture at large. It may also reflect troubling sexual scripts that stereotype, pigeonhole, or limit women sexually. Though pleasure is difficult to analyze because of its elusive nature, women's sexual pleasure is nevertheless a relevant and understudied subject of analysis. Pleasure can show the extent to which women simultaneously *internalize* and *resist* their oppression.

Pleasure is a diverse, tricky, gendered, and multifaceted part of women's sexual lives. The chapter circles around two contradictory goals: 1) understanding and narrating the kinds of pleasure that might resist contemporary sexual scripts and empower women and 2) deconstructing these narratives of empowerment in light of how pleasure can *reinforce* the status quo. In short, do women's accounts of pleasure reveal empowerment or disempowerment discourses or both? Because women's bodies and their bodily pleasures are *gendered constructs*, beholden to power dynamics that privilege men's desires and needs over the desires and needs of women, how do women's performances of pleasure bespeak these conflicts? Consequently, this chapter takes up questions raised so far by Goffman, Irigaray, and Foucault, respectively: What pleasures do women feel if sex represents a series of performances? If women serve as the mirror to men's sexuality, what does their pleasure look like (or is their pleasure simply *men's* pleasure)? If power is always already present, is women's pleasure inextricably connected to women's sexual powerlessness?

To discuss these questions, this chapter examines events that women described as their *single best* sexual experiences as a way to concretely discuss pleasure, power, sexual performance, and the relationship between emotional connections and physical pleasure. Because this chapter focuses on women's different, and often conflicting, experiences of sexual pleasure, I specifically examine several cultural phenomena of particular interest, including women's descriptions of love influencing sexual pleasure, women's embodiment as it relates to sexual fulfillment, the gendering of bodies, and the connections between pleasure and power. Key questions include: What specific sexual experiences and stories stand out in women's narratives of pleasure? What do sexual memories of pleasure look like, and why do they matter? How might women's cultural status be communicated via their descriptions of pleasure and sexual satisfaction? How can pleasure simultaneously represent empowerment and disempowerment? Is pleasure even an appropriate site of cultural criticism?

RESEARCH ON WOMEN'S SEXUAL PLEASURE

> Her face would now be, forever, more mysterious and
> impenetrable than the face of any stranger. Strangers' faces
> hold no secrets because the imagination does not invest them
> with any. But the face of a lover is an unknown precisely
> because it is invested with so much of oneself. It is a mystery,
> containing, like all mysteries, the possibility of torment.
> —Baldwin, *Another Country*

Cultural scripts that publicly allow for women's entitlement to sexual pleasure are relatively new, particularly in the United States. Prior to the women's movement of the 1960s, public discourse about women's sexual expression remained relatively silent, and the conversations that did occur focused on keeping women compliant with traditional gender norms. Women had little access to birth control (as the pill did not receive FDA approval until 1960), and representations of nonmarital sex, particularly same-sex eroticism or sex for the purpose of pleasure, were virtually nonexistent. As Risman and Schwartz (2002) argued, "[The sexual revolution of the 1960s] has revised the entire framework of how American society thinks about sex. Premarital, unmarried, and post-divorce sex are now seen as individual choices for both women and men. The revolutionary principle that divorced the right to sexual pleasure from marriage (at least for adults) is no longer controversial" (p. 22). Of course, the past few decades have seen a dramatic increase in women's "hooking up" behaviors (Paul, McManus, & Hayes, 2000), lesbian polyamory (Munson & Stelboum, 1999), and women's lifetime number of sexual partners (Laumann et al., 1994). That said, women are still plagued with more inconsistent orgasmic pleasure and sexual satisfaction (Haavio-Mannila & Kontula, 1997), indicating that more sexual partners and (alleged) sexual freedoms do not always correlate with *better*, more orgasmic, or more satisfying sex.

Research on women's sexual satisfaction and pleasure has yielded mixed results, yet one consistent finding holds that women tend to report lower sexual satisfaction than men (Haavio-Mannila & Kontula, 1997), think about sex less, masturbate less, have fewer orgasms with partners, and fantasize less than men (Baumeister & Tice, 1998; Laumann et al., 1994; Sprecher & Regan, 1996). This may in part stem from living in a culture that still—despite its claims of sexual liberation—promotes the lingering traditional idea that women should only want sex after they marry, that sex should exist solely for reproduction and, if women's pleasure is factored in at all, it must serve the interests of men. Women often carry the burden of these discourses of purity and contamination (e.g., women's virginity is valued much more than men's virginity) and thus may experience less sexual pleasure when living within the context of these social norms. These problems remain particularly relevant for lower status women—women of color, poor women, sexual minority women, and so on—who have largely shouldered the burden of "sexual deviance" for many generations.

The gender gap about sexual pleasure may also reflect a holdover from the Victorian past, where women who enjoyed sex garnered the label of "deviant" or "mentally ill" (Smith-Rosenberg, 1985). "Oversexed" women were thrown in mental hospitals and otherwise shunned from polite society for the many decades leading up to the sexual revolution (Cushman, 1996). As Foucault (1978) said, "Through the various discourses, legal sanctions against minor perversions were multiplied; sexual irregularity was annexed to mental illness; from childhood to old age, a norm of sexual development was defined and all the possible deviations were carefully described; pedagogical controls and medical treatments were organized; around the least fantasies, moralists, but especially doctors, brandished the whole emphatic vocabulary of abomination" (p. 36).

Currently, evidence supports the claim that women's pleasure often serves the interests of sexist and heterosexist institutions. For example, across all age groups, when not accounting for orgasm frequency, heterosexual women continue to report that penile-vaginal intercourse yields the most self-reported satisfaction for them, despite the fact that it leads less often to consistent orgasm than do oral sex or manual stimulation (Costa & Brody, 2007; Fugl-Meyer et al., 2006; Nicolson & Burr, 2003). Further still, heterosexual women often report being preoccupied with satisfying their male partners, either via pleasuring them or by having an orgasm (real or fake) in order to satisfy the male partner's ego needs (Nicolson & Burr, 2003), as shown in chapters 1 and 3.

As further evidence of women deriving pleasure from different scenarios than men, women's sexual fantasies often include elements of romance and physical/emotional caretaking of men or submission to men, while men's sexual fantasies often include elements of casual sex and physical domination over women (Paul & Hayes, 2002), a trend explored later in chapter 6. Many cultural markers of sex also reveal a bias toward men: the definition of sex (e.g., when it begins and ends, whether it "counts") often revolves around male erections (or lack thereof), male ejaculation, and male orgasm. In essence, sexual intercourse in the most conventional sense typically "ends" when men ejaculate, effectively rendering the sexual exchange as complete (Plante,

2006a). Thus, the study of women's pleasure occurs in relationship to norms of lopsided power differentials between men and women.

Correlates to Sexual Satisfaction

Though some argue that pleasure and satisfaction may not always align—as pleasure implies enjoyment during an action, while satisfaction implies postaction evaluation of that act—the two nevertheless inform one another. Also, because this chapter focuses on women's *best* sexual experiences (spoken about retrospectively), pleasure and satisfaction often appear in those narratives as closely intertwined concepts. When looking at the specific data about sexual satisfaction, research consistently shows that women who reported more sexual satisfaction tended to be younger, more educated, and more politically liberal. Women who endorsed sexually repressive belief systems had lower sexual satisfaction outcomes than those who described less repression and sexual restriction, in that more satisfied women reported more sexual assertiveness, earlier first sexual intercourse, and nonreligious childhoods (Haavio-Mannila & Kontula, 1997). They also had less anxiety about the meaning of sex along with fewer intrusive thoughts (Purdon & Holdaway, 2006). Satisfied women also had more variety in their sexual exchanges, more interest in using sex toys and trying new sexual positions (Haavio-Mannila & Kontula, 1997), and more self-disclosure to their partners about what brings them pleasure (MacNeil & Byers, 2005), again confirming the assertion that sexual repression typically does not contribute to sexual satisfaction.

Correlations among sexual satisfaction, emotional satisfaction, and relationship satisfaction have also been repeatedly documented, highlighting the centrality of positive relationships as facilitators of women's sexual pleasure. Women who reported reciprocal feelings of love in their relationships reported more frequent intercourse, more frequent orgasm, and more satisfaction (Gonzalez et al., 2006; Haavio-Mannila & Kontula, 1997; Sprecher, 2002). Similarly, better communication with partners predicted more sexual satisfaction (Bridges, Lease, & Ellison, 2004), as did autonomy without too much distance and ability to manage stress (Kingsberg, 2002). Women's sexual satisfaction also seemed linked to the internalization of different types of gender expectations; more satisfied women reported less body shame (Sanchez, Crocker, & Boike, 2005; Sanchez & Kiefer, 2007) and greater endorsement of non-traditional gender roles (Lottes, 1993; Pederson & Blekesaune, 2003). A study of newlywed women found that those who began their marriages feeling sexually satisfied were more likely to continue feeling satisfied; frequency of sex did not correlate with women's satisfaction (McNulty & Fisher, 2008).

When analyzing what women described as their best sexual experiences, a recent study by Paul and Hayes (2002) found that women reported several themes: interest, attraction, a good-looking partner; an evolving relationship; feeling wanted and cared about; and feeling comfort, security, and trust. Compared to men, women cared less about the enjoyment of the sexual behavior or an appreciation of their partner's body. These findings indicate that women derive pleasure most centrally from *highly satisfying and comforting* connections with a partner rather than from the sex itself or their partner's physical features.

As established in chapter 1, correlates between sexual satisfaction and orgasm appeared consistently in the literature (Hurlbert, Apt, & Rabehl, 1993; Young et al., 1998), though it raises the question of why women prioritize orgasm (i.e., for themselves or their partners?). One recent study attempted to answer this question and found that heterosexual women reported a desire to experience orgasm less for *themselves* and more for *the sake of their male partners*, thus suggesting that women's sexual pleasure remains deeply connected to their ability to perform sexual scripts that reinforce the status quo (Nicolson & Burr, 2003). That said, the contexts within which women · experience pleasure, orgasm, and satisfaction must be examined in order to more fully understand this finding.

Sexual Behavior and Pleasure

Women do "sex" in many different ways, and each approach yields different levels of pleasure and satisfaction. Not surprisingly, women derived sexual pleasure from a wide variety of behaviors, including masturbation, sexual fantasy, touching, oral sex, anal sex, penile-vaginal intercourse, and "foreplay" in general (Rye & Meaney, 2007). Masturbation has consistently represented a reliable pathway to sexual pleasure for women, even while the cultural lexicon often prohibits women from discussing it publicly. Over two-thirds of women have masturbated at least once, and women are particularly likely to masturbate if they perceive social norms in support of masturbation (Pinkerton et al., 2002). Importantly, studies show that more sexually active people masturbated more often, indicating that masturbation does not likely substitute for other sexual activity (Davis et al., 1996). Compared to men, women reported more varied masturbation techniques (Masters & Johnson, 1966), more vibrator use, more multiple orgasms from masturbation (Davis et al., 1996), and more emphasis on relieving sexual tension as a key feature of physical pleasure (Laumann et al., 1994). Women with more knowledge of the clitoris were more likely to have pleasurable experiences with masturbation than those with less knowledge of the clitoris (Wade, Kremer, & Brown, 2005). Thus, masturbation seems to reliably contribute to women's pleasurable sexual experiences.

Studies indicate that women also derive pleasure from external aids during sex. Both during masturbation and during partnered sexual activity, women described pleasurable experiences with sex toys. Approximately a third of women said that they used sex toys (Rye & Meaney, 2007), and other research has shown that education is highly correlated with use of sex toys (Laumann et al., 1994). Lesbian women were slightly more likely to use sex toys than bisexual and heterosexual women, and close to 80% of women who owned a vibrator used it during partnered sex (Davis et al., 1996).

Women described a variety of avenues to pleasure while having sex with a partner. During partnered sex, women typically believed that mutual masturbation felt pleasurable (Pinkerton et al., 2003), as did oral sex, anal sex, and vaginal intercourse. Approximately 73–83% of women have received oral sex (Mosher, Chandra, & Jones, 2005), while 80–85% of women have performed oral sex on a partner (Rye & Meaney, 2007). University women ranked oral sex as second only to vaginal intercourse as the most pleasurable activity they engaged in (Barrett, 2004; Pinkerton et al., 2003). Research has shown that heterosexual women prefer "woman on top" position over other sexual positions during intercourse as the most pleasurable method of having sex, likely because it allows for control of movement and more frequently contributes to orgasm for women (Browning et al., 2000). Further, approximately one-fourth to one-third of adults have had anal sex (Browning et al., 2000; Mosher, Chandra & Jones, 2005), yet approximately 1–5% of participants rated anal contact (including stimulating a partner's anus, having one's anus stimulated by a partner, or anal intercourse) as "very appealing" in a 1994 national survey (Laumann et al., 1994). No studies have directly addressed this discrepancy of activity and satisfaction with anal contact.

Importantly, while research has typically addressed the frequencies of these behaviors, including masturbation, oral sex, anal sex, and penile-vaginal intercourse, little research has been conducted about the relationship between these sexual activities and *why, or under what circumstances,* women find them pleasurable. Very few studies have qualitatively addressed the experiences women derive sexual pleasure from, and even fewer have directly asked about women's pleasurable experiences with anything beyond penile-vaginal intercourse. For example, studies have rarely examined, even tangentially, women's pleasurable experiences with oral sex, and no studies have qualitatively addressed women's pleasurable experiences with anal sex. While more is known about what people *do* sexually, little is known about how women *feel* while engaging in these actions.

Though little research has addressed women's pleasurable experiences with "mainstream" sexual behavior, research about correlations between pleasure and sexual domination has expanded in recent years, though often without differentiating men's and women's pleasurable experiences within the BDSM community. Studies show that some women reported pleasurable experiences with sadomasochism, including the administration of pain (e.g., spanking), deliberate humiliation (e.g., face slapping), physical restriction (e.g., handcuffs), and fetishistic play (Alison et al., 2001; Rye & Meaney, 2007). About one-quarter of women enjoyed being bitten during sexual activity (Kinsey et al., 1953), many women enjoyed spanking (Plante, 2006b), and about two-thirds of people in a recent study reported having fantasies of tying up a partner or being tied up (Renaud & Byers, 1999). Still, most S&M research tends to focus almost exclusively on men, and little research has examined women as an S&M subculture or women's pleasurable experiences with S&M (Levitt & Moser, 1987; Sandnabba, Santtila, & Nordling 1999).

Thus, even though research discusses the *activities* that women engage in, surprisingly little research has addressed the specific qualities of women's sexual pleasure, particularly in a qualitative sense. While the kinds of behaviors women enjoy have been catalogued, themes of what constitutes pleasure and satisfaction continue to be understudied. In particular, little attention has been paid to the nuanced stories women have about their pleasurable sexual experiences. Little is known about women's *best* sexual experiences, which provide a unique window into *intense* and *memorable* sexual pleasure, or their routine or everyday pleasures, which, while less memorable, still constitute a central part of women's sexual lives.

NARRATIVES OF SEXUAL PLEASURE

> The concept of the 'body' has traditionally denoted the finite, a material limit that is absolute—so much so that the juxtaposition of the terms "concept" and "body" seems oxymoronic. For the body is that which is situated as the precise opposite of the conceptual, the abstract. It represents the ultimate constraint on speculation or theorization, the place where the empirical finally and always makes itself felt.
> —Doane, "Technophilia: Technology, Representation, and the Feminine"

During the interviews, when studying women's sexual pleasure and asking women what they find enjoyable or satisfying, their ambivalence about asserting their sexual needs or claiming pleasure for themselves became immediately visible. During conversations with women, confusion about how to claim or value pleasure became immediately apparent even on the level of language (e.g., ambivalent statements such as, "I don't know, I like it when he's happy I guess," said Carol). In my interviews with women, I asked them, "How would you define sexual satisfaction for yourself?" and "What is the most important aspect of physical pleasure for you?" Such questions often led to various preconceived and socially sanctioned abstractions about love or emotions while failing to give texture to these experiences. In between their words and phrases, they repeatedly said, "*I don't know,*" even as they tried to articulate their ideas about these questions. Apparently, figuring out how to *define* sexual pleasure seemed quite difficult.

Conversely, when I asked women about their best and worst sexual experiences, these narratives had a richness and specificity that brought to life women's astonishing range of memories about their sexuality. Their descriptions of pleasure when recalling a particularly pleasurable event—as compared with the more abstracted question of what they *wanted* or how they *defined* pleasure—conveyed vitality and vividness. As such, this chapter focuses primarily on women's best sexual experience narratives as a microcosm of larger conversations about pleasure, satisfaction, and fulfillment. Notably, with only a few exceptions, women rapidly and easily recounted their best sexual experience narratives, perhaps because the *intensity* of pleasure from women's "bests" leads to stronger associations with memory, emotions, and words. As Doane (1990) noted, it is *here*, in these explorations of the body and its pleasure, where the empirical makes itself felt. While these descriptions might not give a sense of women's general, day-to-day relationship to pleasure, they highlight the sexual highs women have experienced and thus reveal stories of intense, textured, and tangible pleasure.

Best Sexual Experiences

Women's best sexual experience narratives fell into four primary categories, each of which speaks to the complex interplay between gender and sexuality. First, many women described their best sexual experiences as involving intense emotional connection between themselves and their partners along with, at times, an emotional healing element. Recognition of love, shared experience, or even recovery from a painful past relationship via a new relationship appeared in these narratives.

Second, women described their partner's *attentiveness* and kindness as central to their best experiences. This description closely corresponded to women having intense physical pleasure along with *embodiment*, where they felt fully present and focused on the experiences of their bodies (i.e., not distracted, bored, disconnected, fatigued, or "absent"). Some of these descriptions highlighted women discovering their bodies as sexual, and most described the experience of intense orgasm(s) as memorable and significant in defining their best experiences.

Third, women frequently described their best experiences as related to a feeling of experimenting or trying something new, particularly behaviors that they perceived as originating from their own desires and fantasies. These descriptions presented notably different experiences from, say, performative bisexuality, where women perceived *others* (primarily observing men) as nudging them toward same-sex desires. Women's pleasurable new experiences included experimentation with heightened power relationships, new positions or sexual acts, or acting out fantasies that they had always wanted to try (notably, though, this latter point also frequently emerged in women's worst experiences, as botched attempts at novelty translated into humiliation, shame, and disappointment).

Finally, in the fourth category, women enjoyed the experience of "being away," either mentally or literally. Some described comfort and pleasure from having vacation sex, while others described getting away from the mundane or routine as intensely erotic, particularly as they escaped the demands of their domestic and work life. Also, some women described feelings of losing themselves or even the intensity of an extramarital affair as pleasurable versions of being away.

Theme 1: Pleasure as Emotional Connection

Women's beliefs that intense emotional connection heightened their sexual experiences appeared frequently in conversations with them, as they repeatedly said that feelings of love, understanding, and connectedness led to sexual pleasure. This raises several questions: Do these instances reveal a true departure from the (largely male-generated) pressures to orgasm frequently, perform sexual acts with women, and medicate their desire (presented in chapters 1–3)? When women eroticize love, does it represent an internalization of prescribed gender roles that women *should* eroticize love (versus men, who may internalize social scripts to enjoy sex as "just sex")? Or does it reflect something else, perhaps related to the perception of their partner's kindness or care for them as contributing to women's pleasure? What does this suggest about the subversive potential of these sex-with-love narratives?

The texture of women's responses helps to highlight the complexity of these questions. Notably, women frequently reported that an emotional connection with a partner either deepened or intensified their experiences of pleasure. Niko, age 23, said, "I think the best sexual experience for me is when two people love each other and when they're really committed, and it feels like it's more than just sex. It has a whole new meaning. I think that's the most emotional and physical thing that feels really good." Courtney, age 23, also echoed these sentiments about the importance of emotional connection: "The best was with someone that I really cared a lot about and was really, really attached to, and it brought me to the conclusion through my tests and trials that it's good to have sex with someone you care about. That's the best sex, when you have the best connection." When I asked her what she found the most pleasurable about her experience, she indicated that comfort and passion led to pleasure: "I was just so comfortable with the person, and I also really, really liked the person, and so I really wanted it as opposed to other times where I'd sort of just said, 'Okay, why not.' It's hard to fake passion or desire so it's pretty obvious when you're not into it, at least for me."

At times, emotional connectedness seemed to trump the physically pleasure aspect of relationships as well. Twenty-four-year-old Fiona described an emotionally intense first love:

> It was the summer, and it was kind of love at first sight style. We got along immediately, in a very intimate deep way, the most I've ever been since then, and that was the most amazing sexual experience in terms of kissing, and just everything felt so much more magical. The actual act of sex wasn't very enjoyable. It wasn't very fulfilling, but the intimacy made up for that. It didn't matter because it was very comforting. I think that I just really connected to her . . . The whole environment part was very poetic, on the beach, much more deep than any man I'd ever been with. I just remember breaking down crying at the drop of the hat because it was so intense.

Priya, age 23, also argued that sexual fulfillment that came through emotional connectedness felt so intense that sex itself became somewhat irrelevant:

> I think my best is like intimacy with someone else, like staying up for a really long time and talking, really feeling comfortable with another person, like if something goes wrong or there's some kind of mishap, then just to laugh about it; those are the experiences which I think of as really positive, just like anything that has that aura of comfort around it . . . I mean being able to be yourself and just expose yourself, so you're kind of in a vulnerable state. You know that you know your body. It's just really helpful to be really comfortable and to have someone that makes you feel comfortable in every way: physically, emotionally.

Thus, while one can read these narratives as subversive in their decentering of "sex" as the dimension within which women find pleasure and fulfillment, these narratives also raise questions about what happens when women prioritize emotional fulfillment over physical fulfillment. In other words, if pleasure is no longer generated via orgasm or physical sensation, does that facilitate women's partners deprioritizing women's orgasms? Does the valuing of emotional pleasure over physical pleasure become a mechanism through which women stop expecting physical pleasure because they have learned that emotional pleasure should be "enough"? What would such a view mean to a feminist politics of sexuality?

These questions became more vivid in the narratives where women sought other emotional connections aside from romantic love; at times, women wanted to feel desired or even objectified. Susan, age 45, described her desire for boundary crossing and sexual objectification:

> Sex has become more of an emotional experience, even though I'm very much into the physical. It's not orgasms necessarily. I like orgasms, but I like having someone pay attention to my body or some part of my body, showing that they care for me and about what we do together. If somebody will care

enough to do the things they know I like, really pay attention to me, I can have an orgasm . . . As I've gotten older, I won't have sex just for the sake of fucking anymore, and also, I think I have another partner who kind of tests my limits, and I think that's fun, just kind of that special trust I have for him . . . He anticipates my needs well, or kind of gets me to explore the edges of what I would like. I feel loved and appreciated and respected by the people I have sex with, but I also like to feel, well, *naughty*, or kind of the opposite of how I am to the rest of the world. I'm looked at as straight-laced or capable, and I think *slut* is a positive word, used in a proper context. There are times when I do like feeling objectification, just like someone really likes the way I feel or the way I look or the fantasy they have had about me and want to make it happen . . . I'm not real thin or textbook, but yet, men find me attractive, which reinforces how I feel about myself.

This description implies that emotional connection need not always map onto a classic and stereotyped ideal of sex in the context of *love*, but rather, sex can fulfill multiple emotional needs, even if women replicate gender stereotypes. In this case, Susan's desire for objectification *both* subverts dominant narratives of women as universally oriented toward romance while also eroticizing a certain degree of powerlessness (or receiving men's attention). These complications speak to the problem of pleasure as, at once, entrenched in patriarchy while also resisting it, as indebted to archaic ideas about gender while also breaking through to something new and different. Many women—regardless of their backgrounds (age, sexual abuse histories, race, sexual identity, etc.)—expressed multiple and conflicting desires to receive romantic attention and other, more power-laden forms of attention such as objectification from partners.[1]

Returning to the question of pleasure and emotional connection, women also described emotional connectedness during sex as a way to heal from painful relationships that were ending or had ended, making "therapeutic sex" a key element to women's pleasurable experiences. These descriptions of sex with a former lover or sex with a new partner show how women use the scripts they have been given at the cultural level (e.g., you should only have sex when in love) to, in essence, partially fulfill their emotional needs (e.g., feeling attractive, wanted, desired; feeling connected to their bodies, etc.). Aya, age 25, mentioned, "I had break-up sex that was really good once, with that guy I told you about. It was because we had been talking a lot and it was very emotionally charged all the way with meaning." Bonnie, age 51, framed her experience as a way to regain confidence following the dissolution of her marriage:

> I was married once, and my first husband just one day picked up and left. So, a couple of weeks or a month after that my friends said, "Why don't you go out with this guy," so we went out on a date, and at this point I'm feeling really low about myself. My husband had just walked out the door pretty much out of the blue, so the second or third date he came over, and we had a very nice time sexually and romantically. It was just exactly what I needed for my self-esteem was to have this great night of romance and sex all night long with somebody. It was just a magical night . . . I was not feeling loved or attractive or wanted, and it lasted all night, and it was just perfect in every way. It was romantic, and we did a variety of things. It was just really a night to remember.

In the context of relationships ending, women also described profound emotional and spiritual experiences with sex, in part based on the emotional release and intimacy that sex allows. Geena, age 51, communicated the healing properties of sexuality when she described her experience with a new lover following a break-up with a long-term partner:

> It was just so incredibly intense and wonderful and emotional. The tears just spontaneously occur, and the other person instantly knows that you're not in pain. They just know. Nobody panics when they see the tears. It's almost like a divine experience sexually, emotionally, tenderly. It's just the combination of the both of us and the energy. There's a healing component to it because there's been something going on with me

and the sexual act with that person has been so emotionally
cleansing and healing and that's where the tears came from. It's
a spiritual thing that comes from the pleasure.

Nora, age 23, explained the emotional intensity of one encounter as the
relationship ended, noting the connectedness she felt to the broader
spiritual universe:

> I cried after sex with him. It was just a feeling of it being so
> huge and overwhelming and tapping into this archetypal per-
> sona of feeling like mother goddess. It sounds a little heady, but
> just these immense feelings of being a creator and this ability of
> being involved with the world and just how dumbfounding
> and amazing it was. The contradiction of our existence, our
> little existence of ourselves, and this huge experience we were
> having, it was like we were creating the whole world in that
> moment. In theory, if you break it down, we could be. It was
> after a lot of intimacy had been built up that it happened. It
> wasn't some arbitrary thing. It was of great magnitude for me.

Another manifestation of this paradigm where women used their
inherited conventional cultural scripts (e.g., sex must involve love, connection, and togetherness) to fulfill themselves in less traditional ways
happened when women framed their best sexual experiences as ones
that occurred during masturbation. In separating women's best sexual
experiences from the context of *men* as partners, masturbation potentially has subversive qualities. Sonja, age 24, told me, "Probably masturbation is still the most satisfying because there is probably for me some
anxiety involved still in having sex with somebody . . . When I masturbate, I am actually able to have an orgasm, whereas other times I can't
really. With a partner, there's just more anxiety. By myself, I feel joy,
some sadness, no guilt though, I guess on the happier side of things."
Describing similar masturbation experiences with even more intensity
and detail, Nora explained:

> Masturbating by myself feels like some of my best experiences.
> I do artwork, and for whatever reason right now art has really

turned me on too . . . It's so freeing because it's like a celebration of my own self, like loving myself. So now, I will fantasize
about making love to myself, and it's amazing actually, like cul-
tivating this whole relationship with myself, and being able to
try to have sex with myself and appreciate myself is really hot
for me for some reason, in lieu of these big relationships,
because I have so many more expectations of relationships. I
want people's *soul* to be involved with their sex now. I want a
huge connection, like physical, emotional, spiritual, and sexual
. . . During masturbation, I get a little fluttery and start to kind
of drift off, and upwards. I want to just breathe deeper. It's like
this invigorating life feeling of vitality and passion.

The cultural imperative for women to experience emotional connection, therefore, may manifest in the more traditional forms (e.g.,
women claiming that they have the best sex when in love; women
desiring emotional connection as a precursor to physical connection,
etc.), or in less traditional forms (e.g., expanding definitions of emotional satisfaction, using sex as a healing force, or embracing emotional
connection in autoerotic sexual experiences). As such, love may serve as
a kind of gendered performance—in that women may anticipate that
they *should* feel in love in order to have pleasure—and/or it may serve
as a way for women to feel appreciated, respected, trusting, and self-
affirming. Like all elements of sex, love, too, can have dimensions of
performance, as shown in these narratives.

Pleasure as Attentiveness and Physical Embodiment

The theme of *attentiveness* repeated itself frequently throughout
women's "best" sexual experience narratives, particularly as they spoke
of partners who treated them with patience, kindness, and care. Interestingly, the actual word *attentive* kept reappearing again and again (e.g.,
over half of the women interviewed used this precise word when
describing their best sexual experiences), implying, perhaps, that
women notice this aspect of a sexual encounter when they feel over-
looked, not attended to, and not *seen* in their lives more broadly. If one

considers the specific qualities of 'attentive,' several dimensions come to light: observant, mindful, patient, watchful, polite, courteous, intent, intuitive, watchful, devoted, giving comfort. Perhaps women experience pleasure in moments when their partners treat them with the kind of attention they want to feel more of, either during sex or in other arenas of their lives. The centrality of attentiveness to sexual pleasure was a major finding in this qualitative work and should be highlighted as a theme that warrants further attention in future research.

Often, narratives of attentiveness and pleasure had an intensely tactile quality, as women remembered the encounter in a detailed, sensual way. Fifty-six-year-old Ophelia described her best sexual experience as, "It was just very sensual, just the smell, the feel, feeling cared for, touching." Esther, age 44, similarly described her best encounter as a vivid and sensual scene:

> He was so attentive. I felt very strongly for him, and then it was also the setting because we found a place right off the freeway that was beside a creek, and we'd found a little area under a tree, like a little grassy area. There was a thunderstorm, and it had stopped thundering and lighting, and it was just starting to rain, but it wasn't really raining, so the whole atmosphere—it was just absolutely wonderful. We were kind of in the mountains, and it was just a really romantic thing. He was really gentle, and he was very soft, with just a gentle, kind touch, and so that made it special too.

Charlene, age 44, described attentiveness as the key to her best experience, even while relaying the pain of her relationship with an exhusband. Notably, her positive experience followed a negative experience with performative bisexuality, revealing the interesting way she drew a divide between exploitation and attentiveness in her narrative:

> We had a threesome the previous night that went horribly, so the following night, I guess it felt good because we were very attentive to each other and took our time, and like I said, he thought he had to prove something to me, so I guess he tried harder than usual. I didn't realize he wasn't trying very hard

before, but that particular time, he seemed to care a lot more about how he made me feel. It made me feel good about myself, attractive, and wanted. He tended to be more selfish other times . . . Usually he wanted me to just do whatever made him feel good, and he would accommodate me sort of, like, "Well here, this is what you wanted, now let's get back to me."

Related to this theme of attentiveness, many women described intense orgasms, combined with how they interacted with an attentive partner, as their best experiences. This indicated a direct relationship between women's orgasmic responsiveness and their partners' awareness of their physical desires and needs. For example, Geena described her first experiences with multiple orgasms as both surprising and exhilarating:

I might have just turned 19, with a boyfriend, and he fingered me apparently internally and found my G-spot over and over and over and over and over again, so I had multiple orgasms. He even left the room we were in to take a phone call, and I had put my clothes back on. He came back and said, "You put your clothes back on?" and I said, "Yeah," and then I took them off, and he did it some more. I couldn't believe my body could do that, so that was pretty exciting, because I felt pretty satiated after the first half dozen orgasms, but then I just kept having them. It was just exciting, just that my body could feel that good. I didn't know that was possible for anybody. I didn't know it was possible for my body, and I had no idea that it could do that!

In this paradigm, attentiveness allowed women to claim their sexual pleasure by involving a partner in their sexual empowerment. While the partners participated, women did not construct their partners as entirely responsible for their pleasure (which differs greatly from the gift paradigm in chapter 1).

In this light, women's descriptions of their first orgasm experiences also appeared frequently, as it marked a turning point in women's sexual lives where they experienced their bodies differently. For example, Sally, age 20, described her first orgasm with an old boyfriend, saying, "I remember the first time we had ever had sex together. The first time I actually ever had an orgasm was with that person. It was the first time that he'd ever had sex, and he was very, very Catholic, and he's very religious. I felt really special that he could confide in me enough and love me enough that he would want to lose his virginity to me." Kate, age 25, who had struggled for years with feeling pressured to conform to partners' expectations during sex, described her first orgasm experience positively:

> I think my best experience would have been this past summer when I was living with my current partner. It was the first time that I ever really experienced what an orgasm is, and it was really wonderful and especially wonderful because I was in the position of control and power, because usually I've had the perception that sex has been something that's been done *to* me, and so, with the person that I'm seeing now, it's been really different because he's forced me to take ownership . . . I've often found in this question of orgasm, there's always been this other me hovering over what's going on and thinking, "Is this what it feels like? Is this it? Is this it?" and what was different this time is suddenly something happened, this kind of sensation happened, and I didn't know where it came from. It wasn't like there had been a buildup. It was just there, and it was really wonderful. It was probably one of the few times when I felt totally like I was feeling something, and I wasn't feeling that I *should* be feeling something.

Kate's last sentence particularly captures women's conflicts about internalizing, and resisting, sexual scripts. She indicated feeling less beholden to the various inadequacies that are communicated to women about sex and more fully embodied in her actions.

Another aspect of this theme of attentiveness and orgasmic pleasure involved the way that women described feeling satisfied through their physical embodiment of pleasure, where pleasure facilitated a closer and more intuitive relationship between women and their bodies. Looking at the narratives of Emily, Dawn, and Lori, three women with vastly different approaches to sexuality, this synthesis of attentiveness, orgasm,

and embodiment is apparent. Emily, age 22, described her best experience as a feeling of performance *combined with* embodiment:

> You know I do adult movies, and a lot of that I really have
> enjoyed. I thought it was a great experience. I just had fun the
> whole time. I had my girlfriend on the sidelines doing little
> cheerleader things, saying, "Oh yeah, you look hot doing that"
> . . . I definitely appreciate an audience, and I mean the films
> that I really enjoyed, I did a couple of scenes with the same
> people that I'm really good friends with . . . I feel turned on
> when I'm in comfortable settings like that. Some people get
> turned on when they don't really know that person or some-
> thing, but for me, knowing the person I was working with
> helped to make it a lot better for me, like crazy lust.

Dawn, age 43, described her best experience as a complicated combination of attentiveness, emotional connection, physical pleasure, and
embodiment:

> I was in a relationship with another woman who I was very
> much in love with, and her husband was involved with us too,
> and that was extremely powerful and good on a deep spiritual
> level as well as a physical level. It didn't last too long though
> because of jealousy, which is really a shame . . . but while it
> lasted, it was really beautiful. There were so many parts of me
> that were met: the potential for a relationship with her, with
> him, with my partner, seeing my partner loving her, those kinds
> of things. It was really open-hearted, you know. It was coming
> from a pure open-hearted place, extremely nurturing, like a lot
> of honoring the body, coming to a place of experimentation,
> and that was extremely powerful.

Finally, 33-year-old Lori's description of her best sexual experience also
reflected an integration of care, attentiveness, and embodiment:

> My best sexual experience was with a man who I was deeply
> in love with. We went to this hotel early on in our relationship,

and he touched me in the slowest and most sensual way. I
didn't feel like he was fixated on my orgasm, or on his, but just
being together and touching and loving each other's bodies.
Everything just worked about that situation, and my physical
arousal was off the charts. I felt like I couldn't stop myself from
moaning. I remember the way he smelled, the way he looked,
the way he undressed me. I don't think I've ever felt as fully in
my body as I did that afternoon, and the orgasms were so
intense.

In this way, a partner's attentiveness may transform the conventional
arrangements of sex that dissuade women from placing their desires and
orgasms at the center of the exchange. By putting (male) partners in a
more giving or altruistic stance, these sexual exchanges may facilitate
women's physical pleasure and allow more space for equality between
partners.

Pleasure as Experimentation and Newness

As a third dimension of women's best experiences, women sometimes
felt excitement surrounding newness and experimentation as the key to
their sexual pleasure, particularly related to the surprises of a new partner or sexual act, experimentation with sexual behaviors, or pleasure
related to acting out their sexual fantasies. These stories were at times
tinged with statements about rediscovering sexuality as essential to a
feeling of life and vitality. With regard to the newness of a mutually sat-
isfactory relationship, several women felt elated when confirming their
mutual attraction with someone else. For example, Janet, age 21,
remembered discovering that her sexual attraction was mutual:

My best experience was in the beginning, and I don't know if
you just call it that puppy love stage or whatever, just the
excitement of that first night . . . It was kind of just one of
those things where we were just talking, and at first I didn't
even really know that she was gay, and I'd known her for a long
time, but I didn't know that she liked girls, so even just the first

time she kissed me, I was like, "Are you fuckin' with me?"
What the hell! It was just complete happiness. It was just crazy,
like I don't know how to explain it really.

Similarly, Diana, age 50, described her first encounter with a woman
she had met online as the fulfillment of her wishes combined with a
major turning point in her sexuality:

> It was the first time being intimate with a woman. It was
> highly arousing, highly intoxicating, and I had developed feel-
> ings for her quite quickly. Every aspect of it was pleasurable
> and loving and satisfying and sweet and sensual, just every
> wonderful feeling. It was a very complete experience . . . that
> liberated me. I knew spontaneously, instinctually, that I was
> never gonna date another man, and I was never going to have
> another sexual experience with a man and that I would con-
> tinue to be intimate with women. It was like a turning point
> for me as far as my sexuality. It was intense, completely com-
> fortable and uninhibited, which I'd never felt with a man. With
> her I felt more in touch with my femininity and being a
> woman than I ever did being with a man.

In addition to newness, women described feeling pleasure about
experimentation with different sexual acts, particularly when they met
partners who encouraged them to explore different avenues to pleasure.
While these experiences definitely referenced the kinds of experimentation discussed in chapter 2 at times—in that women's desire to try
new sexual acts often accommodated demands they perceived from
men—many of these narratives revealed women generating desires and
needs outside of conventional gendered expectations. Recognizing and
connecting with one's own desires enough to act them out appeared
frequently in these narratives. For example, Julie, age 23, remembered a
sexually adventurous partner: "The sex was just so good. He was really
willing to explore things with me—new, adventuresome things that
were positive. He was really in tune to my body and what I wanted and
what I liked, and he really paid attention to the way that I reacted to
things and remembered them." Similarly, Brynn, age 25, recounted a
positive threesome experience: "We basically got to experience a three-

some, which I had wanted, which was kind of exciting. It was something different. You can always bring new things in, try new things, and this just happened to be adding another person to it." Ciara, age 24, described her husband's desire for rougher sex as one of her best sexual experiences because it departed from their normal sexual routines: "I guess it had been a while one time, and he said, 'Come into the bedroom.' We did it rougher, and it was more fun because it was a little different than normal. We both had an orgasm."

Lucy, age 25, who recently got married, explained that some of her early same-sex experimentation felt like her best experiences:

> My favorite one was in college—the whole trying out girls thing at a girls-only party. The party was done where it was an exercise to be open about our sexuality, so everything was done in the nude. It just opened me up to other things. Everyone gave each other a back rub and then we actually made h'ors d'oeuvres together, just talking and having drinks and having a good time. It was a comfortable environment. I guess just going to Catholic school my whole life and my family not immediately being open to talking about sex, I didn't really have people to talk to about it. All of a sudden I guess I felt it was more acceptable to be open about that sort of thing . . . Everyone I think was probably turned on that there was probably a lot of sexual energy there.

Along these lines, three women described feeling pleasure when they acted out their domination and submission fantasies directly, particularly if they had been in relationships with people who had not recognized or validated their desires. Many of these narratives involved direct elements of power, fetish, domination, submission, and control (chapter 6 further explores themes of women's sexual submission fantasies), often without the mentioning of attentiveness and love. Melanie, age 21, described a strong connection to a man who shared her fetish as her best experience:

> My partner at the time had a blood phobia. I have a blood fetish. My friend in New York also has a blood fetish. When I went out there, I was on my period . . . I don't know whether

you can call it sex or not, but we got into like really, really
heavy duty blood play, lots of power stuff, though I didn't actually have intercourse with him. It came in a period of my life
where I had really stopped following my intuition. I was not
expressing myself. I was not expressing my emotions. The long
term relationship that I had been in—and this was a five-year
relationship—had become actively repressive.

Jill, age 32, who reported intense eroticization of dominance/submis-
sion play, also described her best experience as a time when she acted
out these once-repressed desires directly:

It was probably the first time I had been noticeably, shall we
say, roughly manhandled to mutual enjoyment. At some point I
was tied or handcuffed to a table leg. I liked being tied up and
forced to do it . . . It's the first time I can really recall that I was
actually playing out some of the kinky shit that goes on in my
head to any substantial degree.

As a vivid example of acting out a direct fantasy or sexual wish that
involved a more powerful man, Edie, age 19, described her best experience as a casual sex encounter with a celebrity:

I had sex with the lead singer of my favorite band in New York
City in an "alleyway" type situation . . . Just the complete animalistic, savage way it happened and that it was like completely
devoid of conversation at all, 'cause he was obviously the lead
singer of a band, which allows him to just pick and choose
from a group of women. He was significantly older than me
and foreign. He was just an absolutely insane person . . . That
whole experience is just like the pinnacle of what you imagine
when you would go to a show and become completely in a
trance by the other person, and you absolutely fall for them, for
their music, but never really can imagine transcending that bar-
rier of security guards to actually talk to the person or touch
the person or take a photo of the person, you know, so getting
to be able to have sex with him after probably about five years

of me being absolutely obsessed with the band was amazing . . . It would be like losing your virginity on prom to your high school sweetheart. For some people, that's the dream, and for me, it was always, you know, getting fucked in an alleyway somewhere by him.

Thus, while only a few women reported themes of acting out fantasies of power in their best sexual experiences, these stories suggested that some women eroticized dominance in their partnered sexual behavior. It raises the question, which I take up in chapter 6: How do women liking domination scenarios complicate notions of sexual autonomy and power, and does the eroticization of dominance translate into women's sexual fantasies? And if *newness* leads to sexual pleasure for women, how might certain kinds of newness validate and empower women while other kinds of newness disempower women? Is this distinction even useful? Newness and attentiveness might overlap at times, particularly at the beginning of a relationship, but they might also diverge, particularly as a relationship evolves over time. The interplay, then, among domination, newness, and attentiveness represents a compelling and complicated mixture of factors that contributes to women's positive sexual experiences, particularly when considering the contexts of the performances they internalized. In fact, domination, newness, and attentiveness might each represent a different *kind* of performance, in that dominance could symbolize women's performance of their powerlessness, newness could symbolize women internalizing "youth" and "freshness" as essential to good sex, and attentiveness might symbolize a performance of closeness and love. The distinction between pleasure and performance thus loses its dichotomous qualities.

Pleasure as "Being Away"

The concept of 'being away' represents the final category within which women conceptualized their best sexual experiences, both in terms of feeling mentally or emotionally relaxed and, in a more litcral sense, when women embraced "vacation sex" or even an extramarital affair that took them away from their marriages. Women described getting away from the ruts of their daily lives, the boredom of monogamy, or the limitations of a dependent relationship. Sometimes women even described a mental state of feeling "lost" or "outside of oneself" as the most pleasurable, as great sex meant an escape from the mundane. For example, Mitra, age 29, described her best sex as a sensation of letting go and being outside of herself:

> I think my most positive sexual experiences have been those where I felt completely comfortable with myself and with the other person. I had an experience with someone where I felt he took me out of myself. That doesn't necessarily mean I had an orgasm, but just passion and heat. I wasn't feeling like I was performing. It just felt very erotic and sexual and relaxed. I don't think that it's something that I can really put into words. It's just that feeling of being able to totally let yourself go, because that was more of my mindset . . . I was not self-conscious, not feeling like I was performing or had to be a particular way for somebody. I was just transported outside of myself.

Pam, age 42, described sex while on vacation as having a particular erotic charge for her:

> He just surprised me by coming by, getting me, and taking me to a very nice, sweet hotel for the weekend. It was just out of the blue, just like, "Come on, let's go." The sex was great because it was all in the moment. He had taken the time, put a lot of effort into it, and then there was not anything that I had to ask for. Maybe it was the whole getaway thing, because most of the time, I'm just on the go, busy. School, life, work—I just want to take my mind away.

Ruth, age 46, reported similar sentiments, saying, "We've always had really good hotel sex. Usually I brought some things with me, and we went away for the weekend or whatever. I can recall a lot of good experiences, just going away, just being away from the house needing to be cleaned or whatever. I never have a rushed feeling or never worry about letting the dogs out or whether the sheets were clean or whether the phone would ring." Thus, women reported that leaving the stale confines of their houses and finding a new enthusiasm for their current partner in a different setting created a positive and memorable sexual experience for them.

Finally, being *away* from a husband or partner by having an extramarital affair also seemed to tap into women's impulses to construct pleasure from escape, though only a few women mentioned this. Marilyn, age 54, described a pleasurable extramarital affair:

> In 1978, I did have an affair with someone I met at work. That was the best intercourse because it was unexpected, secretive, and it was something for me, not for the family or the home relationship. The gentleman was very attentive towards me. We explored different avenues that were never done in my marriage, like anal sex. He made sure every part of the body was centrally touched, so I guess I felt like he was there for me, as opposed to the marriage where I was there for him. He wanted to make sure that I was pleased. It was the first time it was all about me. I didn't have to share it with my family. When you're a mother and a wife and you work, it seems like you're divided up and going in many different directions, and when you're married at such a young age, it's always been instilled in you that family comes first. When someone gives you attention outside of the family and those obligations, I think it's very satisfying.

Collectively, these narratives of being "away" indicate that the regular performance of gender, during sex or outside of sex altogether, may feel taxing to some women, particularly those in long-term relationships. The recognition of sex as a means to escape everyday concerns or, more importantly, to escape certain *productions of gender*, reveals a connection between sexual pleasure and nonhegemonic expressions of femininity. While women may feel competent and confident in their regular lives—including their ability to care for their partners—the fact that they find sexual pleasure outside of their regular lives suggests that they may *not* eroticize traditional gender roles. Thus, removing oneself from "real life" may indicate both that women derive pleasure from new social roles and/or experiences *and* that women find "real life" somewhat dissatisfying, particularly in the sexual realm. They want a different scene to feel sexual within. Being away may provide women with a way to focus exclusively on sex outside of the demands of other aspects of their lives. In this way, vacation sex may also allow them to act out different versions of themselves (e.g., the relaxed woman, the nonmother, etc.) that they cannot access in their ordinary performances of gender.

CONCLUSION

When examining the four categories of women's sexual pleasure—emotional connection, attentiveness/orgasm/embodiment, newness, and escape—the diversity of women's lived experiences comes alive. Tying together these four categories of sexual pleasure, consider the following argument by Deleuze (1989):

> The body is no longer the obstacle that separates thought from itself, that which it has to overcome to reach thinking. It is on the contrary that which it plunges into or must plunge into, in order to reach the unthought, that is life. Not that the body thinks, but, obstinate and stubborn, it forces us to think, and forces us to think what is concealed from thought, life . . . To think is to learn what a non-thinking body is capable of, its capacity, its postures. (189)

When questions are asked of the body—in this case, what sexual experiences women remember as their best and most pleasurable—this very dilemma is tapped into: How is *meaning* (something largely constructed as "of the mind") theorized from the lived experiences of the (non-thinking) body? How is the body a site from which people *know* or *experience* or *feel alive*, particularly if the body also performs and acts out social scripts dictated by others?

To better illustrate this concept of the 'unthought,' consider Edie's comment after I asked her what emotions she typically feels when having sex with a partner:

Really it's like the one thing that humans can do to completely lose that ability to define your emotions, you know? I feel, uh, very animalistic, like an evolved monkey that I am. I'm sure I feel emotions. I love him, but I don't know if I'm feeling that at the time. I think I'm not thinking or feeling in a describable or definable way.

Part of pleasure, it seems, is the pairing of the mind/body connection. Women felt pleasure from their emotional connections to their partners, the attentiveness their partners paid to their bodies, the newness and experimentation with different sensations or feelings, and the concept of being away. While these are dramatically different, in many respects, they all relate to the sexualized pairing of the mind/body in different and nuanced ways. Some women rely upon sexuality to help them ground themselves in their bodies, while other women look to sex as a way to make concrete the emotional connections they have to others (and sometimes even to themselves). Some women seem to enjoy the *sensation* of sex, while others enjoy the discourse around sex. Some use sex as a means to heal, while others seek out pain and domination in order to achieve pleasure.

Certainly, the question of pleasure is as complex as any in this book. Pleasure can be *cerebral*, in that women may have certain individual standards they seek to fulfill via pleasure; for example, in order to respond sexually to another person, women may require that that person excite them intellectually and emotionally or that the conditions of the experience itself meet an ideal they have about place, interaction, and sensuality. Moreover, pleasure can be *hedonistic* (Deci & Ryan, 2008), in that, despite the cultural admonishments that women should not shamelessly seek pleasure as a form of bodily gratification, many women described pleasure as a quest for physical fulfillment without regard to the more cerebral or intellectual aspects of pleasure. Still more, pleasure can reflect a desire for *constancy* or, in direct contrast to constancy, as a *break* from one's daily existence. Some women described the consistency of their positive sexual interactions with their partners as central to their experience of pleasure, in that the familiarity and connectedness that emerged from long-term sexual relationships felt more fulfilling than any one particular act. These women wanted a

consistent stream of pleasurable experiences within which to experience themselves and their partnership. Contrast that with the opposite
point of view, where women described intense pleasure as a moment of
difference from their normal sexual lives (whether via a new experience
or a new partner or a new place), and one can start to see the enormous complexities of theorizing and thinking about pleasure.

Added to these overarching problems of theorizing pleasure in a
multifaceted way, consider the fundamental problem of *subalterity*, or, as
Homi Bhabha (1996) states, an oppressed group "whose presence was
crucial to the self-definition of the [dominant] group" (210).[2] How
does one read women's pleasurable experiences in light of the fact that
nearly every major cultural institution women interact with (e.g.,
work, education, media, marriage, economics, etc.) tries to actively distance them further from the knowledge produced by the body, to strip
them of the power that arises from embodiment, to objectify and distort their sources of sexual joy? In short, should women's accounts of
pleasure be trusted, given that they are oppressed people? Going back
to the problem that runs through this book, if women learn to *perform*
their sexualities, how might this inform the concept of, and liberatory
potential of, pleasure? Growing evidence suggests that women defer
their ideas about pleasure to the definitions provided by others, particularly those found in the media and/or those articulated by partners
(Brown, Steele, & Walsh-Childers, 2002). In chapters 1 and 2, it seems
that, because women's sexuality so often serves the status quo, finding a
space outside of that becomes increasingly difficult or even, as some
would argue, *impossible.*

This elicits another central question: Do performances of pleasure
empower or disempower women? When looking at women's best
sexual experience narratives collectively, several viable interpretations
come to mind. First, embedded within anything women construct as
pleasurable, there are traces of both empowerment and disempowerment. Even when examining women's descriptions of emotional connectedness as a precursor for intense sexual pleasure, it seems likely that
emotions *can* and often *are* performances with multiple goals. If American culture teaches women that they cannot have sex without love,
they learn that emotions like love are not just expected but demanded,
in order to allow space for their sexual expression. Emotions like love

and care and connectedness become compulsory rather than optional for some women; their socialization teaches them that sex without love makes them "sluts" or "whores," so they construct pleasure around the *avoidance* of these stigmatized identities. Women want to avoid being constructed outside of "good girl" femininity; they can only engage in socially sanctioned sex if they perform the proper emotions. This is not to say that they do not *feel* love for their partners, but rather, it suggests the ways that women's options are often limited by the cultural terms within which they operate.

Women also experience pleasure while conforming to cultural expectations (just as, perhaps, *anyone* might feel validated when he or she meets societal expectations placed upon him or her, whether conforming to the norms of a workplace, fitting in with a group of friends, or conforming to various body image and grooming norms). If gendered scripts demand *conformity*, it makes sense that some women find pleasure *in conforming*—a position both Goffman and Irigaray have argued. This appeared when women eroticized their own objectification (e.g., Susan), when they became aroused *because* they were performing (for example, Emily) or when they felt acutely aware of the sex act as a fulfillment of fantasy (e.g., Edie).

Women also enact performances of empowerment and disempowerment in a variety of seemingly innocuous sexual events. For example, this tension might be at play when women described their first orgasm as their best sexual experience; pressure to orgasm underlies much of the anxiety women have about their (in)ability to orgasm prior to the event. These tensions might also contribute to women's descriptions of masturbation as fulfilling, as, in the case of Sonja, she felt she *should* be sexual but could not orgasm regularly during sex with another person. The wide variety of performances associated with masturbation represent a vastly understudied area of women's sexual lives; for example, despite there being no cultural lexicon for women to speak about masturbation with each other, women described *naming* their (phallic) sex toys and personifying them as male in gender (e.g., Carol, who said, "I joke with my husband that 'Jim' and I have our own special relationship," when speaking of her vibrator). Tensions between empowerment and disempowerment exist in abundance when examining women's sexual pleasure.

That said, these narratives provide a rather convincing indictment of contemporary cultural scripts about women's sexual pleasure by revealing the many ways that women derive pleasure from nonnormative, nonscripted actions. American culture ascribes caretaking tasks to women, and it teaches them to value others' pleasure above their own, to accept not being heard or seen (except when being objectified), and to love and nurture others. Women spend an enormous amount of time being *attentive* to others' needs—often at their own expense—as part of their prescribed roles within a patriarchal society. So, when women say, clearly, that they feel sexual pleasure from rejecting this script (i.e., from receiving that same care and nurturance from their partners that they have typically provided), this suggests that the rejection of this gendered performance contributes to intense sexual pleasure. While women may derive pleasure from embracing their social roles (e.g., sex in the context of love, pleasing one's partner, etc.), they also derive pleasure from rejecting those social roles (e.g., receiving pleasure from a partner, engaging in sex for other reasons besides love, finding a non-traditional male partner, rejecting heterosexuality, etc.). Women's partners may also reap the erotic benefits if they treat women in an attentive, nonstereotyped manner, as research shows that egalitarian relationships yield numerous social and psychological rewards for both partners (Risman & Johnson-Family, 1998).

When considering this concept of 'attentiveness'—where partners treat women with patience, mindfulness, and care—it reveals the mythologies of much contemporary discourse on women's sexuality. Rarely did women describe intense and dramatic power imbalances as their best sexual experiences; rarely did women describe being "overpowered" or "taken" or "done to"—themselves images and stories repeated again and again in pornography—as a sexual high. Rarely did women describe bodice-ripping clichés as their most memorable sexual moments. Rather, these stories reveal, most basically, a call for partners to treat women with *kindness*, to pay attention to them, to look for, explore, and recognize their active desires, to make them feel seen, to let them exist both within and outside of their prescribed roles. This manifested itself in a wide range of scenarios, including attention to women's bodily reactions (Marilyn), encouragement for women to take ownership of their pleasure (Kate), an intuitive sense that one's body is understood (Lori), and a unification of emotional and physical intimacy (Dawn). Consequently, pleasure may reveal the politics of sexual performance, conflicts about empowerment, and a more utopian vision for social and sexual justice for women. It may also show the ways that women cannot fully escape from power and deference to heterosexist and sexist norms, and in fact, the study of pleasure may reveal that women *internalize* certain stereotyped scripts about gender and sexuality. Pleasure can be, simultaneously, subversive and oppressive, revealing and disguising, empowering and disempowering.

Still, in these best sexual experiences narratives, women consistently rejected the social script that calls for them to eroticize their own domination. This is not to say that women do not eroticize submission (and this will become more evident when considering sexual fantasy narratives in chapter 6), but it does suggest that women's most intense pleasure does not typically arise from contexts that reinforce cultural fantasies of women as dominated by others. Only a few even mentioned domination/submission as one of their best sexual experiences. Rather, women derived the most sexual pleasure from four dimensions: emotional connectedness, attention to women's desires and experiences of their bodies, news ideas about what is possible or pleasurable sexually, and taking women away from the gendered demands of their everyday lives. The study of pleasure, then, reimagines women's relationships with themselves and others, even while pleasure remains mired, to a certain degree, in the trappings of performance and power.

CHAPTER FIVE

THE CULTURE OF DOMINATION

Sexual Violence, Objectification, and Access

> This reality of being owned and being fucked—as experience, a social, political, economic, and psychological unity—frames, limits, sets parameters for, what women feel and experience in sex. Being owned and being fucked are or have been virtually synonymous experiences in the lives of women . . . Women live inside this reality of being owned and fucked; are sensate inside it; the body learning to respond to what male dominance offers.
>
> —Dworkin, *Intercourse*

THE COMMONLY HEARD statistics about violence against women—which typically hold that roughly a third of women have experienced sexual assault of some kind in their lifetime—fail to do justice to the complexity, nuance, and depth of coercive sexual practices women encounter in their sexual lives. While statistics show the pervasive extent of systematic violence toward women, they do not capture the way that nearly *all* women confront components of a culture of domination both inside and outside of their sexual relationships with others. While most women do not endure violence on a regular basis, coercion nevertheless informs women's sexuality in a consistent way. This chapter offers an analysis of how the various manifestations of culturally validated dominance over women—including sexual violence, sexual objectification, sexual harassment, and street harassment—inform, alter, and at times distort women's sexual consciousness. Women's stories reveal that, by simultaneously encouraging women to perform as liberated and empowered, yet barraging them with messages of fear about their physical, mental, and sexual vulnerability, this culture indoctrinates women into a kind of *double consciousness* where the performance of empowerment comingles with the performance of sustained vulnerability.[1]

This chapter explores this tension in women's lives by first examining women's worst sexual experience narratives. In listening to women's descriptions of memorable negative events, their statements and impressions illustrate the range of coercion women encounter and how they react to coercion. The enormous ambivalence women describe about their worst sexual experiences informs the later discussion of women conflating flattery and repulsion when men objectify them, particularly during street harassment (e.g., wolf whistling) and sexual harassment. Women express both willingness and reluctance to label sexual assault as "rape," which informs their relationships and sexual health. While this ambivalence may reflect a resistance toward labels (particularly labels that blame victims for the aggression) and an effort to desexualize or destigmatize violent sexual experiences, these performances also normalize and mainstream sexual assault in relevant ways (i.e., first denying its existence and later by minimizing its significance, downplaying the violent implications of coercion and refusing to acknowledge survivors).

By interrogating women's double consciousness about sexual coercion, this chapter centers on the idea that the sheer pervasiveness of sexual violence in women's sexual lives leads to a variety of performances, many of which serve as protective mechanisms. This chapter poses that 1) it is not a matter of *if* women have experienced coercion but rather, a matter of *how, in what context*, and *what the coercion meant to them*, and 2) *regardless of its manifestation, women learn that they must provide sexual access to men in order to receive sexual and personal validation*. This sexual access is scripted both in contradictory messages about women performing empowerment by having sex (i.e., "You should have *more* sex, in *more* ways, and with *more* people to be a fully liberated woman") *and* in messages that men can sexually violate women if women misbehave (i.e., "If you wear certain clothes or don't watch out for yourself, you will get into trouble"). In both of these constructs, men's right to have sexual access to women remains constant.[2] Consequently, this chapter argues that women's *performance of providing men with sexual access to them*—whether via normalizing coercive practices, prioritizing male desire, eroticizing domination, having sex without being fully emotionally present, or a host of other behaviors—is one of the primary manifestations of the culture of violence.

By asking women about their worst sexual experiences, a range of stories arose, most of which implied various kinds of coercion. Such stories point to the complexities of thinking about and understanding women's worst sexual experiences as illustrations of sexual violence. As such, key questions in this chapter include: How does coercion appear in women's lives, and how do women respond to it? What do women's stories about their worst sexual experiences reveal about the gendered aspects of power and performance? How is women's sexual access to men normalized and demanded by conventional scripts of gender? What does this "double consciousness" between empowerment and domination look like for women? How do women experience the conflation of repulsion and flattery while being sexually harassed or objectified? Finally, how is women's relationship to domination a performative relationship, particularly as they construct meaning from coercive sexual experiences?

RESEARCH ON THE CULTURE OF VIOLENCE

Rape and Sexual Violence

Many sexuality researchers today have identified a "continuum of sexual violence" rather than distinct categories of "rape" and "not rape" that often occur in legal and medical settings (Kelly, 1996; Odede & Asghedom, 2001; Plummer, 2002). Such a continuum makes visible the range of ways that women experience sexual violence, sexual assault, coercion, and harassment, thus providing a fuller picture of how power relationships—particularly between men and women—function with regard to women's sexuality. Issues of consent take center stage in the language women use about sexual violence. Rape has long been a focus for feminist activism and feminist theorizing about the body, as the

gendered components of sexual assault speak not only to the sexualization of violence but also to the larger issues of how women are treated
in this culture. Throughout the process of fighting to combat violence
against women, feminists (not without conflict among themselves) have
identified the phrase *culture of violence* to describe the ways in which,
even though all women are not targets of direct sexual assault, all
women cope with, and struggle against, the construction of their bodies
as physically and sexually vulnerable to attack. Not only does this
change women's relationship to space, but it also inscribes women as
receptive, passive, and susceptible to "damage," while constructing men
as penetrative, active, and physically and sexually infallible. This construct led to several decades of research that focused primarily on
women as victims and survivors of rape; men as perpetrators have only
recently taken center stage in rape research, as more and more studies
examine rape behaviors by focusing on men (Berkowitz, 1992; Viki,
Abrams, & Masser, 2004). Studies of same-sex sexual violence against
women are still in their infancy.

Rape and sexual assault against women represent some of the least
recognized human rights issues in the world today (Rozee, Biaggio, &
Hersen, 2000). For industrialized nations, rape prevalence hovers around
21 to 25% (Koss, Heise, & Russo, 1994), with the United States having
the highest rate of any industrialized nation (e.g., four times higher
than Germany, 12 times higher than England, 20 times higher than
Japan, per Rozee, 2005). One in four women reported that men had
raped them in their adult lifetime (Campbell & Wasco, 2005), though
this number tended to be higher for certain at-risk groups like women
with sexual abuse histories (Parillo, Freeman, & Young, 2003; Sarkar &
Sarkar, 2005), those under age 18 (Tjaden & Thoennes, 2000), those
who identified as Native American or Alaskan Native women (Tjaden
& Thoennes, 2000), or women in college who used drugs, lived in a
sorority, drank heavily in high school, or attended a college with normative heavy drinking (Mohler-Kuo et al., 2004). Indeed, *nearly half* of
women in college reported a history of some type of sexual victimization (Koss, Gidycz, & Wisniewski, 1987), and most rape perpetrators
were men women knew intimately rather than strangers (Marx, Van
Wie, & Gross, 1996). While women represented 91% of rape victims,
men committed 99% of rapes (UCSC, 2008). At least four in 10 rapes

occurred in women's homes (Tjaden & Thoennes, 2000), and the vast majority of nonconsensual sex acts remained unreported (Tjaden & Thoennes, 2000).

Research on the degree to which women label coercive events as rape varies dramatically, revealing the slippages women have about themselves and others when naming sexual experiences. Nearly half of college women who reported a rape experience did not label it as rape (Bondurant, 2001; Kahn et al., 2003; Koss, 1985). This may stem from an overly dichotomous view of rape as either having "occurred" or "not occurred," when in actuality, research supports a multidimensional model of women wanting or not wanting sex. The use of the term *rape* seems contingent on the qualities of both the perpetrator and the victim. Women who labeled their experience as rape more often experienced forceful assault by an acquaintance, awakening to someone performing a sexual act on them without consent, or experiencing the assault as a child. Women less often called their experience rape if they submitted to a whining or begging boyfriend, gave in to an emotionally needy man, were assaulted by a boyfriend, were severely impaired by alcohol or drugs and unable to resist, were forced to engage in oral or manual sex rather than penetrative intercourse (Kahn, 2004), or reported that they initially wanted the sexual intercourse more (Peterson & Muehlenhard, 2007). Further, some research suggests that women did not label rape when their scripts about the rape experience did not match the events where rapes occur (Littleton, Rhatigan, & Axsom, 2007).

Many women expressed difficulty labeling certain behaviors as rape and more often labeled the event as rape if more violence and less alcohol use took place. Women who felt less stigma about their sexual assault experiences also felt less likely to label the act as rape than did those who experienced more stigma (Littleton & Breitkopf, 2006). When judging other women, women also resisted the label of rape more often if the victim had an extensive sexual history or if they had engaged in a lot of foreplay (Flowe, Ebbesen, & Putcha-Bhagavatula, 2007).

The way victims defined the sexual violence that they endured can have long-term consequences on their well-being. In general, however, the label itself did not correlate with a lower or higher likelihood of recovering from the rape experience (McMullin & White, 2006), but the label *rape* correlated with higher incidences of health complaints (Conoscenti & McNally, 2006). This indicates that the labeling of rape experiences is not an inconsequential factor in both mental and physical health outcomes of sexual violence. Narrating rape experiences can improve women's well-being.

Studies consistently show that women underreport rape and that rape statistics may reflect less than a third of actual rape events. The reporting of rape also varies in relationship to women's feelings of shame, guilt, and embarrassment; concerns about confidentiality; and fear of not being believed (Sable et al., 2006). Women's experiences with reporting rape tend to be met with varied reactions ranging from highly supportive and nurturing to complete disbelief (Guerette & Caron, 2007). Studies show that women have much more positive mental health outcomes if they reported rape within one month of its occurrence when compared with those who waited longer than one month (Ruggiero et al., 2004). In cases where women did report rape, the relationship between the victim and perpetrator, whether the victim had consumed alcohol (Tellis & Spohn, 2008), and the victim's demeanor and dress (Jordan, 2004) affected the legal outcomes of rape trials, perhaps indicating that certain "blaming the victim" ideologies are enhanced by the perception that the woman drank too much or otherwise "asked for it." This may help to explain why women resist the label *rape* and why they underreport rape in general.

This variability in labeling rape as rape may also stem from America's longstanding history of failing to criminalize marital rape. The cultural script for married couples' sexuality tends to hold that men can have sexual access to their wives and that women should not (and sometimes legally could not) resist their husbands' efforts to initiate sex. Marital rape only became illegal in all 50 states in July 1993. Studies show that 10–14% of all married women experienced rape by their husbands, while 40–50% of married women were battered by their husbands. Marriages in which marital rape occurred had significantly higher rates of nonsexual violence and marital dissatisfaction as well as lower ratings of marital quality. Most marital rape victims felt unable to or afraid to resist sexual aggression by their husbands and often reported depression, PTSD, gynecological problems, and negative physical health symptoms (Martin, Taft, & Resick, 2007).

Research consistently shows that rape survivors experience a range of mental health consequences, including Post-Traumatic Stress Disorder, depression (Wolitzky-Taylor et al., 2008), anxiety, mood disorders, sexual disorders (Faravelli et al., 2004), and Borderline Personality Disorder (Clarke, Rizvi, & Resick, 2008). Negative social reactions from others and avoidance coping correlated most strongly with PTSD symptoms (Ullman et al., 2007). Unfortunately, studies have consistently shown that women overwhelmingly did not seek mental health treatment following sexual assault (Ullman, 2007) and most often suppressed the event or resorted to self-blame and self-loathing following sexual assault (Littleton & Breitkopf, 2006). Many rape survivors also reported more risky sexual health behaviors, including increased frequency of sex without the use of condoms and increased use of drugs and alcohol during sex (Campbell, Sefl, & Ahrens, 2004). Compared to women without sexual assault histories, sexual assault survivors also had more marijuana use, diet pill use, eating disordered behaviors, suicidal ideation, and were far more likely to experience sexual victimization again (Gidycz et al., 2008).

Feminists have long argued that rape functions as a way for men to exert power over women and, as such, is *not* a *sexual* outlet per se. Studies linking the rape of women with antigay violence support these claims (Franklin, 2004), as do cross-cultural studies of cultures that do not construct the penis as a potential weapon but rather see the penis as inconsequential and incapable of violence (Helliwell, 2000). Feminist social scientists have long argued that rape allows men to dominate and terrorize women, and it does not represent an extension of men's libido. Rapes occur more often in contexts that encourage more stereotypically masculine behavior and attitudes; such environments promote the acceptance and perpetuation of "rape myths," a set of beliefs related to just-world theory (Lonsway & Fitzgerald, 1994) that hold that good things happen to good people, and bad things happen to bad people. People who believe in rape myths rationalize why women might get raped, arguing that they might have brought the event on by wearing certain kinds of clothes or otherwise "asking for it" (Workman & Orr, 1996).

Rape myth ideologies are often interwoven with other sorts of ideologies that condone the subordination of minority groups. Rape myth acceptance correlated significantly with racist, sexist, homophobic,

ageist, classist, and religiously intolerant attitudes, indicating that acceptance of power-laden relationships between people contributed to rape
myth ideology (Aosved & Long, 2006). Those who *rejected* rape myths
more often identified as sexual assault victims themselves, came from
egalitarian families, stayed in college longer, rejected modern sexism,
and felt little animosity toward women (Haywood & Swank, 2008).
Men who supported more sexist attitudes and who condoned interpersonal violence against women more often supported rape myths, and
those who generally abhorred, distrusted, and resented women
endorsed rape myth beliefs more often (Chapleau, Oswald, & Russell,
2008; Cowan, 2000; Haywood & Swank, 2008; Lonsway & Fitzgerald,
1995). Similarly, men who supported violence against women also
endorsed beliefs that femininity was inferior to masculinity, women
should hold more responsibility for sexual assault, and alcohol was an
acceptable means to acquire sexual compliance (Burgess, 2007). Even
imagery on the walls in fraternity houses has been correlated strongly
with acceptance of rape myths and acceptance of sexist attitudes
(Bleeker & Murnen, 2005).

Though women far less often supported rape myths or blame the
victim for rape (Fonow, Richardson, & Wemmerus, 1992), their support
of rape myths has correlated with conservative political ideologies as
well as their consumption of pornography, women's magazines, and television; in particular, women who watched more television more often
labeled rape accusations as false (Emmers-Sommer et al., 2006; Kahlor
& Morrison, 2007). Interestingly, one study found that women's acceptance of rape myths was associated with emotional and romantic themes
in their sexual fantasies (Zurbriggen & Yost, 2004). Women who
endorsed rape myths were also less likely to label their own coercive
experiences as *rape* (Peterson & Muehlenhard, 2004). This refusal of the
term *rape* in turn led to greater chances of negative long-term effects
on women. Collectively, these studies reveal that women contend with
significant barriers when internally constructing their coercion experiences as undeserved and unwanted, a pattern that reveals itself in
women's worst sexual experience narratives in the second section of
this chapter.

Cultures of highly stereotyped masculine behavior, combined with
pressure to engage in "male bonding" rituals, also correlated highly

with increased likelihood of committing rape and sexual assault. Fraternity houses have become synonymous with sexual coercion, high consumption of alcohol, sexualized hazing rituals, and boasting about "getting laid" (Sanday, 2007). One study found that over half of sorority women had experienced sexual coercion by a fraternity member, with half of these rapes happening in the fraternity houses themselves (Copenhaver & Grauerholz, 1991). Rapes within the "party culture" of college campuses occurred more often when men expected women to defer to men and when fraternities dominated college parties (Armstrong, Hamilton, & Sweeney, 2006). As another example, rates of sexual assault in the military have skyrocketed in recent years (Murdoch et al., 2004). One recent study of more than 2,000 women in the United States Air Force found that 28% had been raped, a figure nearly twice as high as the prevalence rate in a national sample. Nearly half of the sample had been the victims of rape, molestation, or attempted sexual assault, with 26% reporting rape by a military member (Bostock & Daley, 2007).

Some research has shown that men model after other men's harassing and aggressive behavior toward women, which may help to explain why rates of sexual assault among "cultures of masculinity" remain so high (Mitchell et al., 2002). Following coverage of the alleged Kobe Bryant assault case, for example, rape myths like "She's lying" appeared frequently in articles and segments discussing the case; further, those exposed to such media coverage reported that Bryant was "innocent" and that the alleged victim was "lying" far more often than those not exposed to such media coverage (Franiuk et al., 2008). Further, some research has shown that perceptions of gender equality correlated to occurrences of rape (Martin, Vieraitis, & Britto, 2006) indicating that rape sometimes functions as a kind of punishment for women perceived as feminist or "strong." This research has been contradicted, however, by cross-cultural research that shows that, in countries where women have more social and economic power, rates of sexual coercion are *lower* than in countries where women have less power (Lottes & Weinberg, 1997). Overall, women face enormous pressures to minimize the significance of sexual coercion, play along with messages that inscribe them as vulnerable and easily attacked, and avoid the label *rape* in order to ward off stigma, male hostilities, and disbelief from others.

Street Harassment

Clearly, sexual violence exists along a continuum. Other behaviors aside from the literal act of rape contribute to the culture of violence against women, particularly street harassment and sexual harassment. Gill Valentine's (1989) work on street harassment has shown that women typically change their relationship to public and social space in response to fear of harassment or assault; she terms these spatial changes "geographies of fear," saying,

> This inability of women to enjoy independence and freedom to move safely in public space is therefore one of the pressures which encourages them to seek from one man protection from all, initially through having a boyfriend and later through cohabitation. This dependence on a single man commonly limits women's career opportunities and general lifeworld. This in turn results in a restricted use of public space by women, especially at night, allowing men to appropriate it and hence making women feel unsafe to go out, reinforcing their comparative confinement in the home. Consequently this cycle of fear becomes one subsystem by which male dominance, patriarchy, is maintained and perpetuated. Women's inhibited use and occupation of public space is therefore a spatial expression of patriarchy. (p. 285)

Research on "geographies of fear" has noted that women tend to mentally map out places they deem as safe and unsafe while also heightening their sense of private space as safe and public space as dangerous (Pain, 1997). Given that most sexual assaults occur in private spaces (e.g., inside the home, with acquaintances or partners, etc.), this distinction exists more as a fantasy construct than something grounded in reality. People misidentify the threat level for different locales because they have so long internalized the idea of public space as *dangerous*, private space as *safe*. Still, even accurate assessments can lead to negative consequences: Bowman (1993) argued that street harassment prevents women's full participation in the public sphere and severely limits their sense of liberty, equality, and self-dignity. Street harassment has also been conceptualized as a form of "sexual terrorism," where women experience a dramatic invasion of their privacy while men experience it as harmless fun (Kissling, 1991).

One alarming study argued that women avoid places where they might experience harassment or assault while also claiming that most men who harass women on the street do so in a harmless way (Packer, 1986). This attribution of men as *innocently* harassing women, combined with women altering their relationship to space, normalizes men's harassing behaviors while restricting women's rights and putting the onus on women to change their behavior. This naturalizes men's harassing behaviors as typical while blaming women for their own harassment *because of* their circulation in certain kinds of public spaces.

Looking more specifically at the situations where street harassment most often occurs, some research has shown that, when men accompany women on the street, women experience less street harassment. While alone, when women do fight back, their resistance is often met with anger, hostility, and resentment by men, though some studies show that fighting back is an effective means to stop the harassment (Ullman, 2007; Ullman & Knight, 1992). As Maggie Hadleigh West, documentary filmmaker of *War Zone* said, "There's always a threat of physical or sexual violence . . . The abuse is a very quick incident, but for the women in question, the moment becomes elongated, because they don't know what might happen" (Napolitano, 2005, p. 2). Street harassment correlated with women's perceptions of fear, vulnerability, and lack of personal safety in general. The more women experienced street harassment by strangers, the more they felt unsafe and victimized (Gardner, 1995; Macmillan, Nierobisz, & Welsh, 2000).

While women deemed harassment as offensive and dangerous, they sometimes constructed "catcalls" as complimentary. Surprisingly little research has addressed the conflation of repulsion and flattery that women sometimes feel in response to street harassment. One recent study found that, of 225 women surveyed, 98% had experienced some form of street harassment at least a few times, and 30% reported being harassed on a regular basis. Further, many women felt that the catcalling validated them sexually or made them feel young and attractive. On the other hand, such harassment can lead to physical forms of sexual assault, it can lead to more intensified harassment, and it can teach women to construct themselves as a series of body parts instead of whole human beings (Grossman, 2008).

Sexual Harassment

The pervasiveness of sexual harassment against women has been well documented in recent years, particularly among cultures that nurture and encourage traditional forms of masculinity and thereby sanction perpetrators' behavior. Those who endorsed more hostile sexism and male identity measures more often harassed women than those who admitted to less sexism and less traditional male identities (Siebler, Sabelus, & Bohner, 2008). Sexual harassment has appeared particularly pervasively in stereotypically masculine cultures like fraternity houses (Copenhaver & Grauerholz, 1991), the military (Antecol & Cobb-Clark, 2006; Bostock & Daley, 2007; Street et al., 2007), Wall Street (Roth, 2007), medical schools (Shrier et al., 2007; Witte, Stratton, & Nora, 2006), sports teams (Fasting, Brackenridge, & Walseth, 2007), and workplace settings dominated by men (Berdahl, 2007; Vogt et al., 2007). Interestingly, women who displayed more masculine traits, thereby rejecting traditionally feminine behaviors and presentation, experienced more sexual harassment than women who displayed more traditionally feminine behaviors (Berdahl, 2007). That said, when independent raters judged women as "more attractive," they rated them as experiencing harassment more often than those women judged as "unattractive" (Golden, Johnson, & Lopez, 2001). Further, studies consistently find that men perceive harassing behaviors as fun and harmless, while women perceive harassing behaviors as shaming and emotionally painful; such findings may relate to the degree of performativity expected from men, in that objectification of women and lack of empathy for women is normalized as part of the *production* of masculinity (Quinn, 2002).

Developmental research has shown that women's experiences with unwanted sexual behaviors starts early in childhood and continues throughout the lifespan (Rodkin & Fischer, 2003; Whealin et al., 2007), with harassment coming to a peak in junior high and high school years (Gruber & Fineran, 2007; Pepler et al., 2006). This increase in cross-gender sexual harassment during grades 6-8 has been attributed to pubertal changes and shifting sociocultural models of gendered behavior that occur in early adolescence (McMaster et al., 2002). Some researchers have become concerned with the extent to which online harassment, texting, and blogging may contribute to even more harassment for adolescent girls. Studies have shown that potential for sexual exploitation and harassment correlates with meeting people in person (Mitchell, Wolak, & Finkelhor, 2008) and with substance abuse histories, delinquent peers, a propensity for anger, and poor emotional bonds with caretakers (Ybarra, Espelage, & Mitchell, 2007). While sexual solicitation has declined in recent years, unwanted exposure to pornography has spiked (Mitchell, Wolak, & Finkelhor, 2007).

Research on the intersections between race and gender has also consistently found that women of color experienced more consistent sexual harassment than white women (Berdahl & Moore, 2006). Women of color experienced more pressure to send nude pictures of themselves to others online (Mitchell, Finkelhor, & Wolak, 2007), suffered from the dual oppressions of race and gender when facing sexual harassment situations (Buchanan & Ormerod, 2002), and felt less "buffered" by feminist belief systems as a coping mechanism for sexual harassment than did white women (Rederstorff, Buchanan, & Settles, 2007).

As with other paradigms where sex and power intersect, sexual harassment has consistently led to negative health outcomes such as anxiety, depression, sleep problems, nausea, stress, and headaches (Rospenda et al., 2005; Welsh, 1999); increased rates of eating disorders and self-objectification (Harned & Fitzgerald, 2002; Lindberg, Grabe, & Hyde, 2007); negative work productivity outcomes (Kelly et al., 2005); more organizational withdrawal and lower well-being (Miner-Rubino & Cortina, 2007); and, for active-duty military women, a higher likelihood of dropping out of the military (Antecol & Cobb-Clark, 2006). Women admitted fear of retaliation and retribution and general lack of security when reporting sexual harassment, such that it often went underreported (Wilson, 2000).

Further, the negative health consequences of sexual harassment extend out beyond those who directly experience harassment. Researchers have begun looking at the effects of *hostile climate* as an often-neglected layer of sexual harassment. This research has shown that "bystander harassment," where people observe a man harassing another woman, can negatively affect workplace climate (Hitlan, Schneider, & Walsh, 2006). Women who witnessed sexual harassment without being direct targets of it reported lower emotional well-being and higher organizational withdrawal, particularly for employees in male-dominated work settings (Miner-Rubino & Cortina, 2004; Miner-Rubino & Cortina, 2007).

Collectively, this body of research on coercion, rape, sexual violence, street harassment, and sexual harassment paints a vivid picture of the many barriers women have when holding men accountable for sexual assault and coercion behaviors. In addition to legal and systematic barriers, women confront enormous incentives to minimize the significance of coercion, normalize assault and harassment, and otherwise claim that coercion did not matter, was not a big deal, or was deserved. Further, because sexual assault, coercion, and harassment have become *normal* parts of women's lived experiences, women's outrage, action, and even *labeling* of these experiences occurs relatively infrequently in relation to the occurrence of these events. These trends all appear in women's descriptions of their worst sexual experiences.

Research on Worst Sexual Experiences

Research on women's worst sexual experiences reveals several themes that link up to these findings about rape, coercion, street harassment, and sexual violence (Plante, 2006a). In previous studies, women indicated several themes in their worst sexual experiences: alcohol, forced sexual behavior against their will, feeling used as an object for a partner's physical pleasure, regret and embarrassment, partner being too aggressive, and coercion. Further, women typically did not tell their friends about worst experiences that included coercion, unsafe sexual intercourse, or feeling overwhelmed (Paul & Hayes, 2002). Women also labeled coercion from partners as among their worst experiences. Research has shown that women experience enormous pressures from men to engage in all sorts of behaviors, including kissing, genital touching, oral sex, anal sex, intercourse, and masturbation (Christopher, 1988). Such pressure to engage in nonconsensual sexual behaviors often leads to women's worst and least pleasurable sexual experiences.

The literature on sexual violence suggests that women experience coercion in a multitude of ways, particularly in settings that encourage traditionally masculine behaviors, such as fraternities, the military, male-dominated workplaces, sports teams, and social spaces at night. Such settings emphasize a script already circulating in this culture: *women must provide sexual access to men* as a condition of the demands women perceive about their sexuality. Consequently, women change their relationship to social spaces—by limiting the locations they go to and the time of day they visit them—in order to protect themselves, which directs the burden of safety onto women themselves rather than the men who perpetrate violence against women. Further, coercion seems deeply connected to women's sexuality such that they cannot fully divorce it from their sexual lives; even those women who do not directly experience rape or sexual assault often live under the fear of such attacks, as women's sexual vulnerability is inscribed into the fabric of gendered relationships. Still, the construction of women as sexual victims or passive in sex sustains the active/passive dualism of men and women wanting/not wanting sex. A more accurate representation might argue that women learn to internalize and eroticize messages about their sexual vulnerability. As such, the question becomes: Do women fear and eroticize sexual dominance at the same time, and if so, what does this reveal about gender and performance? If women must demonstrate their sexual openness and availability in a culture that commits violence against them, all while *also* performing as pure and chaste (e.g., mother, child, senior citizen, religious person), how does this translate into women's narratives about their emotional, psychological, and physical well-being? Women's narratives of sexual violence illuminate these tensions and paradigms more closely.

NARRATIVES OF VIOLENCE AND DOMINATION

> The difficulty of articulating physical pain permits political
> and perceptual complications of the most serious kind. The
> failure to express pain . . . will always work to allow its
> appropriation and conflation with debased forms of power;
> conversely, the successful expression of pain will always
> work to expose and make impossible that appropriation and
> conflation.
>
> —Scarry, The Body in Pain

Worst Sexual Experiences

Throughout the interviews, even though I minimally asked about sexual coercion and violence in their lives, women's stories showed that the interplay between sex and violence (or the "sexualization of violence") clearly infected their consciousness on multiple levels. Women's *worst* experiences most often involved violence, meaning that they primarily characterized sexual violence as *sexual experiences* and that they experienced themselves through coercive practices enacted upon them by men. The range of coercive experience women described speaks to these issues: First, many women experienced their *first* sexual encounters through violence (e.g., incest, molestation, rape). Second, women often struggled to attach language to experiences that felt coercive but did not necessarily seem like *rape*, thus revealing a crisis of expressiveness. Without a label for these coercive experiences, society may not recognize the frequency and consequences of sexual assault. Third, within the same relationships, women often experienced both loving, positive interactions and coercive, negative interactions, making it increasingly difficult to label their partner as *either* a perpetrator of sexual coercion *or* as loving and affectionate. In such dynamics, coercion may seem normal or even like a form of love and care (similar to "trauma bonds" discussed in Thomas, 2007). Those who aggress against women may influence the way women interpret and define the violence. Finally, many women eroticized their sexual submission and/or justified sexualized violence as a normative part of their lives; the divide between pleasure and pain, eroticism and domination, and sex and violence becomes incredibly blurry for many women.

Looking at women's worst sexual experiences reveals these complexities and gives texture to the terms *culture of violence* and *sexualized violence*. Evidence for the mandate that women should provide sexual access to men in order to garner sexual validation is typified in women's comments. Women's descriptions of their worst sexual experiences typically fell into four primary categories, the first three of which dealt with issues of noticing, interpreting, and dealing with cases of sexual aggression: 1) narratives of unambiguous coercion and violence, including violent rapes, incest, or other situations where they reported feeling clearly coerced and violated; 2) narratives of ambiguous coer-

cion and violence, including situations where women did not feel entitled to call the event "rape" or "violence" but still felt uneasy about the
event's coercive implications; 3) narratives of performance and domination, where women felt pressured to perform particular acts they were
not prepared for or where they acted out domination in a way that felt
negative to them. The fourth theme, though outside of the context of
aggression, spoke to the ambivalent nature of many sexual exchanges, in
that women described negative feelings about the way sex disrupted
their understanding of their bodies, self-identity, or connections and
obligations to their romantic partners. Collectively, these "worst sexual
experience" narratives speak to the ways that coercion, violence, and
mandated sexual access to men are woven into the fabric of women's
sexual lives.

Narratives of Unambiguous Coercion and Violence

In women's narratives of unambiguous coercion—which appeared in
over a fourth of the sample—the extent to which women *narrated* these
events varied quite a bit. For experiences that happened earlier in
childhood—for example, cases of incest or sexual abuse—the stories
ranged from vague and abstract to detailed and vivid. Similarly, for
experiences that happened as adults—for example, date rape—some
women spoke about these experiences with texture and detail, while
others could only access fragmented feelings about the events. This
range of descriptive detail speaks to previous research that has shown
that the traumatic experiences people *retell* and narrate have stronger
potential for recovery and emotional processing than do stories that are
kept secret or are not narrated (Ahrens et al., 2007). Further, these stories of unambiguous coercion and violence reveal how, regardless of the
severity of the events themselves, women struggle to claim language
about sexual violence when speaking to others. From conflicts about
feeling sexually aroused in the context of sexual abuse, to confusion
about how to respond or feel about oneself during or after the experience, the struggle to make meaning of coercive experiences (and to *persist* in restructuring one's sexuality following these events) appeared as a
central dilemma in women's worst sexual experience narratives.

Several women described early sexual abuse and incest as their worst sexual experiences, yet the detail or meaning they ascribed to the abuse varied greatly. Some women had revealed these experiences to others before, while others had not. In looking at Diana, Esther, and Geena's descriptions, a range of detail and texture emerges. Diana, age 50, who had not discussed these experiences before, had little detail or precision in her stories, while Esther, who had discussed her abuse history before, had more detail. Geena, age 51, who had, prior to the interview, discussed her abuse history frequently, provided a detailed narrative of her incest experience.

When asked about her abuse experience, Diana told me about the long-term effects it had on her: "I had nightmares about the incest for a long time after that. It wasn't physically painful. I was traumatized to the point where I was probably frozen up, but I think what I've heard (and it's true) is that you detach." When I asked her how she felt about the experience, she said, "Definitely sadness. I mean, I don't feel it or think about it all the time, but you're asking me, and if I sit here and think about it, then yes, the emotions that come up would be embarrassment, shame, trauma, and pain. It was emotionally painful." Diana's lack of precise or well-developed language exemplified women's loss of expressive language around sexual trauma, particularly if she sheltered these memories from full consciousness.

Esther, age 44, who reported sexual abuse by her father at age 3, described her experience in slightly more detailed ways, though she focused most on the relational consequences of the abuse:

> He'd want to me to give him a hand job. He would touch me, and basically it was a play kind of thing that went on until I was about twelve. My father was not a very loving person, but after that, he would allow me to go into his change drawer and get money, or he would do a lot of extra things for me. He treated me a lot nicer because I did that, so what that taught me was that that was a way to get close to men. My mom never knew though.

In comparing Diana's description to Geena's description below, the role of previous narration in processing and healing from past sexual abuse becomes evident:

I was abused sexually by my uncle, who would sit in such a way with his robe open. He would expose himself and fondle himself in front of me, and he managed to do this in front of his family without anyone else noticing but me. I remember feeling that it was gross, definitely gross, and I wanted to ignore it and not be affected, but I was upset. There was a part of me that didn't want to have a strong reaction one way or another so that I was impervious to what was happening to me. Then, when I was 16, in a family cottage in the middle of the night, he actually raped me. It was the first day of a weeklong vacation. There was no pain involved. He spent a lot of time touching me inappropriately. I was on a couch with three sides, and I couldn't really get off the couch. There were people sleeping. It was a cottage that had no roofs but there were walls. There was somebody sleeping like 10 feet away, and you know, he had kids and a wife, and I had my parents . . . I remember feeling trapped, and I was angry because I knew that this was wrong, and he was doing this to me. I did not ask for this. I was 16, and my body was responding, but I'm feeling nauseous and sweaty and I want to throw up, so you know, there's a definite conflict.

A similar range of vividness and detail was found in women's descriptions of rape experiences. Twenty-one-year-old Maria, raped by a stranger at age 19, struggled to recall any details of her rape and had rarely discussed it:

It was very bad, very degrading. I got knocked out in a parking lot on school grounds, so I went to official people, and they didn't really seem to do anything. They didn't care. It was kind of horrible. I left town for a couple of weeks to go to a safe house. It was an awakening experience for me. I always knew that rape and domestic violence were issues, and violence against women was real, but when it happens to you, it changes you.

Forty-two-year-old Pam, who was date raped at age 17, described her experience in slightly more detailed terms, showing how her

emotional processing of the event—and her labeling of it as rape—
helped her to recreate what happened, label it as coercive, and emotionally heal from the trauma:

> When I was in high school, I had sex with a young man in the
> backseat of a car. He wasn't going to take me home unless I
> had sex with him. The word[s] *date rape* didn't exist back then,
> you know? I wasn't a dumb girl, so it's not like I was just naïve.
> He threatened me, and we had sex, but I never talked to him
> again. I was very disturbed and upset, but there's not much you
> can do. I felt very violated even though he didn't understand
> that and kept asking why I wouldn't talk to him anymore. I
> look back on it now and know that it was date rape.

Finally, 23-year-old Julie's rich and nuanced description of her rape
experience more fully rounds out the range of details that women
recount when talking about sexual violence. Note also the fluctuations
between self-blame and blaming her perpetrator for the rape, as she
switches between feeling guilty for providing him with sexual access, to
feeling indignant that this happened to her:

> The sexual experience that I remember being the worst was
> when I was 20. This guy I know who was an artist had me over
> to his house, and we had done some work together. He wanted
> to draw me and do a nude of me. I really felt like that was okay.
> I felt really safe about it. He was drawing away and had been at
> it for maybe an hour, and he jumped on me. He was much
> bigger than me, and he raped me. The thing that made it so
> terrible was that he had probably like six or seven piercings on
> his penis that went around and were pointed, so he tore up my
> vagina completely. I had to have it sewn, almost like an epi-
> siotomy, because the piercings had torn me so badly. I have a
> lot of scarring, and I lost so much blood that I passed out, and
> he left; somebody found me in my own blood hours later. It
> was terrible . . . At the time, I felt very shameful about it
> because I had really internalized it and felt responsible, you

know, that I had been naked and had put myself in this vulnerable position with this man. I don't think that any more at all, but at the time, I felt depressed, and I felt like the hospital was shaming me. I just remember going unconscious, really numb, really confused, really sad. I would cry for hours and hours, and it never felt like enough.

Collectively, these narratives of unambiguous coercion suggest two things: first, it is significant when women construct violent experiences as frankly and unambiguously coercive. When women use words such as *rape* and *incest*, it places the experience in categories that facilitate emotional and psychological processing without denying the event's significance or assimilating it into their everyday sexual lives. These events were *different*, *unlike* other events in their lives. Labels pathologize sexual violence and place the experience(s) outside of the context of their normal sexual existence, though whether such pathologization is protective or harmful is debatable. Second, the range of detail women had when describing violent sexual experiences suggests that narrating these events has significance both to their recovery and to their reclamation of language about sexual violence. Those who spoke about sexual violence with more texture and detail were, not coincidentally, women who had had more psychotherapy and who had disclosed these experiences to others prior to our interview. The narration of sexual violence—perhaps a kind of performance—helps women to process the event(s), particularly in a culture that often prohibits such frank discussions of men's violence against women. When women narrate these stories to others, friends, family, and coworkers, can help survivors challenge their abuse by listening to women who have survived such events. Finally, women struggled to claim their outrage at others without blaming themselves, in part because they felt they *should* give men sexual access to their bodies. Just as labeling and narrating rape matter in a social justice context, so does the shift from self-blame to other-blame for instances of sexual coercion. These conflicts about access appeared even more dramatically in cases of ambiguous coercion and violence, where the texture of sexual *performance* starts to clearly emerge.

Narratives of Ambiguous Coercion and Violence

Compared to narratives of unambiguous coercion and violence, over a third of the women described coercive experiences that they refused to fully label as "rape." These experiences collectively revealed several complexities and dilemmas about women's framing of sexual violence. First, when women are generally robbed of a language to speak about their sexuality, it makes sense that they also often cannot directly label or categorize their negative sexual experiences. Second, the same sexual encounters often contain competing elements of both positive feelings (e.g., arousal, excitement, love, attention) and negative feelings (e.g., pressure, coercion, violation, injury, being "on stage"), making it difficult for women to categorize certain encounters as "rape" or "not rape." Third, this culture encourages women to eroticize their own submission, both in an explicitly performative way (e.g., playing around with submissive costumes and roles) and in an implicitly performative way (e.g., finding sexual arousal through the enactment of their own powerlessness). Thus, ambiguous experiences of coercion play into all three of these dimensions, and in doing so, reveal coercion as widespread and as inducing complicated emotional responses for women.

The conflicts women internalize between messages of empowerment and liberation compared with messages of fear, mistrust, and sexual vulnerability—what I have termed "double consciousness"—appeared most clearly in women's descriptions of ambiguous sexual violence. Often, women initially agreed to something that felt "liberating" or "empowering" or "sexy" only to regretfully discover that their partners did not respect their subsequent discomfort with the activity. For example, Aya, age 25, felt pressured to have anal sex:

> I think that when you're actually in the act of something, it doesn't feel bad, but when you think about it later on, it becomes magnified in your mind, like, "That made me feel like shit," but at the time, somehow I wasn't as hurt by it as I am now. With my first boyfriend, he tried to have anal sex with me a couple of times, but I thought it was gross. I would be on my stomach and he would kind of rub it there, and I would say no repeatedly. It was several times where he wouldn't listen to me,

and he would keep trying and trying. I thought I should try it if he wanted to, but I felt violated and humiliated. Because of that, my image of him became worse.

Charlene, age 44, talked about a threesome experience that did not feel good to her, evoking the discourses of pressure and coercion without explicitly labeling it as coercive:

We had a threesome, and I wasn't really that interested in it in the first place. It was something he wanted to do for years. I went to a bar in town and found a guy, and I flirted with him and pretended to be interested in him. I basically used the guy and brought him home. After that, my ex wasn't even aroused by it; he was more jealous. He was angry with me and wouldn't speak to me for over a week. He wanted to do this, and then I did it and then it was sort of like a slap in the face. It was abusive basically.

Women's resistance to using the word *rape* also reveals this double consciousness, as they blame themselves, refuse the label of rape despite clear evidence of sexual violence, or justify the coercion because it occurred with a long-term sexual or romantic partner. Such lack of labeling may also play into neoconservative discourses of individual responsibility for one's actions, again situating women as personally responsible for violence committed against them (Bay-Cheng & Eliseo-Arras, 2008). Self-blame appeared in 54-year-old Margaret's narrative of her sexual assault, as she told me, "I got really drunk, went to a country club, and got taken advantage of. I remember feeling pretty grimy and not wanting anyone to know about it. I wanted a good scrub down when I got back home and realized what had happened. I didn't want to get into that situation again. I shouldn't have drunk like that and expected everything to turn out okay."

Resistance to labeling rape in light of frank sexual violence also revealed women's loss of language and expression combined with pressures to normalize and justify sexual assault. For example, Brynn, age 25, described a painful coercive experience that she still did not define as rape:

The worst sex I would have to say would be forced sex, not actually rape, but not so nice. I was in a relationship once where I kind of got put into a situation I did not want to be in. I was handcuffed and put over the side of a jeep. We were driving out to the middle of nowhere, in the middle of the day, just out and about, and we wound up at the river bottom. Fooling around, we went from one thing to another to me being halfway over the back end of the jeep, handcuffed. He decided that he thought it would be fun to cram a "penis top" inside of me to see how it would feel, and it got stuck behind my pelvic bone. When he went to yank it out, it pulled out the whole inner wall, and it was just painful like no other. I went to the hospital and was in bed for a day and a half. Thinking about it now, I feel small, belittled by the fact that I knew that I didn't want him to do that, and I allowed somebody to do that to me.

When I asked her why she did not define the experience as rape, she blamed herself for the event, citing her lack of protest:

I didn't really protest, but we were kind of playing around, and it stopped being fun real quick. I was scared and wanted out of there, but it wasn't rape. My body tensed up, and it was just not fun anymore. He was rough with me all the time too, or at least a lot of the time. It was one of those things I kept saying we should work on, but it never really happened that way. From that experience now, I can't get pregnant because of everything it ripped from inside and all the scarring.

As a slightly less violent example, Fiona, age 24, described an encounter where she was coerced into sexual acts she did not fully consent to, yet she resisted the label *rape* as well:

The night before my sister's wedding, I was drinking with one of the groomsmen staying in our house. We started fooling around in the guest room, and he did not want to have vaginal sex because he got a previous exgirlfriend pregnant. He just wanted to do anal, but I'd never done anal before, and he was very forceful. He asked me to suck his cock, and I did that, but I refused to let him come because that felt too intimate to me to have him come in my mouth. He was angry that I made him get all messy. It was very rough and violent feeling, and I felt disgusted. Of course we had to take lots of pictures together at the wedding, which made it all the more negative. And after it all happened, he says to me, "You're not going to want anything more from this, right?" Wow, yeah, of course a *man* is going to think that a female is automatically going to be wanting it to continue!

Repeatedly, women expressed resistance to labeling coercion as rape when a romantic partner sexually coerced them. The resistance to labeling sexual violence in the context of relationships plays into the long history of women not having control over their sexual person: women could not prosecute marital rape for a long time, others often do not believe women's reports of sexual assault, and women may feel inclined to stay with abusers due to lack of financial resources or the belief that they should "keep their man" in order to be a "good woman," and current cultural scripts mandate that women provide sexual access to male partners while in relationships or marriages. For example, 20-year-old Sally told me about an experience where she had been held down and forced to have sex against her will by a partner who was physically much larger than her: "It was hurting me, and he just kept going, and he just held me down. I was like, 'Stop! Stop! It really hurts,' but he kept going. I was still with him for two months after that, justifying the kind of person he was." When I asked her whether she considered this rape, she minimized the coercive dimensions of the event:

I don't consider it rape. I felt scared, and I felt like he wanted to dominate me. I bet he wouldn't even remember to be honest. I wouldn't say it was rape because I don't feel that he intended to do that. I don't feel that he did it on purpose. I think that he was just being arrogant . . . I was really scared and sad because I guess I wasn't a strong enough person to get up and leave. I trusted him a lot, and I couldn't even talk to him about it afterwards, but I felt belittled.

Women's conflicts about tolerating coercive experiences despite feeling that they deserved better—or tolerating exploitation despite a feminist belief system—revealed the disconnect between women's internal narratives and the power they can exert in their sexual relationships. Again, the fact that these coercive experiences occurred in the context of long-term romantic relationships greatly heightened women's sense that they could not directly label the experiences as rape or exploitation. Kate, age 25, described this minimization quite eloquently:

> I'm angry at myself that I let it go on as long as I did. I didn't tell my friends what was happening. There were just a lot of coercive incidents, typically around oral sex. He would force me to perform oral sex on him, and since then, I just can't do it to anyone. It was a feeling of wanting to please him because I had a strong desire to please, like a feeling that I should be having these experiences because I'm an adult now, and this is part of being an adult, part of being an independent woman. You've gotta do all these sexual things.

When I asked her what emotions the experiences made her feel, she told me, "There was this rational side of me saying that if this person really cared about you, they wouldn't make you do these things. But at the same time, if I don't do these things, I could lose him, and why don't I want to do this in the first place? I felt a sense of betrayal and generally a lot of bitterness."

The cultural script that encourages women to put their (male) partner's pleasure above their own also contributed to women's narratives of sexual coercion. As with Kate's previous example, she felt trapped between doing sexual acts she did not personally find appealing in order to "save" her relationship while also feeling violated and belittled. She felt compelled to *perform* as a liberated woman by minimizing the coercive implications of forced oral sex. Susan, age 45, described a similar problem when discussing coercion, though she did not fill in the details about what she was forced to do, again revealing both the loss of language and the normalization of coercive sex:

I think the worst sex that I had was in an emotionally abusive relationship where sex was used as a reward for me being compliant. I had sex because I felt like I needed to do that for him, and I was hoping to feel connected to him. It always felt like he was pretending I was someone else, so I felt really used and emotionally distant. It's really sick because when he wanted to have sex with me, I felt like I had done something right because of that, but at the same time, if I refused sex, there were times I was afraid about what would happen. It's like I went along with his desires to keep things going. He never told me I had to do them, but I did them because there would be hell to pay otherwise, even if it wasn't explicit. I coped with this, of course, by blanking out a lot. I feel so embarrassed and disgusted and disappointed in myself that I allowed myself to be treated that way.

One of the more extreme examples of normalizing and reconciling rape experiences was articulated by Ruth, age 46, who described feeling raped on her wedding night, followed by decades-long marriage to that same partner:

It was our wedding night, and I said no, but he didn't listen. It was just so unlike him, because he's a very sweet, gentle man and always puts me first. I told him, "I don't want this tonight." I wish that our wedding night hadn't happened that way. I was dead tired and stressed out and my husband had been waiting for sex, you know? We went ahead and had intercourse that night, but I did not want to. I've suffered from depression most of my life, and I remember one time I snapped at him that I felt raped on my wedding night, and he was like, "Whoa, where did that come from?" That's been kind of hanging out there, and we've talked about it over the years. I feel deeply sad when thinking about it. If we had just waited one night, I think it would have just been better. Both of us were virgins, and neither of us had a lot of sexual experiences and such.

In this example, Ruth describes the immense difficulty in choosing whether to label a particular event as rape and her dilemmas about how to heal from it in light of her partner's subsequent actions. Unlike most women's experiences—where they can divorce coercive experiences more readily from their present day context—Ruth had to integrate that experience into her (mostly positive and loving) marriage. Collectively, these narratives reveal that coercion thus becomes *woven into* the fabric of women's sexual lives in surprising and sustained ways and that it often requires women to engage in certain kinds of performances, cognitive realignments, and justifications in order to tolerate and understand its occurrence in their lives.

Performance Norms and Domination

Returning to the more explicit context of performance, women's worst sexual experience narratives also highlighted subtle pressure to perform acts they were not fully prepared for or interested in, even if these acts did not feel directly coercive. Pressures to comply with partners' demands led to women's negative feelings about the event. For example, 56-year-old Ophelia described pressure to have sex while she had pneumonia as her worst experience: "I felt forced into it. I was very mad and hurt that someone would be so unfeeling towards somebody that was ill, that they would just kind of say, 'My needs come first.'" Additionally, women described pressure about bondage, dominance, and submission as uncomfortable—a striking similarity to other semicoercive sex practices (e.g., pressure for threesomes, pressure to fake orgasm, etc.). Mitra, age 29, described *pressure to perform* unwanted sexual acts and her discomfort with domination in general:

> I had one sexual relationship where he was into this whole S&M thing, and I think it just never felt natural for me, so I was trying to act like something I wasn't, and I always felt like I was on a stage. I had nightmares about it where I was on stage and trying to be sexy and just not feeling sexy. It's just that bad cycle, and I think it made me really self-conscious for a while. I really loved this person, and so I wanted to be into it so desperately that I tried to be someone that I wasn't. Sometimes he wanted to call me names, or he wanted to cheapen me or make

me look slutty in a way that just did not feel like me. That felt very degrading.

Nora, age 23, also mentioned degradation and violence as she described an experience where domination went too far, and she did not stop the encounter, which highlighted her conflicts about allowing domination in light of her feminist identity:

> I had a friend of mine who I really cared about who almost always wanted to role play these fairly violent things. I had a huge conflict with him once because he totally pushed me down on the bed and ripped off my underwear and made it this rather extreme thing, which was so out of character for him. I guess I felt like if he had asked, it wouldn't have been something I was opposed to, but it was so demanding and male-dominated. It felt like he was a friend, but then all this anger towards women he had dated starting coming out . . . I view myself as a strong feminist woman, but at the same time, in these very hetero relationships, I still am surprised to find this subconscious thing where I want to please the man or something, and I will end up succumbing to it.

As a self-described artist, Edie, 19, rationalized sexual domination as something that inspired her art:

> I was really a masochistic person then. I definitely went along with things sexually that I shouldn't have. I had given up cutting myself and piercing, so I think that maybe I had had sex with him just to feel like shit about myself. I'm an artist, too, so it's like that kind of conflict or trauma or disgust with yourself or self-loathing that drives you. It's inspiring to put yourself in completely horrible places. I did the best art that I've ever created in my life following horrible, forced experiences.

Thus, women frequently justified domination and violence despite articulating clear intellectualized sentiments that rejected this kind of rationalization.

Shifting Meanings and Emotional Numbness

In addition to instances of unambiguous, ambiguous, or performative coercion, many women also described lack of investment in the sexual encounter as their worst sexual experiences. Though not a form of sexual violence per se, these experiences reveal the culture of domination women encounter. In part because women often live in social milieus that demand their sexual access to men (husbands, boyfriends, etc.) as a condition of their sexual worth or value, women often engage in sex without being fully present or interested. When women provide sexual access to men when they do not feel fully present, this represents a version of sexual performance consistent with some societal expectations. Whether women act out sexual victimization by emotionally disconnecting from sex, or whether they internalize the idea that "good women" do not like sex, mental disengagement during sex speaks volumes about the cultural investment in performance. Women *should* have sex even if they do not want to (as in chapter 3, when drug companies medicate desire and physiological responses).

Many women described negative sexual encounters where they felt emotionally distant from the act or where their partners deprioritized women's pleasure. For example, Ciara, age 24, felt that her husband consistently valued his pleasure over hers:

> Sometimes we might have intercourse, and he might get done and then just kind of forget about me, and he forgets to pleasure me afterward. I feel neglected and forgotten. He'll just want to go back to watching TV or sleeping. He doesn't care about me, not as much as he used to.

Women sometimes expressed similar feelings when discussing new partners or one-night stands, in that the lack of emotional connectedness made it feel empty or shallow. This directly contrasted with the emotional connectedness narratives presented in chapter 4, again revealing the paradox that sex with love may have elements of performance, but sex *without* love appeared far more often in women's worst experience narratives. Dorothy, age 19, described a disconnected sexual experience: "It was kind of a rebound thing, and I realized that it was just a bad idea. We hooked up too fast, and it became physically painful from my dryness, probably because I wasn't emotionally with it, and that manifested as not really being able to enjoy it." Similarly, Courtney described a one-night stand experience as devoid of emotions and, consequently, as demeaning:

> With this one guy, I was drunk, and we ended up having sex. I'd never had a partner where there wasn't at least some kind of emotional connection, even if it wasn't the deepest, strongest thing. With that one, I felt like it was purely just sex for sex, and there wasn't anything satisfying from it. There was just nothing there, and to me, that just felt almost like borderline prostitution. It's really demeaning and really cheap.

Though some women disliked sex with unfamiliar partners, other women described longer relationships as distant, particularly when a relationship had transitioned from emotionally connected and present to emotionally distant and disconnected. Having sex with a former partner heightened this sense of loss even more, as women lamented both the loss of emotional connection and the loss of the relationship. Dawn, age 43, explained her anxiety and sadness while having sex following the dissolution of her long-term relationship:

> With my third husband, who's really good friends with me now, after we had pretty much parted ways romantically and sexually, he said to me, "Let's just try to have sex one more time. I would really like to do that." It just didn't work. Even though we had been partners before, it just wasn't good because I didn't feel present with him. It just wasn't a happy situation. I was participating without having my heart in it, and vice versa. It wasn't satisfying to each of us. It was just kind of mechanical.

In addition to postbreak-up sex, women described sex with friends or acquaintances as sometimes unpleasant, showing the possible detrimental effects of the "friends with benefits" scenario. Some women felt confused and upset when trying to adjust their emotional connections in friendships that had turned into sexual relationships. Emily, age 22, described a negative situation where she had sex with a friend, citing the emotional complexity of the encounter:

> I had this weird, complicated relationship with one of my guy friends when I was 17, and he was 20. I took his virginity. He's really religious, so he feels guilty about anything sexual, and it's been years since then, but there's still a lot of tension about this. I can sense that he feels guilty and then I feel guilty.

Thus, in a culture that romanticizes and demands women's emotional investment in sex as a condition of their participation (e.g., prohibitions against women having one-night stands are not only layered with messages about emotions mattering but also enforce *avoidance* of becoming a "slut"), it makes sense that many women construct their worst experiences as related to a lack of emotional investment in the exchange. At the same time, it also speaks to women's prioritization of a mutually agreeable emotional connection as a condition of satisfying sex. Rarely did women describe their worst sexual experiences as ones where they felt physically dissatisfied; rather, worst sexual experiences typically involved varying degrees of *coercion* in a physical and emotional sense. Whether through literal coercion (e.g., rape, incest, violence), ambiguous coercion (e.g., pressure to engage in anal sex, rape that is not called "rape"), the performance of domination and submission (e.g., women feeling pressured to engage in S&M, domination play "going too far"), or shifting the terms of the emotional relationship (e.g., unfulfilling one-night stands, postbreak-up sex), women overwhelmingly confronted and coped with the cultural demand that they comply with the wishes of their (male) partners. Interestingly, *not a single woman* described a worst sexual experience that involved a female partner, despite the majority of participants having engaged in at least one (and often many) same-sex sexual encounters. While many factors may contribute to this finding, it does suggest that men's literal enactment of patriarchy onto women's bodies affects women negatively. It also suggests that men's gender role socialization can make men oblivious to, or more likely to disregard, what women want from sex. Coercion and the conditions of mandatory sexual access to men together form the crux of women's worst sexual experiences on the whole.

The Ambiguities of Harassment

Women's double consciousness about understanding sex as a means of empowerment and liberation as well as an avenue to exploitation and violence appeared not only in women's worst sexual experience narratives but also in their stories about street harassment and sexual harassment. Though these stories have less direct intensity than the worst sexual experience narratives, they round out the picture of women's experiences with double consciousness. Toward the end of the interview, I asked women,

> Most women report that they have had the experience of being treated as a sexual object. For example, many women have been sexually harassed at work or have been whistled at on the street, stared at inappropriately, etc. What are your experiences with being treated as a sexual object?

Responses to this question illustrated women's *simultaneous tendencies* to feel both repulsed *and* flattered by harassment, as harassment validated their sexual attractiveness while also oppressing them.

In fact, *most* women constructed street harassment experiences as both flattering and repulsive, in that street harassment made them feel special/attractive *and* degraded. For example, Ophelia said,

> Sometimes it's okay, it's flattering, and other times it's not. It just depends on what kind of mood you're in that day. If you're in the mood where you need an ego boost, then it's flattering, and if you're not, then it's disgusting.

Melanie, age 21, expressed similar feelings of both flattery and repulsion, differentiating experiences where she felt more or less threatened:

> Sometimes it's frustrating, and sometimes it's flattering. I think when the advances are from people that I feel no rapport with or interest in, and they're presented rather gracelessly or even with a kind of predatory sense to them, then it bothers me. A hooting car of drunkards barreling down the highway while I'm walking along is not going to make me feel very good

about myself. A wolf whistle from a construction worker on a rooftop is probably going to be neutral. If it's somebody at a party who doesn't really know much about me, but I can see he's checking me out from the side of the room and is kind of cute, then I feel good.

Some women appreciated the sexual validation while disliking the power dynamics of street harassment, such as Mitra, who said:

> Sometimes it makes me feel threatened, not like I have to fear for my life, but it's intimidating. I also think it's flattering to a certain degree, like if that stops happening altogether, I think that would be kind of sad. It's someone letting you know that you're sexually attractive, so it's fine. If someone is literally making me feel like a piece of meat, then that's not really flattering, but if someone is just checking you out, or even saying something that's not too lewd, I think that makes you feel good about yourself.

Many women felt *more* positive than negative about street harassment, noting that its validating qualities sometimes outweighed the negative or harassing implications, particularly when women did not feel threatened or when they sensed mutual attraction. For example, Pam liked to brag to her husband when other men sexually objectified her. Emily felt invigorated by sexual objectification even while maintaining a critical lens about it:

> For the most part, I associate pretty positive things with being sexually objectified. When I do movies and photo shoots, that was the kind of thing I was looking for. There's something extremely flattering about being looked at in that sense. If it's unwanted attention, as long as it's not persistent, it doesn't bother me. I'll be flattered to the point where I've told someone to back off, and they won't. It was definitely difficult in my last office job when they found out that I did porn. That was *not* how I wanted to be looked at around the office.

For Emily, the attention during the filmmaking seemed exciting, while attention that brought stigma with it felt disempowering and negative. In a somewhat similar manner, Edie, who admitted that she thrived on male attention, said that sexual objectification excited *and* frightened her. She specifically layered a racial analysis of street harassment into her response:

> This stuff just happens to me really frequently, and I know that I attract it because I'm an artist. I'm a peacock, and I like colors and weird things, and I know it fits, but *shit,* it makes me feel bad sometimes. Sometimes, though, it makes me feel good. Yesterday these guys came up to me and said, "You look good. You just made my day." They're so fucking nice to me. If it's someone my own age that speaks my own language, it's fine; if it's someone significantly older who speaks another language and immigrated to this country, I don't like it. I can understand the intentions of boys at school because I come from a black neighborhood, and I just like black people. They just tell women how they feel, and I think that's a good thing.

Still, other women reacted negatively to street harassment and discussed the way it humiliated or insulted them and did not provide flattery or affirmation. Rather, themes of anger, resentment, fear, bitterness, powerlessness, and rage appeared. For example, Janet, age 21, responded with anger and rage when experiencing street harassment:

> Men will stare at my boobs or say, "Hey chick" or whatever, and it's like, don't talk to me like that. I'm a woman, not some object that you can just throw around and talk crap about or think that you can just look at whatever way you like. It's not going to work that way. It makes me angry. It makes me want to sock 'em. Of course, in my mind, I'm like, "Cut their dicks off," you know? (laughs) It's because they're rude or disrespectful.

In contrast, Dawn's responses included more themes of shame and invisibility:

It really has affected me much more than I would like to say. It
has bothered me tremendously being whistled at. Mostly I'd
just kind of slink away, feeling shameful. Sometimes now I will
turn back and call him on it, which feels more powerful, but it
used to make me feel really bad, very ashamed, like something
was really wrong with me.

The degree to which women fought back against street harassment
when they constructed it as negative varied greatly, from small acts of
resistance (e.g., talking back, removing oneself, telling the man he was
behaving inappropriately) to more aggressive acts of resistance (e.g.,
shoving, kicking, spitting). Twenty-five-year-old Kate, who admitted
having problems with self-assertion, responded to street harassment by
directly confronting it using "maternal code," whereby she invoked
nonsexual female roles to ward off men's sexual advances toward her.
She said,

I remember one incident where someone in his truck passed
and said something, and when I saw him later, I just asked him,
"How do you think this is an appropriate way to speak to
women? How would you like it if someone said that to your
mother or your sister or something?" He just didn't know what
to say and just shrugged it off, but at least I felt like I said
something.

Nora, who typically resisted men's efforts to commodify or otherwise objectify her, responded aggressively to street harassment:

I want to look nice for myself and then suddenly the whole
world feels the need to comment on it. Growing up around
here, we used to experience that with the frat boys, with
people shouting inappropriately and hollering at you. We used
to pick our noses and yell back and make barf noises and stuff.
You kind of learn to get over it and ignore it, but it's there.
Even walking over here, there were two or three cars that
honked. Sometimes I don't know what to do because it's so
engrained in our culture, this whole cat-calling and lewd comments and whistling. I don't go out to bars and places because

that happens. I had to quit a job because I felt uncomfortable walking near all the titty bars. Sometimes people will directly solicit me, and I'm like, "Who the fuck are you?"

As a more extreme example of resistance and fighting back, Jasmine, age 37, directly confronted harassing men by talking back and being physically aggressive. Jasmine also touched upon the way that women resisting men's harassment provokes hostilities and rage, indicating that *men* likely do not engage in this behavior to flatter women, but rather, to dominate them:

> I see men look me up and down like they're shopping, and they'll look at you like a piece of meat, like you got dressed up and looked good so they can just choose you, like *they're* the whole purpose *you* went out that night. Sometimes I'll tell them to fuck off. Then you see the real man. He treats you like shit, and he's going to cuss you out, and he's going to fight with a woman who's half his size because she just told him off. I've actually pushed other men around. I'm pretty aggressive. I don't like men belittling women. It makes me queasy.

Women's varied responses to street harassment ranged from the conflation of flattery and repulsion, to the more positive response of feeling affirmed or sexualized, to the more negative response of feeling belittled or shamed. This speaks to the ambivalence women have about their relationship to cultural discourses that sustain their simultaneous vulnerability and objectification. While women want affirmation or approval, they also sense the coercive, patronizing dynamics of street harassment. In fact, most women changed their relationship to space as a result of such harassment (e.g., quitting a job, not walking certain routes, not visiting certain bars, etc.). Regardless of how flattering it might make women feel, street harassment ends up dictating women's ability to have full rights to themselves in public space. Women also internalize the contradictory messages that they must present themselves as hegemonically beautiful and desirable and that, when they do this, they risk "eliciting" harassment and violence. Again, the implications for men's sexual access to women are overwhelming, as men reject women who refuse to play along (in terms of beauty standards, sexual norms, etc.), but at the height of women's obedience to cultural norms, women's risk for sexual violence potentially increases.

CONCLUSION

Coercion and sexual violence pervade women's lives, as shown in the available research on these subjects as well as in women's narratives of their worst sexual experiences. Even those women who have not directly experienced rape or sexual assault often nevertheless construct parts of their sexualities around such concepts, whether by internalizing messages about the fear of men and/or their own sexual vulnerability or by tolerating and accepting norms that allow for eroticized domination. Women expressed awareness of *other* women's experiences with sexual violence as well, indicating that secondary victimization may also support the culture of domination (just as women's secondary exposure to performative bisexuality—as seen in chapter 2—maintains its relevance in women's lives). Clearly, violence informs the erotic and thus distorts and alters the way women experience their bodies, their sexualities, and their relationship to others, particularly men.

When considering the broader impact of coercion on women's sexual lives, several points should be reiterated. First, *coercion is everywhere*. From women's accounts of feeling pressured to have sex while they were sick to women's descriptions of direct sexual force, coercion is not merely a possibility but an *inevitability* in women's erotic lives. Whether physical, psychological, or emotional, coercion informs women's sexualities in a nearly universal way. This group of women testified that sexual violence affected all demographic groups equally, as white women and women of color, older and younger women, heterosexual and queer women were all equally likely to experience sexual violence. At times, coercion is built into women's relationships with current partners (e.g., staying in relationships where coercion exists), women's new or short-term stints with sex (e.g., one-night stands, single-incident violence), or it infects otherwise positive dynamics between partners (e.g., pressure to participate in anal sex or S&M without women's full consent).

Second, women's fear of sexual violence changes their relationship to public space, as shown in the research literatures and in women's stories about street harassment. Women's experiences of their sexual vulnerability literally inform the way they move through the world, as they avoid certain places where they fear sexual victimization. In addition to the victim-blaming qualities of such spatial arrangements, fear of coercion literally limits women's access to the world both directly and indirectly. This has direct and serious consequences: women may not enter certain professions, may not take night classes in college, and may rely upon men to ward off perceived external threats (thus ironically placing them at greater risk for sexual assault, given that male romantic partners most often perpetrate violence against women).

Third, women internalize and sometimes eroticize their own submission, thereby confirming stereotyped expectations of women as powerless. When women respond to street harassment by feeling validated or flattered, this indicates that paradigms of imbalanced power serve as habituated and normal ways for men and women to interact. When women accommodate their partners' desires for sex that causes women discomfort, this shows that women's compliance with submission matters more than their pleasure. As such, women's general reluctance to report sexual harassment or to reject sexual powerlessness aligns with these cultural priorities. As a key part of performing sex, women are quite adept at shaping their desires to serve the purposes of hegemonic masculine power, as shown in chapter 1 (faking or exaggerating orgasm), chapter 2, (women performing as bisexual), and chapter 3 (medicating sexual desire and arousal).

Fourth, embedded within all of the narratives in this chapter, the same message appears: women must always provide sexual access to men, whether by choice or by force. Perhaps as a condition of women's oppression, women's physical and sexual access to men informs much of their lives, sexual or otherwise. This mandated sexual access thus distorts women's sexual autonomy, self-determination, and consciousness by making it increasingly difficult for them to determine when, and with whom, they have sex. Even women who have sex exclusively with other women often felt pressured or forced to give men physical and sexual access to their bodies. Street harassment, the eroticization of lesbian sexuality by heterosexual men, and the high rates of overt sexual violence against queer women all support these claims (Kite & Whitley, 2003; Valentine, 1989). Similarly, women who refuse sexual access to men often meet men's hostility and violence toward them, as women who do not comply often confront intensified harassment and scorn. This fits well with the tenants of hegemonic masculinity, as men demand compliance with their wishes and sexual desires.

Finally, in relation to the previous points about sexual access, the culture of violence demands the *performance* of women's sexual availability. As evidenced by the impact of pornography on women's sexuality (chapter 6), women experience tremendous pressures to perform as sexually vulnerable, available for sexual access, and willing to submit to male dominance. These performances dominate the landscape of women's sexuality, from the way they dress to the bars they frequent, from the sexual positions they engage in to the way they move through physical space, from the way they use language about rape to the self-blame they have about "allowing" coercion to happen. These performances indicate that they not only participate in cultural fantasies of women's subservience and submission but also perpetuate and normalize, in language and in practice, the imbalanced power relationships between men and women. They not only *externally* experience the consequences of the culture of violence—via rape experiences, street harassment, and enforced compliance with men's sexual scripts—but they also *internally* validate and conform to these norms of eroticized violence. This raises the question: Can women resist the performance of their eroticized powerlessness? This question is taken up more closely in the next chapter, which considers the meaning of women's sexual fantasies as they map onto, and diverge from, the metanarratives of pornography. If women are trapped in a system that dictates their compliance with male fantasies in practice, how do they mentally construct their own fantasies?

CHAPTER SIX

IMAGERY AND IMAGINATION

Pornography and Sexual Fantasy in Everyday Life

> The system is constituted as system or whole only as a
> function of what it is attempting to evade and it is within
> this process that the woman finds herself symbolically
> placed. Set up as the guarantee of the system she comes to
> represent two things—what the man is not, that is, differ-
> ence, and what he has to give up, that is, excess.
> —Rose, *Sexuality in the Field of Vision*

THERE IS PERHAPS no more poignant example of the interplay between patriarchy and performance than the symbolic content of women's sexual fantasies. Within the imaginary, the conflict intensifies between women internalizing their own passivity, receptivity, and sub-mission even as they desire mutuality and emotional connection with partners. An analysis of women's conscious sexual fantasies strips away the partnered context of women's sexual lives and reveals the more private and internal context where different kinds of performances thrive. Similarly, in moving beyond women's internal fantasies, this chapter also addresses the way women interpret, filter, and frame the social cues found in pornography. By looking at the way women con-sume and/or reject pornography and its messages, the space between women's lived experiences and the realm of fantasy becomes apparent, particularly as it relates to women internalizing oppression. As Catharine MacKinnon has said about pornography, "Pornography does

225

not simply express or interpret experience; it substitutes for it. Beyond bringing a message from reality, it stands in for reality ... Pornography makes the world a pornographic place through its making and use, establishing what women are said to exist as, are seen as, are treated as, constructing the social reality of what a woman is and can be in terms of what can be done to her, and what a man is in terms of doing it" (Butler, 1997, p. 66).

Examining narratives of pornography and sexual fantasy invokes the following questions: Does liberation mean that women no longer need to confront and consume representations of themselves as debased or degraded? Or does liberation mean that women can have total freedom to express their sexuality in whatever form they choose, whether by acting out extreme power differentials (e.g., sadomasochism), engaging in nonreproductive sex (e.g., oral sex, anal sex, lesbian sex), widening the range of acceptable sexual practices (e.g., sex toy use, different positions, using strap-ons), or using their bodies in nonstereotyped ways (e.g., refusing to have children, etc.)?

This chapter examines two groups of related material: constructions of sexual fantasy in women's lives and the performative narratives of pornography. Certainly, with the viewing of pornography growing more frequent, the context of pornography affects women's private fantasy lives. This chapter analyzes these parallels, particularly the ways that women's fantasies reveal and draw from these pornographic constructions of women. At the same time, this chapter also interrogates fantasies that veer away from mainstream pornographic representations and story lines.

To contextualize women's narratives about fantasy and pornography, the chapter starts with a review of the debate between sex-negative (or protectionist, prowoman) and sex-positive feminism and then considers the recent research about sexual fantasy and pornography. The narrative analysis examines six different categories of women's fantasies that reveal the range of fantasies women embraced; because themes of coercion, objectification, and dominance appeared most prominently in these fantasy narratives, those fantasies receive the most critical attention. Women's political perspectives on pornography and their conflicts about consuming pornography are then considered in light of their fantasy constructions. Collectively, these analyses situate women's sexual fantasies as an *extension* of the kinds of sexual performances demanded in the rest of their sexual lives.

Key questions in this chapter include: What are the different types of women's sexual fantasies and how do these fantasies both collude with, and resist, the impositions of patriarchy? What does it mean that there is such an enormous amount of coercion in women's sexual fantasies? How prevalent is pornography viewing among women, and as such, do women appropriate or reject pornography narratives? What does the distance between literal pleasure and sexual fantasy say about the gendered politics of performance? What emotional narratives and cultural scripts do women attach to their sexual fantasies? Are fantasies politically relevant, whimsically interesting, or primarily a reflection of deep-seated internalization of male fantasy narratives? What is gained or lost by considering these fantasies as literal representations of power or by seeing them as playful flights?

SEX-NEGATIVE VERSUS SEX-POSITIVE FEMINISM

> Contradiction is the stuff of revolutionary struggle. The
> point is not to deny the reality of contradiction, but to uti-
> lize the space of contradiction to come to a greater under-
> standing.
> —hooks, "Tough Talk for Tough Times"

Though pornography has technically existed since the advent of photography, the meaning of sexual fantasy and pornography must be contextualized within the historical development of sex-negative (or protectionist, woman-centered) feminism and sex-positive (or prosexual expression) feminism. In the 1980s, a major shift in views about sexuality occurred within the feminist community as the debates between these two camps intensified. Conflicts surrounding the discursive position of sex—that is, sex as violent and oppressive versus liberatory and empowering—have historically represented some of the fiercest battles between feminist scholars, particularly as they assess the role of pornography within the movement. Following the "free love" movement of the 1970s, feminists started to disagree about the role of sex within the women's movement, as those who valued the political significance of lesbian communes and nonmale spaces argued for separatism, while others, who had embraced ideologies of free sexual expression, argued for a total destigmatization of sexuality. While sex-negative feminists located women's oppression in the act of intercourse itself (i.e., sex as inherently coercive) and specifically found fault with the circulation of pornography (e.g., feminists should promote censorship in the name of equality), sex-positive feminists embraced pornography as well as a range of sexual acts, fantasies, and desires. Sex-negative feminists argued that fantasies of domination and power seeped into women's sexual consciousness and prevented them from being fully agentic about their sexual lives. Sex-positive feminists located women's primary barriers to sexual freedom in the repressive climate of this culture, arguing against the denial of women's sexual expression. Instead, they suggested that encouragement for women to have sex, fantasize, consume pornography, and experiment with their sexuality constituted a progressive break from the repressed past.

Sex-negative Feminism

Paradoxically, sex-negative feminists' advocacy of sex as violent and oppressive—along with their frank revolt against pornography's stranglehold on the culture of sex—in some ways managed to entrench women in a trap of silence, rejection, and denial about sexuality even while offering them strategies of empowerment. Susan Brownmiller (1975) argued that men's sexual access to women laid out a system of sexual exchange whereby women underwent the repeated experience of rape. Similarly, Andrea Dworkin (1997), longtime opponent of pornography and coauthor of civil rights legislation recognizing pornography as sex discrimination,[1] argued that oppression stemmed from the act of heterosexual intercourse. In her view, equal or loving sexual relationships between men and women could not exist because of the inherent power inequalities built into the act of sex.[2] She wrote, "The normal fuck by a normal man is taken to be an act of invasion and ownership undertaken in a mode of predation: colonializing, forceful (manly) or nearly violent; the sexual act that by its nature makes her his" (p. 63). Dworkin argued that male desire arose from the eroticization of dominance, from the act of asserting power over women. As such, she positioned women's sexual freedom as possible only to the extent that women rejected sexual exchanges altogether.

Aligned with these views, MacKinnon (1987) also viewed intercourse as inherently power-imbalanced and oppressive and took particular issue with representations of intercourse portrayed in pornography. She called the pornography industry "an exemplary synthesis of the eroticization of dominance and submission with capitalism's profit motive" (p. 52), adding that the pornography industry made unbelievable profits and represented the largest internet business in the world. (Sexually explicit websites are currently trafficked more often than *all other websites combined*.) Similarly, Gail Dines (1998), another prominent antipornography advocate, asserted, "One outcome of this type of work is a construction of pornography as a free-floating sexual fantasy that belongs in the realm of the private, rather than as an industry that is historically located within a specific matrix of economic and cultural conditions. To examine the text outside of its politics of production is to miss how the pornographic text is itself shaped by the different ways production is financed and organized" (p. 37). In essence, both MacKinnon and Dines constructed pornography as *hate speech*, as a medium devoted to the male gaze and invested in inequality as its fundamental tenant. This gaze, MacKinnon said, "eroticizes the despised, the demeaned, the accessible, the there-to-be-used, the servile, the child-like, the passive, and the animal" (p. 54). Women internalize such a gaze, constructing their own sexual pleasure around the desire for debasement. MacKinnon argued that women consistently derive sexual (orgasmic) pleasure from subordination, which then defines femininity as wanting male dominance.

Sex-negative feminists such as MacKinnon located the problem of pornography in its ability to *generate, not just reflect* actual hostilities and violence against women, particularly as it affected men's sexual socialization. As Judith Butler (1997) has said,

> The problem, for MacKinnon, is *not* that pornography reflects or expresses a social structure of misogyny, but that it is an institution with the performative power to bring about that which it depicts. She writes that pornography not only substi-

tutes for social reality, but that that substitution is one which creates a social reality of its own, the social reality of pornography. (p. 66)

If pornography creates, reinforces, and perpetuates patriarchy, this presupposes that pornography *intends* to imitate the real, a position later disputed not only by sex-positive feminists but by Butler as well. This position also assumes that pornography acts as a *causal* agent (rather than correlative) on behavior, a fact also disputed by a number of social scientists (for a full discussion of this, see Boyle, 2000).

MacKinnon drew parallels between the context of pornography and sexual fantasy, on the one hand, and women's lived experiences, on the other. She used the example of faking orgasms to represent this connection, saying, "They want us to have orgasms; that proves they're virile, potent, effective. We provide them that appearance, whether it's real for us or not" (p. 58). Moreover, she argued that women perform their sexual satisfaction because "it is far less damaging and dangerous for us to do this, to accept a lifetime of simulated satisfaction, than to hold out for the real thing from them" (p. 58). Additionally, she warned of the dangers of a performative culture, saying that men should worry that women do not experience the sexual pleasure they claim to experience. After all, "their power to force the world to be their way means that they're forever wondering what's really going on out there" (p. 58). By reconfiguring heterosexual intercourse and pornography as oppressive and inexorably tied to systems of power and inequality, Dworkin and MacKinnon implicitly promoted asexuality (or at the very least, avoidance of heterosexual penetration) as a kind of sexual ideal (see Barry, 1979; Russell, 1993; and Wynter, 1987 for other examples of those who promoted abolition of all sexual exchange).

Sex-positive Feminism

At the other end of the feminist spectrum, sex-positive feminists advocated a view of sexuality as expressive and expansive. Sex-positive feminists wanted to allow for "multiple differences within each gender: the differences of race, class, and sexual practice among women, but also similarly varied relations to power among men" (Pitchford, 1997, p. 6). By recognizing that women have different ways of conceptualizing sexuality, and different means of achieving pleasure, sex-positive feminism argued against the "severely constricted" (p. 6) views of antipornography feminism. In particular, sex-positive feminists took issue with representations of women as falsely unified by their degradation, equally oppressed, and universally situated in power-imbalanced heterosexual relationships. To counteract these claims, sex-positive feminists such as Carol Queen and Annie Sprinkle argued that women should have multiple subject positions and participate in different forms of sexual expression. To prevent women from being sexual, they argued, would further oppress them. Sex positivity included openness to pornography, particularly woman-friendly pornography that subverts traditional pornographic scripts (Smith, 2007), acceptance of different forms of sexual desire (particularly queer sexuality and other sexual subcultures), anticensorship activism, experimentation with different sexual acts, and social and public health support for those in sex work professions.

Though sex-positive feminists differed in their definitions of acceptable sexual practices, they generally advocated openness to sexual expression. Some feminists argued for an acceptance of alternative sexual practices such as sadomasochism, prostitution, and pornography, while others drew the line more rigidly against sexual acts that involved direct displays of aggression (rape fantasy, rape simulation), dominance (sadomasochism), and capitalist exchange (prostitution, stripping). Jill Nagle (1997) located feminism in the marginalized spaces of sex work, including strippers, prostitutes, porn actors, writers, producers, professional dominatrixes, and phone sex workers in the United States. She argued that, because mainstream feminism advocates for many different oppressed groups (e.g., racial/ethnic minorities, sexual minorities, working-class, etc.), it should also advocate for sex workers, particularly surrounding health care and destigmatization. She wrote, "Most public discussions about sex work fail to distinguish between voluntary and coerced sexual exchange, a distinction every bit as salient (and problematic) as that between consensual sex and rape" (p. 3).

Importantly, Nagle also argued against the distinction between prostitution and "implicit sexual-monetary exchange" (p. 4) present in marriage and long-term cohabitation, saying that many women behave like sex workers in their relationships by exchanging sex for money, so an absolute dichotomy is therefore false. She particularly lobbied against the cultural dichotomization of women as either virgins or whores, saying that distinctions between privileged and stigmatized identities (e.g., white women versus women of color; heterosexual women versus lesbian/bisexual women) have a long history within the feminist movement.[3] As Nagle said, "Women can *choose* the less socially sanctioned of the good girl/bad girl boxes, and can do so out of liberation rather than compulsion, or can refuse the dichotomy entirely" (p. 6). Pendleton (1997) added, "The 'good wife' as a social category cannot exist without the 'whore,' whether she takes the form of a prostitute, an insatiable black jezebel, a teenage mother, or a lesbian" (p. 73). Other sex-positive feminists shared these views, advocating that sex work be included in the repertoire of feminist acts (e.g., Nina Hartley, Annie Sprinkle, Carol Queen, Gayle Rubin). Some have illustrated, for example, that strippers engage in emotional labor and interaction and are not merely sexual objects that men look at (Barton, 2006; Wood, 2000). In addition, some sex-positive feminists even condoned and promoted extreme power imbalances during sex and sexual fantasy, such as those found in sado-masochistic sexual practices, as way to enhance pleasure and satisfaction (Nagle, 1997; Réage, 1965).

This debate between sex-negative and sex-positive feminism illuminates some of the core conflicts within the feminist movement regarding sexual fantasy, pornography, and expressions of sex outside of the mainstream. Disagreements about how to best liberate women's sexuality—either from the oppressive context of patriarchal domination (sex-negative), or from the repressive power of patriarchal silence (sex-positive)—form the center of this debate. While some feminists have called for an end to the sharp dichotomization between sex negatives and sex positives, particularly because it reinforces the "virgin/whore" dichotomy (Russo, 1987), these debates still permeate much of feminist sexology. These conflicts extend into the research literatures on women's sexual fantasies and pornography as well, particularly as movements against sexual repression garner increasing amounts of power and momentum. That said, the question remains: What kinds of empowerment and liberation are possible in a in a "postrepression" paradigm?

RESEARCH ON WOMEN'S SEXUAL FANTASIES AND PORNOGRAPHY

Research on Sexual Fantasy

We are what we masturbate to.
—Jensen, *Getting Off: Pornography and the End of Masculinity*

To introduce the research on sexual fantasy, consider this quote from 43-year-old Dawn: "I grew up in a culture of the late 1970s and early 1980s where just the *idea* that women could have fantasies was like 'Wow!' It was a big deal back then." While the last three decades have ushered in a dramatic proliferation of images, representations, and possibilities for women's sexual fantasies, research on sexual fantasy has queried men's sexual fantasies far more often than women's fantasies, thereby portraying women's sexuality as less present and relevant than men's sexuality. Feminist research has rebelled against this by taking up, both directly and indirectly, questions like: What kind of sexual fantasies do women have? Why do women's sexual fantasies often represent regressive cultural fantasies of women as dominated, abused, and submissive when they have clearly gained ground in their fight for equality with men? Why do patriarchal fantasies of women tend to seep into women's consciousness, and as such, can women fantasize outside the context of patriarchy? What does it mean, particularly about gender scripts, when women fantasize about romance and relationships? In particular, feminists have interrogated the meaning of women's fantasies in a culture that generates imagery of women's powerlessness, bondage, submission, domination, and control juxtaposed with women as romantically driven, emotional, nurturing, and pure. In using the existing literature to address such concerns, the following section first addresses the ways that advertising and the broader media may shape the sexual fantasies of women. Later sections address the ways that women *internalize* their own submission and passivity.

An analysis of women's sexual fantasies would be incomplete without considering the context of advertising and media imagery surrounding women's sexualities. Many have argued that Americans now live in a "sex-saturated media culture" that blurs the lines between fantasy and reality; as such, women regularly consume images of their bodies and learn how to think about their bodies in relationship to these images (Bufkin & Eschholz, 2000; Jochen & Valkenburg, 2007; Ward, 2003). As Jean Kilbourne (2007) has said,

> Sex in advertising and the media is often criticized from a puritanical perspective—there's too much of it, it's too blatant, it will encourage kids to be promiscuous, and so forth. But sex in advertising has far more to do with trivializing sex than promoting it, with narcissism than with promiscuity, with consuming than with connecting. The problem is not that it is sinful, but that it is synthetic and cynical. (p. 229)

Jane Caputi (2006) has also argued that "everyday pornography"—or that kind of pornographic impulse that has crept into so-called normal life—has generated a new kind of cultural lexicon surrounding women's bodies, desires, and needs. Because of the strong association between sex and violence, aggressive words take on sexualized connotations:

> We might also ask what does this contempt for the feminine role simultaneously reveal about common male attitudes toward intercourse with women? *Fucking, screwing, banging, having, taking, possessing, scoring, nailing*: all these terms indicate an association of penetrative sex with violence, humiliation, conquest, and domination. (p. 437)

This association intensifies the bond between men's domination over women, women's submission to men's domination, and violence as a key connector between the two. As Caputi has said, "Pornography and everyday pornography construct feminine and masculine subjectivities based in gender inequality, conditioning us to eroticize domination, subordination, violence, and objectification, even when, as in some contexts, a woman takes the masculine role or the man the feminine" (p. 434). As such, Caputi argues that the frequency with which women take on roles of submission in their sexual fantasies directly reveals the role of "everyday pornography" in women's lives.

Popular magazines and websites have occasionally discussed women's fantasies, often in relation to men feeling aroused by, or interested in, these same fantasies. For example, a recent online article on askmen.com posited that women's top ten sexual fantasies included domination (her dominating you), domination (you dominating her), teacher/student, sex with a stranger, threesome with another woman, threesome with two men, voyeurism, rape, exhibitionism, and private dancer (Snow 2008). While the author provides no methodologies for arriving at these conclusions, she quickly points out, when speaking about rape fantasies, "She'll protest as he tears her clothing off and expertly arouses her body, but on the inside, she'll love every minute of it." Though the article does not pose any critical questions about these fantasies, the article implicitly raises questions about how men and women might feel about such intensified power dynamics.

Cosmopolitan, another popular women's magazine, also normalized fantasies that fit into the dominant cultural narratives about gender. For example, one article explicitly gendered sexual fantasy by noting: "'[F]or women, often the most potent essence of a fantasy is the emotion it can evoke.' For instance, he's peeling off your clothes—dwell on how sexy you feel when he looks at you like you're a goddess" (Get Revved, 2009). Another column minimizes the possibilities that women may actually desire sex *exclusively* with women; when a woman asked whether she is normal for fantasizing about lesbian sex, *Cosmo* responded, "There's a difference between thinking about doing something and actually wanting to do it. However, if you *are* considering turning your fantasies into reality, or you do experiment—but you still sleep with guys—you may simply be curious, or it's possible that you are bisexual" (Love Advice, 2009). Or consider this comment about the relationship between women's cognitions and their sex lives, implying that women should stop thinking in order to become sexually aroused: "Scientific research has revealed that during sexual arousal, areas of the female brain . . . need to shut down in order for a woman to have an orgasm, and fantasizing plays a key role in facilitating that process of mental deactivation" (Kerner, 2008). Sexual fantasy, at least as represented in women's magazines, ensures women's *conformity* with stereotypes about proper femininity, whether via fantasizing about romance, ensuring continued sex with men, or deactivating their (annoyingly active) brains.

Regardless of whether popular culture *causes* women's fantasies, women internalize a variety of stereotypically gendered roles in their sexual fantasies. Most studies discussed sexual fantasy as something that occurs *while awake*, during either masturbation or partnered sex and sometimes with the aid of pornography. Within the social science literatures, one study found that women reported four primary categories of sexual fantasy: exploratory (e.g., group sex, promiscuity, homosexuality); intimate (e.g., kissing, oral sex, outdoor love); impersonal (e.g., watching others, fetishism, using objects for stimulation); and sadomasochistic (e.g., whipping or spanking, being forced). Compared to men, women reported more fantasies in the "intimate" category and described themselves as more passive or receptive in their fantasies. Those women who fantasized reported higher libido, higher orgasm frequency, and higher sexual satisfaction than those who did not fantasize (Wilson & Lang, 1981). Studies also showed that most people fantasized about people other than their steady partners (Hicks & Leitenberg, 2001) and that many people suffered from shame and guilt about the often "perverse" nature of their fantasies. In particular, bondage, sadomasochism, incest, and voyeurism apparently represented common themes in people's sexual fantasies. Further, while many people fantasized about sexual abuse and rape, particularly women, those with abuse or rape histories fantasized more often about these scenarios and more often required "dominance stories" to become aroused (Kahr, 2008).

Research on women's sexual fantasies has often focused on correlations between women's submissive fantasies and their sexual well-being (Critelli & Bivona, 2008; Davidson & Hoffman, 1986). Consistent with this emphasis, research has found that women internalized fantasies about their own submission, in part due to the larger cultural narratives that mandate women's submission to men in heterosexual sex (Kiefer & Sanchez, 2007; Kiefer et al., 2006). Over 50% of women reported fantasies of submission (Strassberg & Locker, 1998). Interestingly, however, such fantasies did not predict ability to reach orgasm or sexual arousal (Kiefer et al., 2006), indicating that women may cognitively enjoy submission while not becoming physically aroused by submission.

The positive benefits of sexual fantasy have been noted in the literature, as women who reported having sexual fantasies had more sexual and relationship satisfaction and fewer sexual problems than women who did not fantasize at all (Alfonso, Allison, & Dunn, 1992; Byrne & Osland, 2000; Leitenberg & Henning, 1995; Nutter & Condron, 1983).

Research has also shown that over 60% of women fantasized while engaging in sexual activity with a partner, and 93% of women fantasized during masturbation (Rye & Meaney, 2007). Such fantasies may allow women to repair disrupted attachment relationships or act out desires for better romantic connections with others, which may translate into better psychological functioning overall. This may be particularly true for women in sexual relationships with partners who do not fully excite, arouse, or interest them (Birnbaum, 2007).

Correlations between women's fantasies and their sexual behaviors, particularly with partners, have typically been mixed. In general, women's sexual fantasies correlated more strongly with experiences they had actually done (e.g., sex with a current or past partner), while men fantasized more about experiences they had not done (Hsu et al., 1994), suggesting that women's fantasy lives may match up more directly with their sexual practices. Some studies suggest that women's fantasies of submissiveness predicted engagement in sex submissive behaviors (Kiefer et al., 2006), while other studies suggest that fantasies did not predict behavior (Davidson & Hoffman, 1986; Strassberg & Locker, 1998). For men, correlations between pornography, sexual fantasy, and sexual behavior were more evident, as pornography contributed to men's view of a male-dominant society and to men's difficulty in separating sexual fantasy from reality. Men's sexual fantasies may contribute to them initiating sexual abuse or violence against women (Jensen, 1995).

Other behaviors also correlated with having sexual fantasies, including, to varying degrees, casual sex and cheating behaviors. One recent study found strong correlations between women's acceptance of casual sex and their likelihood of reporting sexual fantasies of dominance (Yost & Zurbriggen, 2006). Correlations between sexual fantasies and cheating behaviors have been mixed, as people felt threatened by the perceptions that their partners *could* cheat rather than sexual fantasies of cheating per se (Yarab & Allgeier, 1998). Women who described anxious attachments to their partners also admitted to more fantasies about cheating on their partners than those women who described a secure attachment (Birnbaum, 2007).

In particular, researchers have been troubled by the frequency with which women report "rape fantasies" or fantasies where men explicitly force them to have sex against their will. A recent study found that between 31 and 57% of women had rape fantasies, and for 9 to 17% of these women, this was their favorite or most frequent fantasy (Critelli & Bivona, 2008). Another study found that low sex guilt and high interest in eroticism predicted more forceful sexual fantasies (Shulman & Horne, 2006; Strassberg & Locker, 1998). As such, rape fantasies may represent sexual expressiveness and openness to sexuality rather than sexual repression and guilt. Still, childhood sexual abuse also predicted more force fantasy, more sexually-explicit fantasies, and more fantasies with the theme of being under someone's control (Gold, 1991; Shulman & Horne, 2006), though not all studies have found a link between childhood sexual abuse and force fantasies (Strassberg & Locker, 1998).

Theories vary greatly about why women paradoxically said that they fantasized about an event (rape, coercion) that would clearly be traumatic if it occurred in real life. Some believe that these fantasies stem from culturally inscribed masochism imposed upon women, while others think that rape fantasies allow for sexual blame avoidance (i.e., in rape fantasies, women do not have to take responsibility for their sexual desire and/or actions). A biological perspective holds that such fantasies allow for sympathetic physiological activation and may also reflect women's biological predisposition to surrender (a finding heavily criticized by feminists). Still others argue that rape fantasies represent openness to sexuality or a deep-seated need for women to prove their sexual desirability. To counter these claims, feminists often point out that women live in a rape culture that engenders male dominance in many ways, sexual or otherwise, so it makes sense that this translates into women's fantasies of domination (Critelli & Bivona, 2008).

Aside from rape fantasies, research has found strong gender differences in other kinds of sexual fantasies, in that women's fantasies tended to differ from men's fantasies in terms of content and frequency. Women's sexual fantasies, when compared to men's, included more emotional and romantic themes (Kimmel & Plante, 2005), more emphasis on touching and partners' feelings (Ellis & Symons, 1990; Pelletier & Herold, 1988), more imagery related to submission (Hsu et al., 1994; McCauley & Swann, 1978), fewer images of dominance (Byers, Purdon, & Clark, 1998), less content with multiple partners, more vivid imagery, and more passive words (Kimmel & Plante, 2005). Women's fantasies also involved someone they were in a relationship with, while men's fantasies featured different themes: imagined partners, domination, impersonal exchanges, quick progression to sexual acts, sexual objectification, and partner variety (Ellis & Symons, 1991; Zurbriggen & Yost, 2006). Interestingly, women who had more emotional and romantic fantasy themes articulated rape myth acceptance more often than those who reported different fantasy themes (Zurbriggen & Yost, 2006), casting doubt about the liberatory implications of romance-themed fantasies.

Research has found some differences between heterosexual women and lesbian and bisexual women's sexual fantasies as well. Lesbian women described similar fantasies to heterosexual women except that they typically imagined female partners (Robinson & Parks, 2003) and were less interested than heterosexual women in sexual fantasy (Hurlbert & Apt, 1993). A recent study found that relationship functioning significantly predicted the thematic content of sexual fantasies (Robinson & Parks, 2003). Further, lesbian women fantasized more often about same-sex encounters, performing oral sex on a partner, having sex in natural surroundings, and having sex with a stranger. Heterosexual women fantasized more often about sex with a current partner, group sex, feeling "irresistible" to the opposite sex, being overpowered or forced to surrender against their will, and observing group sex (Price & Allensworth, 1985).

Collectively, the rather chaotic and contradictory research literature on sexual fantasy suggests that the strong cultural norms for women to eroticize their own submission and passivity have translated into the content of women's fantasies. Not only do women eroticize submission, but they also sometimes eroticize rape and coercion scenarios. The political implications of such fantasies are difficult to determine, as some argue that sexual fantasies might predict better sexual and psychological functioning, while others suggest that sexual fantasies might recreate troublingly imbalanced power relationships between women and men. Conflicts about the meaning of women's romance fantasies also reveal these tensions. Because social scripts normalize women as nurturing, emotional, and caretaking, their romance-themed fantasies are also difficult to fully analyze or understand, particularly for their political implications. Taken together, women's sexual fantasies offer some interesting insights into the relationship between gender and power.

Research on Pornography

> [W]hat pornography delivers is what it recites and exaggerates from the resources of compensatory gender norms, a text of insistent and faulty imaginary relations that will not disappear with the abolition of the offending text, a text that remains for feminist criticism relentlessly to read. To read such texts against themselves is to concede that the performativity of the text is not under sovereign control. On the contrary, if the text acts once, it can act again, and possibly against its prior act.
> —Butler, *Excitable Speech*

Pornography has long represented a key site of contention among feminists, as it can potentially advance the goals of sex positivity while also normalizing dominance over women. As seen in the debates about pornography (as "bad") versus erotica (as "good"), in the woman-produced porn (as "good") versus man-produced porn (as "bad"), or in the sex-positive versus sex-negative debates described earlier, concern for what liberates and empowers women is a central concern of the feminist movement. Questions that circulate in the debates about pornography include: Can women claim "the gaze"? What does pornography imply about the relationship between men and women and, alternatively, between women and the culture at large? While some of these questions have already been addressed in previous sections of this chapter, the research on the consumption and circulation of pornography reveals much nuance about the interplay among performance, power, sexuality, and the media.

The history of pornography underlies some of the conflicts women have about using and watching it today, as early 20th-century pornography originally started out as a genre that poked fun at the overly repressive and uptight mainstream of American society. In this way, the mocking, subversive qualities of early stag films at times line up with the aims of the feminist movement. As Constance Penley (2004) stated, "Stag films are full of humor, and the narrative . . . is often more vignette than fully developed story, itself structured like a joke. And here we are talking about really bad jokes, ranging from terrible puns to every form of dirty joke—farmer's daughter, traveling salesman, and Aggie jokes" (p. 314). Pornography, at least historically, made fun of the restrictive sexual mores of the day by using humor and wit, a fact in many ways forgotten in the modern day manifestations of pornography.

Still, others argue against American pornography's origins as benign and silly. While pornography may have its roots in humorous and somewhat harmless stag films, it also has its roots in the racist exploitation of low-status groups, particularly women and people of color. Patricia Hill-Collins (1997) pointed out that modern pornography is based on the exploitation of black women's bodies that occurred in 19th-century Europe. In this way, paradigms of objectification, domination, and control are largely based on the iconography of black women's bodies (e.g., Hottentot Venus). Hill-Collins argued,

> Black women were not added into a preexisting pornography, but rather . . . pornography itself must be reconceptualized as an example of the interlocking nature of race, gender, and class oppression . . . for African-American women pornography has not been timeless and universal but was tied to Black women's experiences with the European colonization of Africa and with American slavery. (p. 397).

Similarly, Alice Walker (2004) argued that "the more ancient roots of modern pornography are to be found in the almost always pornographic treatment of black women, who, from the moment they entered slavery, even in their own homelands, were subjected to rape as the 'logical' convergence of sex and violence. Conquest, in short" (p. 42). The relationships among pornography, gender, and race form a basis for the exploitation of women and their bodies found in pornography today.

In the social science literatures, research on women's consumptions of pornography and other sexually explicit material has varied greatly, with some studies showing that 10–15% of women enjoy consuming pornography (Cooper, McLoughlin, & Campbell, 2000; Laumann et al., 1994), while other studies show that 80% of women used the internet for sexual purposes, with approximately a third of those engaging in cybersex (Daneback, Cooper, & Mansson, 2005). Watching porn images has grown in popularity during the past decade because of the afford-ability of materials, easy accessibility of pornography, and the fact that people can access pornography anonymously online (Cooper, McLoughlin, & Campbell, 2000). In qualitative studies of women's feel-ings about pornography, women expressed ambivalence about it based on several concerns about the actresses, including the emotional labor required of them, their pleasure and emotional authenticity, their eco-nomic backgrounds, and their history of sexual coercion. Even for women who watched pornography frequently, they expressed deep ambivalence and confusion about its implications for women (Parvez, 2006). In contrast, qualitative work has also shown that, for women, pornography can serve as a source of knowledge, a resource for inti-mate practices, a site for identity construction, and an occasion for per-forming gender and sexuality (Attwood, 2005).

Significant gender differences in use, endorsement, and consump-tion of pornography appear in the literature. A recent study found that 49% of women, compared to 67% of men, believed that consuming pornography was acceptable, while 31% of women, compared to 87% of men, reported using pornography (Carroll et al., 2008). Other studies have shown that men more often approved of pornography than women, that women felt more threatened by pornography than did men (O'Reilly, Knox, & Zusman, 2007), and that women more often labeled pornography as "repulsive and offensive," while men labeled pornography as "arousing and exciting" (Reid et al., 2007). That said, women reported heightened arousal to pornography when imagining themselves as participants, while men reported arousal regardless of whether they imagined that they observed or participated in the pornography (Janssen, Carpenter, & Graham, 2003). Compared to men, women first viewed pornography at an older age, consumed less pornography, and used pornography less often during masturbation (Hald, 2006). Still, researchers point out that significant numbers (upwards of 49%) of women like and enjoy pornography, while signifi-cant numbers (at least 33%) of men dislike and are offended by pornog-raphy (Carroll et al., 2008; Johansson & Hammarén, 2007), casting some doubt upon the highly stereotyped claims that men like pornography and women do not.

While men often serve as financiers and directors of pornography, an emerging number of female directors who make porn for both heterosexual and lesbian audiences have gained popularity in recent years. Questions of whether women enjoy pornography made specifically by and for women—often involving more plot elements, less "gonzo" imagery, less violence and degrading imagery, and more themes of romance and love—have had mixed results. Some research has shown that women who watched pornographic videos made "for women" reported more subjective sexual arousal than those who watched male-oriented films (Pearson & Pollack, 1997; Quackenbush, Strassberg, & Turner, 1995). Another study found that women who watched videos intended for men experienced more negative feelings; when watching videos intended for women, they described more sexual arousal, more positive feelings, more absorption, and more frequent intercourse after viewing the films (Mosher & MacIan, 1994). Some caution should be taken about these findings, however, given that this culture socializes women to associate sex with love; consequently, pornography involving more romantic themes may very well simply reflect the social demands placed upon women to eroticize love and relationship scenarios.

Studies on the concrete *effects* of pornography are fraught with conflicts over proper research methodologies and competing findings, with some studies showing that women's use of pornography correlated strongly with risky sexual behaviors and substance abuse (Carroll et al., 2008), while others showed that use of pornography had no clear negative effects on women's lives (Hald & Malamuth, 2008; McKee, 2007). In particular, research has shown that, for men, the correlation between acute alcohol intoxication and sexual arousal to violent pornography contributed to greater likelihood of sexual aggression (Davis et al., 2006).

Related to this, ongoing debates rage on about whether pornography *causes* violence against women or whether it simply represents one cultural manifestation of the culture of violence that already exists (Boyle, 2000; Seto, Maric, & Barbaree, 2001). Recent research has indicated reliable associations between men's pornography use and sexually aggressive behavior towards women, particularly for men who watch violent pornography or for men at high risk for sexual aggression already (Malamuth, Addison, & Koss, 2000).

Other research has focused on the relationship between pornography consumption and attitudes about gender and sexuality. Research shows that sexual explicitness itself did not negatively affect people's attitudes about women, but sexual explicitness combined with degrading imagery produced hostile thoughts and antipathy towards women. Also, the more anonymous the women were in the pornographic films, the more likely people were to express antipathy towards women and to request more extreme types of sexual stimuli (Shim, 2007). Compared to women, men admitted to more arousal from degrading imagery toward women and aggressive imagery of men (Glascock, 2005). Pornography also affected people's judgments about women: both women and men labeled women who watched pornography as more "loose" than women who did not watch pornography (O'Reilly, Knox, & Zusman, 2007). Further, women pornography watchers more often accepted rape myths that blamed women for sexual assault (Shim, 2007). In general, negative attitudes toward women were predicted by older age, right-wing political identification, living in rural areas, and less education (McKee, 2007), which may, when combined with consumption of pornography, correlate with hostilities toward women.

Collectively, this research suggests that women experience intense conflicts about their use of pornography, as it had a diverse range of effects on their lives. Debates about sex-positive versus sex-negative feminism appeared in full force when looking at the different arguments about what pornography means for women. For some, pornography can expand one's repertoire of sexual activities and facilitate them questioning or considering their gender roles; for others, pornography can contribute to more victim blaming, tolerance of violence, and risky sexual behaviors. As seen in the next section of this chapter, women's stories about their relationship to sexual fantasy and pornography also reveal these conflicts.

WOMEN'S NARRATIVES ABOUT SEXUAL FANTASY AND PORNOGRAPHY

> You know, it's not the world that was my oppressor, because
> what the world does to you, if the world does it to you
> long enough and effectively enough, you begin to do to
> yourself.
>
> —Baldwin, *A Dialogue*

In the interviews I conducted with women, their narratives about sexual fantasy and pornography reveal not only the power of gendered performances but also their conflicts about how to assimilate or reject messages they receive about femininity, passivity, masochism, and submission. These conflicts appeared as they discussed their sexual fantasies, particularly in light of the fact that their fantasies differed substantially from their lived experiences of pleasure (discussed in chapter 4). Similar conflicts arose when women discussed their political attitudes about pornography, as most women disapproved of censorship, yet felt concerned with the messages and implications of pornography. In order to provide a window in the range of fantasies women described, this section highlights the six most prominent categories of women's sexual fantasies. An analysis of coercion and dominance fantasies particularly illuminates the ways that women internalize patriarchal ideas about performance. Women's views about pornography also emphasize their conflicts about consuming and using pornography in their everyday lives.

Sexual Fantasy Narratives

Notably, several women reported *no* sexual fantasies at all. A variety of competing explanations may account for this: women who do not fantasize may have less interest in sex and masturbation; they may feel reluctant to disclose fantasy scenarios due to embarrassment, shame, or need for privacy; they may avoid fantasy because they do not prioritize it in their sexual lives; or their lack of fantasizing may protect them from internalizing sexism. This fits with previous research that has shown a "missing discourse of desire," or, more precisely, a variety of erotic silences women face around their sexuality. Not surprisingly, sexual fantasy may, for some women, represent one of these "missing discourses" (Fine, 1988; McClelland & Fine, 2008; Tolman, 2002). For those who did fantasize, six primary categories appeared, many of which confirmed the findings of previous research in this area. Women's fantasies prioritized submission at the expense of romance or dominating others, though both of the latter categories appeared, to a lesser degree, in women's fantasy stories. Moreover, women's fantasies illuminated a great deal of relatively unprocessed baggage about gender, race, and power.

Women typically fantasized about content that fell into six categories. First, women frequently described fantasies about threesomes and group sex, including a substantial amount of content about same-sex eroticism with men in the room. Second, women described fantasies about romance and sexual caretaking, including content featuring current and previous partners. Third, women fantasized about inaccessible people who often had status, power, or authority, including celebrities, men in uniform, married men, teachers, strangers, and men of different races. Fourth, women fantasized about having sex in taboo places, often with the risk of getting caught or being otherwise publicly humiliated (e.g., dressing rooms, public parks, elevators, etc.). Fifth, women occasionally mentioned an interest in dominating or exploiting others, including voyeurism, talking dirty to partners, or having sex with someone who would not remember it. Finally, and most prominently, women described themes of being subjected to sexual force and coercion in their sexual fantasies, including rape, sexual objectification, prostitution, stripping, physical injury, masochism, bondage and dominance (BDSM), and pain.

Themes of sexual access figured prominently in women's sexual fantasy narratives, even when women fantasized about other women. Women's fantasies about group sex most often included threesome scenarios where women had sex with two other partners (at least one man) or scenarios where women had sex with another woman while a man watched. At least one-third of the women interviewed expressed an interest in threesomes as a sexual fantasy, particularly threesomes endorsed by their male partners. For example, Ciara, age 24, described a threesome fantasy that would satisfy her husband:

> I fantasize about threesomes with another girl. My husband wouldn't mind having one, so I think it would be fun because I'd be with somebody that I love, and since I like girls, it would be fun. We could do it together, and he'd be into it, I think.

Lucy, age 25, also felt interested in a threesome fantasy yet felt her husband would *reject* her desire for this:

My most common reoccurring fantasy would have to be a threesome with two women and one man. It would give me the opportunity to try both worlds at once. That sounds good. My husband hasn't been very comfortable with me actually having sex with another woman. It would hurt his feelings. I guess I do fantasize about having sex with people other than my husband, like men I've dated or have been attracted to. I told my husband that I have dreams about other guys, and he's okay with it as long as it's not while I'm awake (laughs). If I told him I dreamt about another guy while I was awake, he'd be insanely jealous.

Occasionally, both heterosexual and lesbian women described an interest in having threesomes with two men. While such a fantasy still provides figurative sexual access to men, the stories sometimes prioritized women's pleasure over men's pleasure. For example, Ruth, age 46, described her most recurrent fantasy as focusing on her pleasure:

I fantasize about two men just giving me pleasure. It's something that I feel I never would have in life, just that much attention, where their only goal was to pleasure me for that particular moment or whatever. I feel fortunate to have found someone who's like that and is so loving, but I occasionally think about having sex with someone else. I'm in a monogamous, Christian-based marriage which I love. I can't see upsetting the applecart for anything in the world.

On the other hand, threesome fantasies about two men also reinforced men's right to have sexual access to, or power over, women. Lesbian-identified Jasmine, age 37, described such a threesome fantasy about two men:

I fantasize about a threesome with two guys because a little forcefulness is nice. When it comes to sex and my fantasies, I like pain and pleasure, where it's a little bit of pain but mostly pleasure. I like when men get a little more aggressive and after you're totally in the mood and you're way past hot and heavy,

they're just pretty much having their way with you and being
very aggressive. That's nice.

Twenty-three-year-old Niko described a more ambivalent sense of
gender in her group sex fantasies, saying several remarks about shifting
gender dynamics:

> Usually it's like me with a lot of other guys or seeing someone
> (other women) having sex. It's more just lesbian sex and groups
> of people with one girl, like a group of guys with one girl.
> When I masturbate or fantasize, it's never with any men
> though. It's always just women. I think [it's] women's bodies
> that arouse me.

At times, group sex fantasies shifted into a realm without men,
where women sometimes discussed same-sex encounters with multiple
partners that did not include men, though these occurred less often
than scenarios involving men. Only *two* women (both heterosexual)
described fantasies about same-sex encounters that did *not* include men
(e.g., men watching, men involved in the sex, etc.), again reinforcing
the earlier findings in chapter 2 and chapter 5 about the compulsory
quality of *men's sexual access to women*. Kate, age 25, told me about her
same-sex group fantasies but also indicated that these fantasies felt
increasingly less pleasurable to her:

> I have fantasized about being with several other women, but
> I've just never met a woman that I've been attracted to. I think
> I get frustrated by how routine my fantasies become. I wish I
> could be more creative with them sometimes, but my mind is
> so occupied with other things.

As a second category of women's sexual fantasies, themes of
romance, caretaking, and being "swept off of one's feet" appeared regularly, particularly for the older women I spoke with. These fantasies
ranged from going on a lavish vacation to having sex beneath a water-
fall to reliving an experience with a current or expartner. Romance
fantasies were the *only* fantasies that correlated strongly with the pleasurable experiences women mentioned in chapter 4, perhaps indicating

a parallel between fantasy and lived experiences for these particular women. Pam, age 42, described her fantasies of leaving her ordinary life by running off with a special man:

> For me, fantasy is not having to think about the everyday life, so I think that's why I enjoy the getaway sex. The greatest fantasies that I have are stuff that I see on TV, like having a room filled with 20 dozen roses and then having sex to express my gratitude for those roses. Also, faraway places, with the drapes down, people serving me—anything that takes me away from regular life.

These fantasies typically included content about escaping familial and work obligations, indicating that mental escape from *gender roles* fulfilled some women similar to chapter 4's findings.

Fantasies of romance also often included content about relationship satisfaction, where women described men taking care of them in ways they did not experience in their actual lives. Esther, age 44, described a romantic scene where a man prioritized her sexual needs:

> I think about being beside a creek, feeling emotions toward a man, noticing the scenery, being with this person, looking at his face, and the raindrops on my face. Usually they're the romantic kind, where somebody comes and sweeps me off my feet, treats me like a queen, just really takes care of me and is sensitive to my sexual needs. Whatever I tell him, that's what he's going to remember to do, so my fantasies tend to stay around the idea of being fulfilled or him being there for me instead of looking for me to be there for him . . . It's kind of sad when I think about them because to be 44 years old and still looking for that man that's going to do those things, and to wonder if such a man exists, that makes me feel sad. At this point in my life, I should have been married for 20 years with 2 or 3 kids and be happy with the big house and all the things we wanted in life.

Similar themes of wishing for better caretaking from men appeared also when women thought longingly about a past partner who they no longer had contact with. Marilyn, age 54, constructed her fantasies around a man she had an affair with years before:

> The only fantasy that I have is about the gentleman I had the affair with. I would think about him after that, after we weren't together anymore, and I'd think about him during intercourse with my husband. It got me through the act of having intercourse with my husband, just thinking of him and the times we had together that were satisfying. It would help me climax.

Still, a few women fantasized about their current partner and positive experiences they had with that partner, such as 33-year-old Lori: "I fantasize about my boyfriend all the time, like him going down on me or sucking on my nipples. I think about things we've done where I've had incredible orgasms, and that usually sends me right over the edge."

While most romance fantasies involved men (regardless of women's sexual identities), women occasionally described romance fantasies about other women. For example, Diana, age 50, elaborated on a lesbian romance scene:

> My fantasies are in water, being with a woman on the beach at night, stripping our clothes off and running into the ocean in the moonlight and making love in the ocean. A lot of times a visual fantasy happens like a lagoon in Hawaii with a waterfall and ferns, like something sensual and romantic. Most of my fantasies are all with women, in various locations like elevators or stopping along Topanga Canyon road to go into a pool. I like things that aren't traditional.

Collectively, these romance fantasies bring up a central question about fantasies in general: Do fantasies help women fulfill something that they do not otherwise experience in their real lives? Or do fantasies represent extensions of, or more extreme versions of, things that they have experienced in their real lives? Women who generated these romance fantasies typically did not feel satisfied by the amount of romance in their lives. Notably, no younger women described romance fantasies, as older women exclusively reported romance fantasies. This may reflect the different kinds of media messages women receive in their lives. For example, if younger women consume pornography more often, while older women consume romance novels more often (Miller, 2007), this disparity in fantasy constructions makes sense. For older women, fantasies of a passionate, attentive, caring lover might have more relevance if they have lost some of the spark, freshness, or passion in their current relationships or interactions. Also, older women may have had more past partners who did not show them consideration, so the fantasy component helps them to construct a different narrative about sexual partners (especially male partners).

As a third category of fantasies, women frequently described imagining sexual exchanges with men whom they could not access in their lives. Such men often had particular social roles laden with different sorts of privileges and taboos, including celebrities, men in uniform, married men, strangers, or men of different races. Often, women described these nameless men as having more power than them both socially and sexually. For example, lesbian-identified Maria, age 21, described her fantasies about male sailors: "I like their outfits—those tight, white suits with the bell bottoms. I like that they have power and how they have that swagger." Charlotte, age 34, described her intense fantasies about celebrities in a similar manner: "I've had quite a few dreams and fantasies about certain celebrities, like Marshall Mathers, 50 Cent, Tobey Maguire. I mean, they are just hot!—their build, their body language, their whole attitude, their personalities."

Women also fantasized about men who seemed unreachable. For example, several white women mentioned fantasies about men of color as "hypersexual," replicating racist cultural narratives that oversexualize people of color. Twenty-three-year-old Courtney (a white woman) described highly stereotyped fantasies about Latino men: "I fantasize about romantic, hot, sweaty, passionate lovers, like Antonio Banderas or someone with a Spanish accent who is a very passionate person. I've always fantasized about Latino men just because I like the idea of having really good, hot, passionate sex." Edie, age 19, also white, mentioned fantasies about black men, tapping into and furthering old racist stereotypes in her sexual fantasies (Bobo, Kluegel, & Smith, 1997; Hill-Collins, 2005), by saying, "Even with ethnicity, it's like a different species when having sex because I'm white so having sex with a black

man sounds exciting. I have never seen a black penis before." Such fantasies recreate racist stereotypes circulating in the broader culture and
indicate that women not only internalize *sexist* fantasies but also *racist*
ones as well. A few women also fantasized about married men, such as
38-year-old Carol: "There's something appealing about married men. I
imagine them running off to be with me and then having incredibly
hot sex." Still others described married men as inaccessible and a relative turn-off for them sexually.

Another classic fantasy—the stranger fantasy—also predictably
appeared in women's narratives, as the "no strings attached" paradigm
appealed to women's sense of wanting emotionless, uncomplicated,
physically passionate sex. Interestingly, however, while stranger fantasies
often met women's need for emotional distance, these same fantasies
also inspired a great deal of shame and guilt. For example, age 29, Mitra
described personal conflicts about stranger fantasies:

> My big fantasies are stranger fantasies, threesomes, and being
> forced to have sex. With the stranger thing, it's almost like the
> lack of emotional responsibility and just being able to com-
> pletely sexualize the situations. Sometimes I fantasize simultane-
> ously about the stranger fantasy and the force fantasy, but I don't
> know why I do this. I had a boyfriend who wanted to have
> more domineering sex, and I tried it and didn't like it at all. The
> reality of it did not feel like a positive experience, and I don't
> know if that was just a personal issue or if it was him, but it kind
> of turned me off when I did it in a real way. I'd also never have
> sex with strangers, but I like to think about it sometimes.

When I asked her how her fantasies made her feel, she said, "I feel
guilty sometimes, like something is wrong with me." Thus, perhaps
stranger fantasies tap into women's guilt about not providing emotional
labor and caretaking for partners, even while it (ironically) accesses their
desire to avoid such emotional caretaking by eroticizing disconnection
from a sexual partner.

As a fourth category, fantasies about having sex in taboo places, particularly public places with a high likelihood of getting caught,
appealed to several women. For example, Priya, age 23, combined a
fantasy that included both sex in a public place and sex with an author-

ity figure: "I've always wanted to have sex in a public place, and I fanta-size sometimes about doing that with this really good-looking professor I had in college." Anita, age 46, who also fantasized about sex in public places, said, "I fantasize sometimes about this thing I saw in a movie, where people were having sex on the street, like right on the corner. It wasn't like people were around. It was a very empty place, but it was so passionate and in the moment, right out in the open."

Some women described their public sex fantasies with more speci-ficity, claiming that dressing rooms and public restrooms had particular appeal for them. Dawn said, "I really find fantasies to be entertaining, and I enjoy them. I fantasize about having sex in a public place, like in a department store dressing room, because it's semipublic, you could get caught, it's a little bit naughty, things like that." Diana also described an interest in restroom and dressing room sex, saying:

> I have this one fantasy of meeting a woman in the restaurant and not knowing each other, being strangers, and then follow-ing each other into the bathroom where we make out and do other things in a clean bathroom at a really nice restaurant. I also like to imagine doing that in a department store dressing room or at a bar. These fantasies make me feel exhilarated, intoxicated, excited, aroused, and liberated. It's emotionally intense to imagine these things.

Edie also fantasized about public sex, citing the likelihood of being watched as a turn-on:

> If I'm masturbating or having sex, I'm definitely fantasizing about things. I fantasize about public sex but would never do it. Fantasizing about being watched is a common fix for me. It's just like this state of being so immersed that you don't care about what's happening around you, and people can just stand there in awe of your shamelessness and be jealous of it and wish they were that free, you know?

Collectively, these taboo places fantasies suggest a need for intense spon-taneity during sex, combined with a disregard for social norms about sex being private. In these fantasies, women ignore the public/private split about sexualized spaces and instead violate those social norms as an erotic stimulus. If fantasy indicates what women do not have in their real lives, such fantasies may fulfill women's needs for less cognitive or planned sex and/or the desire to involve others in their sex life (e.g., voyeurs, authority figures, the "public" broadly speaking, etc.). They also provide men, in the most abstract form, with sexual access to women, as onlookers and those who watch often have male characteristics.

As a fifth category of sexual fantasies, a few women discussed dominating others, constituting another reversal of stereotypical gender roles for women (i.e., passive, receptive, emotional caretakers). Interestingly, with only *one* exception, *all women who described a desire to dominate others identified as butch lesbians and wanted to dominate their female partners.* For example, Leigh, age 21, said, "Usually I fantasize about being the dominating one, like thinking about the girl I'm dating right now. I think about dominating her, but she's not really into that, unless she's been drinking. I get upset about that." Janet, age 21, also described an interest in dominating her female partner:

> I guess my fantasies are like where I get so frustrated with her that I just want to pick her up and throw her on the bed and kind of have my way with her, but I would never hurt her or rape her, you know? But the fantasy is that I feel kind of angry and I just have this picture of picking her up, throwing her on the bed, taking her clothes off, and having my way, but the other part of me is like, I want to do it in a happy, playful mood at the same time, and kind of lightly throw her on the bed, not with so much force. I just want her to give in.

This relationship between butch-identified lesbian women and fantasies of domination suggests that women who played a more masculine role in same-sex relationships more often adopted traditionally masculine sexual fantasies of dominating, controlling, or harming women. This raises several questions about the meaning of such findings: Does this represent an internalization of patriarchal norms, where lesbian women serve the role of the forceful, aggressive partner while fantasizing about other women's submission? Is this a mechanism for a disenfranchised group (butch lesbian women) to take power, at least in their fantasies?

How do gender roles translate into women's fantasies? Such questions warrant further attention and study.

As a sixth and final category, fantasies of being raped, forced, coerced, dominated, and objectified represented the most common sexual fantasy reported by the most number of women. Notably, the disjuncture between dominance fantasies and women's descriptions of lived experiences with sexual pleasure (chapter 4) indicates a chasm—at least in terms of sexual pleasure—between fantasy and reality. While women may fantasize about their own submission and mistreatment, they rarely claimed these acts as literally pleasurable. As Slavoj Žižek has said, "We have a name for fantasy realized: nightmare" (as quoted in DeCarlo, 2009).

Regardless of women's actual experiences with sexual coercion, women reported rape fantasies at high rates. Nearly a third of the sample directly reported rape or force fantasies (a finding slightly lower than other research that has shown over half of women reporting force fantasies—see Strassberg & Locker, 1998); nearly as many reported guilt, shame, confusion, or dissonance about such fantasies. For example, Charlene, age 44, who had married her husband following what she called a date rape, said: "I've always fantasized about the whole rape fantasy thing, and I've always thought that was weird because being in that situation isn't very arousing. I guess I like the excitement of a stranger or just the mystery." Thirty-two-year-old Jill expressed similar conflicts about the content of her force fantasies and her analysis of those fantasies:

> My fantasies are mostly of me being dominated in some way by a partner. One that I use for masturbatory purposes frequently involves basically an arena full of people where the rules involve that the guys can do pretty much anything they want to the girls. I'm not really *me* per se here, but I'm a person who is being played by me. Another one I've been doing lately involves someone who is somehow able to force me to do whatever he tells me to do and renders me helpless and either has sex with me a lot or sends me out to do various sexual tasks or roles or quests so to speak. Most of these fantasies are an exaggeration of what I might actually want to do . . . I

fantasize about being raped a lot. I think there is part of my brain that is the good girl and good girls don't do nasty horrible things like that, but if somebody forces me to do them, then I can't help it. I think part of it also is that if somebody else is in charge of you, in control of you, then whatever happens is not my fault, not my responsibility. I just lay back and take it so to speak. I'm just there to have things done to me.

When I asked her what emotions she had about her fantasies, she responded with concern about herself: "To some extent I worry about my mental health because of them, kind of on the level of, 'Is this normal? Am I really fucked in the head?'" Still, both Jill and 21-year-old Melanie had a fairly sophisticated analysis of how these fantasies helped them to reconcile guilt and shame about their own sexual agency. This rationale was similar to Melanie's feelings about sexualizing werewolves:

I think about sex with trees and werewolves and stuff like that. I don't project myself into fantasies, but I think about what that would feel like. I fantasize about being forced to have sex with werewolves, and I think, if I was forced into it, I did not have to be held accountable for the consequences.

If rape fantasies allow women to embrace sexuality despite a variety of cultural prohibitions against women doing so, their analysis makes sense. If women cannot express themselves sexually, they fantasize about others forcing them to explore their sexual feelings, desires, or bodily sensations, even if that requires violence. Force fantasies may directly stem from the culture of sexual repression that still looms large for many women.

Force fantasies may also speak to women's earlier rape and abuse experiences, as women compulsively recreate them in their fantasy lives, though the research on this presents conflicting findings (Gold, 1991; Kahr, 2008; Shulman & Horne, 2006; Strassberg & Locker, 1998). Sally, age 20, who described some severely coercive incidents in her adolescence, fantasized about men sexually attacking her. Her lack of agency in fantasies recreates her earlier coercive experiences while also giving her permission to feel sexual:

Sometimes I like it very sweet and gentle, and sometimes I would like it where the man is more aggressive and more dominating. I fantasize about being attacked, where someone is holding me down or like pushing me down on the bed or just like kind of taking control of it all. I imagine that I really didn't have to do anything, and he did everything and held my hands up and was more forceful during the sexual experience.

Emily, age 22, who has described several experiences with rape, reported fantasizing about forced sex as well, though her scenarios involved more playful coercion rather than violent rape fantasies:

There are definitely things that I fantasize about and that are appealing that I would never want to do in real life, like being forced. In real life, there's nothing about that that would appeal to me. I'm usually really selfish, and I have to be the one that's always in control, but I'd definitely fantasize about what it's like to not be in control. My favorite one is, well there's this Mexican food place that my girlfriend and I always go to, and they always mess up my order, and I have to send it back. I think about different fantasy scenarios about the angry chef coming out and getting offended about having to remake my order every day. I also fantasize about gang bang scenes and anal sex and fetish stuff.

These descriptions of rape fantasies support the theories that rape fantasies represent: 1) women giving themselves permission to be sexual when they otherwise do not feel allowed to express their sexuality; 2) women internalizing cultural narratives about their submission and passivity; and 3) women reverting to regressive stereotypes about gender roles. Rape fantasies have seeped into the consciousness of women regardless of their experience with sexual assault, revealing that rape fantasies permeate many women's mental space.

In addition to rape fantasies, many women described fantasies about being restrained or otherwise engaging in sadomasochistic play with a partner, again speaking chapter 5's discussion of the pervasive qualities of coercion. For example, Edie said, "I definitely fantasized about masochism because pain for me is just like pleasure. Pain stimulus is the basis of what an animal is thinking, and pain inspires adrenaline, and adrenaline feels really good, so that's where it comes from." When I asked her what it was like to try S&M in real life, she responded, "I didn't enjoy the way I felt, and I guess I'm not shameless enough, free enough. I just didn't prefer it over just having sex with a lover in a loving kind of setting."

Sonja, age 24, described her fantasies in a complicated way, often halting to say that she did not know how to describe them fully but eventually admitting to feelings of guilt about her coercion fantasies:

> Being tied down somehow is arousing, just being tied down and being seduced slowly or something. I'm kind of a sensitive person, so the combination of being tied down and the slow seduction thing is arousing, probably because it's a contrast or combination or something . . . I've probably had a ton of fantasies that were just really dirty. I wouldn't even know how to talk about them. Kinky, talking dirty, power differences of some kind. The power differences are really arousing. I don't think I go very far—just kind of being slapped or something. That's not something I like to talk about, but I do like when there's some kind of struggle where one person has control. I have embarrassment about my fantasies, embarrassment and guilt.

As another form of coercion fantasy, some women described an interest in imagining themselves as strippers or prostitutes because sexual objectification aroused them. For example, 25-year-old Aya justified her stripper fantasy: "I'd feel really sexy and desired. You're on display. I'm really inhibited normally. I don't go to bars or parties, and I feel kind of shy, so these fantasies help me I guess." Brynn, age 25, also fantasized about feeling objectified by her female partner: "I like thinking about the high heels, the bowties, the little outfits, being in a pair of stilettos, with a whip. I like thinking about her looking at me and getting turned on." Here, women internalize the gaze and learn to feel satisfied not only by others objectifying them in real life, but even by *fantasizing* about objectification. None of the realities of these professions—where women often face controlling pimps and the potential for sexual violence—informed women's fantasies about stripping and prostitution.

Guilt about the dissonance between sexual fantasies and feminist identities represented another common theme for women. For example, Julie, age 23, who coordinated a domestic violence program and identified strongly as a feminist, mentioned such conflicts:

> I fantasize about bondage and discipline and things like that. I do have fantasies sometimes about forced sex, but it's not real. I think because I really know the difference. Because I've been raped myself, it means I can safely have those fantasies, and it doesn't necessarily mean that I want to be raped. It just means that I like the idea of playing with power dynamics and relinquishing control . . . I feel conflicted and shameful about it sometimes, particularly because I have my women's studies degree, and I coordinate an assault response program. I'm not sure how my liking of BDSM squares with my feminism. That's hard to do.

Nora, age 23, another self-described sex-positive feminist, also admitted to serious conflicts about her fantasies and her feminist beliefs:

> I like a lot of sexual fantasies. I enjoy fulfilling men's sexual fantasies. My own personal fantasies have been these forced sex things, almost prostitute-esque fantasies, and these weird things, these very sex slave type things. I've also had fantasies about art, fantasies about voyeurism, fantasies about being objectified basically . . . I am sort of perplexed still about the appeal of really getting off on this sex slave, totally dominated stuff. I'd look at it with this rosy lens trying to transform it into a positive thing, but maybe that's just to squelch some of the dissonance and make it so I don't have to feel guilty or shameful about it. This is what gets me off, but it is kind of weird for me with the political views I have.

Forty-five-year-old Susan, another self-described feminist, also admitted confusion and guilt about her S&M fantasies:

> I fantasize about being told what to do, being tied up a little bit, a little spanking, that kind of thing . . . Thinking about the

S&M thing, I realize I'm on the late end of the feminist thing, and it can be degrading to women. I do a lot of work with domestic violence, and it's like, how could I think that it would be fun to get spanked when I'm totally against people hitting each other? How is that different? It's different because it's consensual, and it's not designed to have pain as much as a sensation, but sometimes I have a hard time reconciling that. How can I be so publicly against this thing and then have this whole private life?

When feminist women report rape fantasies, this directly contradicts the earlier argument that rape fantasies allow women from sexually repressed environments to express themselves via rape fantasies. In this case, with women who generally feel quite sexually liberated, aware of their bodies, agentic in their lives as women, etc., how does one explain their relationship to coercion fantasies? Maybe these fantasies signify that they do not feel sexually repressed or held back in their real lives. If fantasies function as a sign of what women do not get in "real life," then fantasies of coercion may reflect that 1) these women feel generally empowered and in control in their lives and 2) the fantasies serve as a way to validate the *differentness* of their cognitions about sex compared with their experiences of sex. In this way, coercion fantasies may indicate the distance and dissonance between women's relationships and their coercion fantasies.

Conversely, feminists reporting rape fantasies may indicate that they were socialized within a framework that encouraged women's submission to male sexual desires and needs, and were then drawn to feminism as a means to understand this and empower themselves. Thus, rape fantasies may serve as a remnant of their earlier sexual socialization rather than a symbol of their distance from oppression in their current lives. In any case, women are mentally oriented toward domination and submission fantasies, a finding worthy of future research.

Coercion fantasies may also represent internalized sexism in a quite literal form. Even those women who felt empowered in most or all other aspects of their lives nevertheless eroticized patriarchal and misogynistic messages found in mainstream media and pornography, even for those women who described strongly feminist belief systems. Coercion fantasies may, in essence, revert women back to a time when their sole sexual purpose was to embrace their submissive, receptive, passive, nonagentic role. Rape fantasies may work to actively situate women within a paradigm of powerlessness. In short, if women make political, social, economic, and sexual progress, their fantasies reflect just the opposite. If women eroticize and condone violence against them, it effectively "keeps them in their place." Much in the same way that the internalization of homophobia keeps the queer community politically deferential to the heterosexual majority and therefore beholden to a politics of self-hatred, the continued generation of coercive sexual fantasies holds women in line with more traditional and regressive gender norms. While both serve as *adaptations* to social inequity, and as such do not suggest "false consciousness" per se, they both reveal that oppressed people *cannot escape* the systems of power (male dominance, heterosexism, etc.) they exist within. Theoretically, then, even if *structural* misogyny was eliminated during sex, women still remain stuck with the power-laden content of their minds. As Aimé Césaire (2000) said, "It is equally necessary to decolonize our minds, our inner life, at the same time that we decolonize society."

Narratives about Pornography

> Sexuality is simultaneously a domain of restriction, repression, and danger as well as a domain of exploration, pleasure, and agency. To focus only on pleasure and gratification ignores the patriarchal structure in which women act, yet to speak only of sexual violence and oppression ignores women's experiences with sexual agency and choice.
> —Vance, *Pleasure and Danger: Exploring Women's Sexuality*

Because sexual fantasy and pornography so often overlap—that is, women's fantasies reflect the same scripts that appear in pornography—both *represent* the paradigms of *power* (male), *powerlessness* (female), and the *complexities of gendered pleasure*. Sexual fantasy and pornography inform each other and point to some alarming parallels in women's lives. For example, the narratives below show that women overwhelmingly recognize that mainstream pornography (especially porn designed for male audiences) degrades women, yet women generate similar images and stories in their own fantasy lives. How should one read such cognitive dissonance? How do women resolve such dissonance, or do they? Might their validation or viewing of pornography function as performance, just as sexual fantasies perform and perhaps further entrench women's powerlessness?

While some women expressed conflicts about their sexual fantasies, nearly *all* women expressed conflicts about their consumption of, and the circulation of, pornography. Over two-thirds consumed pornography at least occasionally, and all expressed clear ideas about the political implications of pornography for women in the culture at large. On the negative side, women worried about young people consuming it (particularly adolescent boys), problematic constructions of gender in pornography (particularly degradation of women), and issues of consent and safety for sex workers. On the positive side, women felt that pornography could expand one's repertoire of sexual behavior, encourage better and more efficient masturbation, enhance partnered sex, and symbolize sexual freedom or liberation. No one described a universally positive view of pornography, for even Emily, who acted in pornographic films for her job, expressed reservations:

> Obviously I'm a porn fan. Larry Flynt is my personal hero. I love that man. But I can definitely understand how so many women would have these conflicted views about porn, just because of how most women are portrayed in porn. Although I decided to go do porn because I like porn, and I like watching it, I just wish that people who enjoyed it had better selections, that there were more female-positive, sex-positive people being friendly with each other in porn. The thing that bothers me the most about porn is the idea that liking different races is a fetish, and how they categorize anything outside of the porn Barbie doll as a fetish. There is definitely positive porn that helps promote healthy sexuality and all, but it's hard to find because it's buried in so much trash. Also, pornography is an easy one to attack and pinpoint because it's so extreme, but I personally feel like I'm more offended just by watching TV, seeing how women and their relationships are defined in mass

media and that's being broadcast everywhere, brainwashing people. Porn isn't any worse than most of the sitcoms on TV right now.

The lack of universal, positive support for pornography suggests that, even for women who did not identify as feminist, they perceived pornography as helping to usher in troubling constructions of gender and power. Women disliked the treatment of women in pornography. For example, Susan said, "Even though I like porn, and I personally sometimes use it, I think that it adds a lot to objectification of women and the idea that that's what we should look like. I think women see it and think that they're supposed to look that way, and that's disturbing." Fiona, age 24, agreed, taking particular issue with the mistreatment of women and the lopsidedness of the pleasure: "I've had mixed views of pornography over the years. Now I'm definitely more critical depending upon the type and how the woman is treated, you know, the submissiveness and high heels and the pain of that versus mutual enjoyment."

Many women reacted negatively to the images of women presented in pornography, expressing a wish for a different sort of pornography that did not blatantly oppress women. For example, Mitra wished for different kinds of representation:

Pornography is not something that I'm into. I think that some of it definitely turns my stomach, and maybe if someone that I was involved with, someone who was really into something that I found incredibly disturbing, that would upset me. It would just be nice to see some different perspectives besides *Hustler* or whatever.

Geena, age 51, also called for *better* pornography:

I think in some ways pornography is a way for women to have their sexual power. However, the way that men use sexuality and exploit women for their sexual power, I think that's perverted. When it's all about women being tied down and men being in charge, it's bad. In my younger days, I would joke about having a women-run company, a pornography company by women, for women, and about women. It would be a way for women to express themselves in that medium without feeling exploited or without feeling used and degraded.

Ciara, who occasionally watched porn with her husband, also wanted more woman-friendly porn available: "I was watching a show today about porn made for women by women and porn made for men by men, and even the people who are antipornography agreed that pornos made for women by women were more acceptable and had better messages. I think so too. The porn we have now is just not very fun. I feel like my husband is just watching it for himself, so he can be erect when we have sex." While women desired more women-friendly porn based on themes of equality and mutual respect, their fantasies most often reflected themes of women's degradation and powerlessness. This contradiction indicates that pornography in its current form *does* correlate with women's fantasies of their own powerlessness, though that relationship might be *causal* too, in that pornography directly influences fantasies (Schauer, 2005). It may also suggest that women-friendly, women-positive porn might not have the market these women expect it would have given the degree of internalized sexism women contend with. If women, let alone men, remain erotically invested in images and stories of submission and powerlessness, this may perpetuate the porn industry as it currently exists.

For issues of regulating and distributing pornography, several women voiced concerns over freedom of expression issues; even if they did not like pornography, they disliked censorship even more. Kate expressed reservations about who would regulate porn:

I don't understand how it's arousing, like I look at a lot of it, and it just seems to me like a lot of these women look very desperate in the sense that they don't look healthy. I don't know what it's doing for men, but obviously there must be some power or control issue here. For me, I don't ever think that you can argue for pornography on its own merits. I think you have to look at issues of censorship, and *that* I have a huge issue with. I don't agree with censorship. I mean, there's the exploitation of children, yes, but at the same time, who gets to decide about these things? Sometimes we censor things because we're homophobic, and that's not right.

Melanie also felt mostly against censorship but wary of pornography and its impact on women:

> What do you consider pornography? How much freedom of expression should you grant to pornography which depicts forced sex? I think that it encourages a kind of predatory view towards women or a demeaning view. I guess it isn't just the rape sites. It's the slew of sites, the majority of heterosexual sites, and I include girl-on-girl sites that target heterosexual males as their audience, straight sites that call women "sluts." Women are presented as dumb bimbos, and all you know about them is that 22-year-old Suzie really, really wants to suck your cock. I don't feel good about that. But do I feel they should be illegal? I don't know. I wish that a lot of them weren't around, but I don't know that they should be illegal. There's some Japanese bondage stuff that I think is some incredibly well-composed, elegant, arousing shit, but that's violence against women, well, maybe not violence but subjugation. That offends me far, far less than "Fill these co-ed sluts with cum." It's so complicated.

On the other hand, Priya also felt partially in favor of censorship because of conflicts about her consumption of pornography:

> Sometimes I feel like censorship might not be a very bad thing in terms of the exploitation we have to see. I don't like things that just totally disrespect women. I'm not saying that all pornos should be of two people falling in love or something like that. I have watched it before and sometimes been aroused by it, but I've also watched things where it's like this guy is taking advantage of drunk college girls, and I look at that, and it gets to me. The girls don't look happy. It rubs me the wrong way.

Ruth also felt more in favor of censorship, drawing a divide between pornography and erotica:

> Even though I've read some erotic literature, I'd rather not see pornography out there. I think it uses and degrades women, and a lot of people make a lot of money on it, which I think is sad because it's the baser part of our society.

Some women expressed concern about the destructive effects of pornography on different segments of society, indicating that pornography summons women's opinions about class-based inequalities (Parvez, 2006). Some women mentioned concern for women's health and safety in pornography, thinking of the issue more related to the workers themselves. Maria's views on pornography revolved around the concept of class consciousness and labor:

> I'm all about porn and porn unions. It's sex work, not sex acts really. It's a job, and as long as the people that are performing in the videos are taken care of, and it's their choice, that's fine. I think we should make it a law to use condoms in porn because a lot of kids watch it, and they see these hot beautiful actors not using anything. That's a bad message.

Brynn expressed concern about the health of the workers, wondering how the lack of routine health care for porn actors has affected the pornography industry:

> I don't have a problem with porn. It may satisfy some people's pleasure or fantasies or what have you. There are some porn stars who, this being their everyday lifestyle, it's not a big deal to them, but I do think that they need to have a much higher medical background check or see doctors more often to get medical treatment because so many porn stars contract AIDS.

Interestingly, some women imagined the porn stars as actual human beings with their own needs, desires, and lives, while others constructed the porn stars as strictly in the realm of fantasy. This may have influenced their ideas about how pornography functions in their lives and in the lives of others.

This difference between seeing porn stars as people and seeing them as fantasy projections may also contribute to women's concerns for *who* watches and consumes pornography. Concern for adolescent boys' and men's consumption of pornography, as well as young women's consumption of pornography, appeared repeatedly in these discussions, as women worried what messages porn sent to the sexually inexperienced. Bonnie, age 51, expressed concern for her son: "My son spends a lot of time on the computer, and he's Googling stuff and was typing in some stuff and doing searches. I'm afraid he'll type in some word and get some strange thing. I'm not for any kind of censorship, but I would like for him to not accidentally stumble across it." Charlene framed her concern more as directed toward young people in general:

> I don't think that there's necessarily anything wrong with looking at pictures of naked people. I guess it's how they're used when people aren't really educated about it. A lot of times pornography affects young people, boys especially. A lot of times for young boys, their first experience of women is seeing them in pornography. If they don't talk to someone about it, they might think that they should be able to treat women in a certain way, or they may see women in a degrading way. Kids need to be educated about it.

Dawn also had concerns about pornography's effects on young people, framing sex-positive sex education as a tool for limiting the damaging effects of pornography:

> I think there's a distortion that happens when somebody of a younger age is exposed to a lot of stuff. As human beings once again we have a wide range of expression, and let's hope we can have some maturity and discernment. We don't let children smoke cigarettes or have alcohol, so let's not let children have access to things in pornography, particularly nonconsensual acts.

If you have a really good foundation of sex-positive education
to start out with, then pornography might not be as damaging.

In addition to these concerns about younger people, some women
expressed concern about the impact of porn on their adult male partners or friends. Edie said:

I do think it allows for more men to get the conscious or sub-
conscious idea that maybe all women should want to have anal
sex, and all women should want to make out with another
woman, and all these things you see so commonly in pornography. There's some porn out there that caters to people who
would be arrested if they actually engaged in these things! I
don't like to think of my boyfriend staring at a screen masturbating to it. It just seems strange or weird, like a lack of emotions or intellect.

Charlotte also worried about pornography's impact on adult men and
women: "I think pornography can warp your sense of reality, and it just
fuels predators, fuels them to be crazier than what they already are."
    Women did not always portray pornography as a fully detrimental
force. Positive constructions of pornography also appeared, even when
paired with various reservations about pornography's impact on sexual
socialization. Most often, women discussed pornography as having the
potential to both entertain and help women explore new ideas about
sex. For example, Niko mentioned that it can enhance women's sex
lives and serve as a teaching tool:

Porn is something where you can know what possibilities there
are, how many positions and things people can do and everything. I use it, and I think if both people are comfortable with
it, it can enhance your sex life, and it's a good thing. I think it
can help people discover more about themselves, like their fantasies and their sex practices. On the other hand, they might
pay more attention to getting off rather than paying attention
to when they're with their actual partner. People should work

on paying attention to how to make their partner feel good, so it doesn't have a negative impact on actual real life sex.

Women also mentioned that pornography can lead to self-discovery and entertainment. Lucy described the ways it could help young people learn about sex:

> I don't see pornography as a bad thing, because I see it as a tool. It's a way for young men and boys to learn for themselves through masturbation what they like, and there are more women looking at porn now as a means of getting sexually excited. I personally have used porn and, when I met my husband, I had more porn than he did. I'm all for it. I think if it works for you, great, and if for some reason it's not your taste, then you don't have to purchase it.

Jasmine also offered a positive view of porn as an educational tool: "It's a nice outlet whether you just want to watch it, get aroused, or watch it with a partner. I think it's good for other people as well because they may not know what to do. They may not have any ideas about what's going on, and this is a way for them to learn things and educate themselves. It's a win-win."

Finally, some sex-positive and feminist women described pornography as a form of resistance to this culture's repressive messages or patriarchal restrictions. Julie, who studied sex and feminism while in college, likened porn to sexual liberation:

> I identify as a sex-positive feminist and sort of contrary to the Catharine MacKinnon and Andrea Dworkin anti-porn camp. I don't subscribe to that. I think that pornography can be a valid form of artistic expression like a first amendment sort of thing. Feminism doesn't have to be asexual. It doesn't have to mean being gender neutral. It can also include femininity and a lot of different things. It's about freedom and about liberation and allowing people to experience fantasy and life as they see fit, not having that be dictated by a dominant paradigm. Pornography

can be really feminist, like a good entryway into exploring one's own sexuality, particularly when you're new to sexuality. It can also be arousing and used in masturbation and self-exploration.

Julie's point about sex positivity and its relationship to pornography presents a compelling question: Are women, particularly feminists, stuck with only two choices—liking pornography or disliking pornography? If women reject the MacKinnon/Dworkin position that pornography oppresses and degrades women and deserves censorship, must they then embrace the position that pornography is a universally good thing?

Problems of the performative appeared in women's discussions of pornography, as they overwhelmingly felt dissatisfied with the available pornographic options they encountered, yet generally disapproved of making porn illegal or censored in any way (except with regard to legal age). This sentiment indicates several recent shifts in women's sexual imagination: 1) Women watch and consume pornography much more readily than they previously did; as such, they expand the existing audience for pornography and largely reject the more radical feminist view that pornography degrades and violates women; 2) in large part because of the internet, pornography has become accessible to those who previously did not have much access to it, including women, young people, and minors; 3) women sometimes say that they learn about sex from pornography, revealing the way that pornography has become not only a socializing tool but also a teaching tool; 4) women may feel pressure to *not* reject pornography, perhaps because they face performative pressures to like and enjoy sex that follow mainstream scripts of gendered behavior.

These shifts indicate that mediated sexuality has an increasingly prominent role in women's lives, resulting in curious contradictions worthy of future exploration. *Women enacted in their fantasies the very stories they criticized in pornography.* Women argued against pornography as a socializing tool for young people, and yet they claimed to socialize themselves with pornography as a good educational tool. Women argued against the expansion of the pornography industry at the same time that they claimed to purchase and consume pornography (both alone and with partners). Such contradictions hone in on the very crux of gendered performance: Women must still restrict their sexual expression, even while acting out and playing along with patriarchal demands placed upon them. This may serve an adaptive function, in that embracing pornography allows them to perform as sexually liberated women who comply with patriarchal demands, or it may represent, as commonly seen with many lower status groups, women directly contradicting their interests. Either way, such dual performances appeared consistently enough to render them normative.

CONCLUSION

> As soon as we regard this femininity as a fantasy-product of conflicts within a field of reason that has been assimilated to masculinity, we can no longer set any store by liberating its voice. We will not speak pidgin to please the colonialists.
> —Le Doeuff, *L'Imaginaire Philosophique*

The dangers of conflating empowerment and liberation with pornography and sexual fantasy are evident in this chapter, as women's fantasy lives (and the fantasy lives they watch and consume with pornography) reveal a great deal about women's social, political, economic, and relational status. These results suggest that most women have some access to pornography, which begs the question: How much does pornography and its accompanying narratives affect women's sexual fantasy constructions? In other words, does the increased use and circulation of pornography affect women's fantasy lives, or does pornography serve as a reflection of the discourses that already exist?

The point can be argued either way and is one that must be taken up in future research. To restate an earlier claim, women's fantasies, particularly dominance and submission fantasies where women submit and men dominate, suggest one of two things: First, such fantasies may reflect what is *not* happening in their daily lives. Dominance and submission fantasies may indicate that women lead more egalitarian lives and that power differentials between women and their partners have lessened (though no evidence directly suggests this from the interviews). Similarly, romance fantasies may reflect the lack of romance women experience as older adults. These claims perhaps offer the more encouraging, hopeful, idealized, and less likely interpretations. A second explanation for the frequency of women's domination fantasies holds that women generate these fantasies in order to keep themselves in positions of powerlessness and submission within their real lives. Fantasies about powerful strangers or group sex may serve a similar function, as women recreate stereotypes about their gender roles in these scenarios. One might imagine that sexual fantasy narratives could offer women the opportunity to reimagine their sexualities outside of the constraints of patriarchal culture; for example, what would it mean to imagine one's erotic life without the requirements of a partner? Could this open up new avenues for self-affirmation and erotic creativity? Yet, consistently, women's fantasies reflected an even more powerful internalization of patriarchal norms than did their sexual practices and behaviors. One must wonder, then: Do fantasies of submission and powerlessness represent an intense form of internalized sexism? Do they reflect the extent to which women are "kept in their place"? Are women simply *performing* their erotic submission in their heads, sustaining themselves as passive, receptive, submissive, and degraded? Further still, are fantasies simply whimsical or silly and therefore not at all representative of "real life"?

These questions illuminate possibilities for why women consume pornography even when they express serious reservations about its negative of women. Much like sexual fantasies of dominance and control, the consumption of pornography fuses together erotic stimuli with the mainstream (patriarchal, misogynistic) message that men have the *right* to consume, use, and exploit women's bodies at will. Indeed, though some pornography escapes these trends, particularly women-friendly pornography, most pornography includes a great deal of content about women's second-class status in sex: the near total lack of regard for authentic female orgasm (apparently, endless moaning now stands in for climax); the performative expulsion of semen onto women's faces at the end of the scene ("money shot" or "facial"); and the explosion of films that depict acts that can physically harm women (e.g., rough anal sex, sex without proper lubrication, fisting, placement of objects in women's vaginas and anuses, scenes depicting double penetration, etc.). So, if women learn about sex from these images or have partners who have socialized themselves into sex via pornography, sex involving more equal power dynamics, mutual respect, or emotional connection fall further and further out of focus.

This is not to suggest that all women enjoy or consume pornography—or that all women enjoy fantasies of domination and submission—but very few women claimed to *not* enjoy dominance/submission fantasies and/or pornography. Only a small handful of women frankly said that those elements of sexuality did not interest them. (Further, only a few women described romance fantasies, and these mostly centered on their escape from domestic life rather than a grounded desire for egalitarian relationships.) Might women's interest in submission fantasies itself signify a kind of performance, where women feel they must express openness to images and paradigms of women's powerlessness?

Some evidence in support of this claim resides in chapter 4, as the striking dissonance between what women actually enjoyed with partners, compared with what they fantasized about, serves as evidence of the complicated paradoxes women experience, particularly with performances of pleasure. A central finding of this chapter argues that *women's fantasies rarely reflected the experiences they found the most pleasurable and satisfying in their partnered sexual lives.* While themes of dominance, coercion, and violence appeared only intermittently in women's descriptions of partnered sexual pleasure, these themes took center stage in their fantasies. What does it mean that women found sexual objectification, physical violence, masochism, and rape satisfying in their fantasy lives, while themes of emotional connection, love, kindness, attentiveness, and newness appeared most prominently as the elements that they found physically pleasurable with partners? Overwhelmingly, women enjoyed mutuality and nurturance when describing their best sexual experiences, yet their fantasies included group sex (often with men present), romance (where men swept them off their feet), sex with men in positions of power (often with racist connotations), sex in taboo places, dominating others (particularly other women!), and being dominated or objectified. Further, women frequently described that when they attempted to act out their sexual fantasies in real life (e.g., attempting to have a threesome; dominance play), they frequently felt disappointed and sometimes even frightened or alarmed (see chapter 5).

Perhaps the culprit for this dissonance, the underlying cause of such a chasm between women's stated desires and their fantasies, stems from women living in a culture that demands precise kinds of gendered performances—as Audre Lorde would say, living from "outward within." Women overwhelmingly described their best sexual experiences as times when they did *not* perform submission, when they did *not* prioritize their (male) partner's needs over their own needs, when they *resisted* the cultural narrative of women as powerless, helpless, and devalued (see chapter 4). In sexual fantasy, however, women could not distance themselves as much from discourses of powerlessness, perhaps because fantasies more rapidly access cultural scripts about gender and power. Consequently, fantasies are more easily sucked into the vortex of gender inequality, fueled in part by the narratives of pornography and given even more momentum by underlying cultural narratives that not only fetishize but mandate women's lack of social, economic, political, and sexual power. However dismal this picture is with regard to the potential for sex to align with liberation politics, remember that women can derive pleasure from experiences other than extreme powerlessness, even if their fantasies often yank them back into submissive roles. This distance signifies an encouraging, albeit small, step toward rejecting conventional sexual scripts of women's sexual lives. After all, fantasy is fantasy—and people should not underestimate the political and social significance of it—but women's lived experiences matter a whole lot more.

CONCLUSION

> As a concept, sexuality is incapable of ready containment: it
> refuses to stay within its predesignated regions, for it seeps
> across boundaries into areas that are apparently not its own
> . . . It infests all sorts of other areas in the structures of
> desire. It renders even the desire not to desire, or the desire
> for celibacy, as sexual . . . It refuses to accept the contain-
> ment of the bedroom or to restrict itself to only those
> activities which prepare for orgasmic pleasure. It is exces-
> sive, redundant, and superfluous in its languid and fervent
> overachieving. It always seeks more than it needs, performs
> excessive actions, and can draw any object, any fantasy, any
> number of subjects and combinations of their organs, into
> its circuits of pleasure.
>
> —Grosz, *Volatile Bodies*

THE QUESTION of *performance*, of living in reference to our cultural
scripts and norms—particularly what it means in women's sexual
lives—carries with it a host of other questions. Namely, in taking up the
problem of women performing sex, we must also consider the associated problems of defining performance, naming and reframing inequalities, and moving toward sexual liberation and sexual freedom. Who
defines resistance, progress, and movement forward? How can people
name and imagine sexual empowerment? Certainly, women struggle to
negotiate the remnants of sexually repressive histories with the
onslaught of new sexual quandaries they now face. Of all the dangerous
patterns I have observed with women and sexuality, the one that seems

275

the most urgently problematic and troubling—and one that my inter-
viewees expressed conflict about—is the cultural tendency to twist and
corrupt empowerment discourses so that they become clichéd, commodified, detrimental, and ultimately disempowering. Over and over,
the various answers feminists and progressives have for sexual oppression—behavioral shifts, cultural shifts, political mobilizations, and so
on—are dismissed, co-opted, and dislocated from their original meanings. The minute people *name* various solutions to women's sexual disempowerment, those solutions enter a paradigm that leads almost
inevitably to their cooptation by dominant discourse.

This is not to suggest that naming solutions and working toward
enacting them is politically insignificant. In fact, the women's movement has historically brought about profound changes for the way society constructs and regulates gender. A little over four decades ago, consider this brief sampling of laws that had *not yet passed*: formal
recognition of marital rape as a form of sexual violence, Title 9 legislation, maternity laws preventing discrimination based on pregnancy
status, women having entitlement to serve as jurors in all states, women
having full rights to their property (as the law still defined men as the
"head and master" of women's property until 1981), and sexual harassment legislation in the workplace. Further still, consider this (nonex-
haustive) list of barriers women faced: women could not seek safe and
legal abortions, want-ads were segregated by gender (with "jobs for
women" earning notably less pay), women could not sit in business class
on airplanes, women faculty could not enter most faculty clubs at universities, doctors prescribed birth control pills exclusively to married
women, women had little access to sex toys and minimal access to
accurate information about sex and heath, institutionalized feminist
publications did not yet exist, women rarely served as politicians, inter-
racial marriages were still prohibited in some states, Take Back the
Night rallies did not exist, women's studies and gender studies programs
did not exist, and the American Psychiatric Association still classified
homosexuality as a diagnosable mental illness. In my study, nearly *all*
women I interviewed said that feminism and the women's movement
had made it easier for them to be sexual, regardless of whether they
personally identified as a feminist. These hard won advances, however
distorted or coopted they have sometimes become, certainly do matter
and have undoubtedly improved women's lives in myriad ways.

And yet, as the previous seven chapters argue, women still suffer from enormous barriers to their full sexual empowerment, even while resistance and empowerment break through in small moments. When observing and recording women's negotiations of power relations through sex, we find that women have fallen woefully short of meeting the idealized egalitarian visions of our foremothers. The picture is, at times, rather bleak: Women struggle to negotiate their sexual needs, desires, and preferences in light of cultural scripts that prioritize men's (and phallocentric) sexuality. Women struggle to feel empowered in sexual relationships, and consequently, many of their performances of sex speak to the conflicts and contradictions they have inherited. They construct their partners as "giving" them orgasms and often pretend to "receive" orgasm in order to satisfy partners. They hook up with other women at parties in order to fit in with their friends and, particularly for heterosexual women, titillate observing men. They express frustration with their waning or underperforming sexual desire and articulate willingness to medicate their sexual responses in order to feel sexually normal or to please others. They argue for the primacy of sex with love and yet have difficulty labeling or fully understanding the coercion they have experienced (particularly if someone they loved committed violence against them). They minimize the significance of sexual assault and sometimes feel flattered by street harassment. They fantasize about submission and powerlessness or construct racist and stereotyped erotic narratives, often with much guilt and anguish. Even when they escape some of these things—by finding new ways of experiencing their sexuality, connecting with progressive and nonstereotyped partners, resisting and fighting back—they rarely escape these conflicts and performances in their entirety. Collectively, these signs do not point toward a liberated sexuality for women; rather, these symptoms speak to the tremendous conflicts women experience when negotiating, on the one hand, the progressive changes they inherited from previous generations of feminists combined with, on the other hand, the newer and more pernicious forms of disempowerment sneaking into their lives.

In experiencing these contradictions, women struggle to resolutely improve their sexual lives. Each potential solution is tainted with the potential for disappointment and destruction, even as it offers glimmers of hope. For example, for years it has been argued that "sex positivity" would serve as an answer to American culture's repressive "Victorian" past. If people embraced sexuality and honored its potential for pleasure and subversiveness in their lives, some argued, they could overcome their antisex, repressed past and instead push forward into the future with erotic gusto. Yet, despite the progress that sex positivity has inspired (e.g., performance art, consciousness raising groups about sex, increasing visibility for sexual communities, better sex education, deconstruction of "normal" and "abnormal" sex, etc.), negative consequences have remained. As seen many times before, the *logic* of the sex positive movement has been mangled and distorted as a means to justify all sorts of antifeminist constructs, particularly a kind of sexual free-for-all that refuses to differentiate, even theoretically, politically suspicious sexual acts from those sexual acts that may facilitate more power for women. The impact of sex positivity is limited by the ways it has sometimes been discursively used to justify rather outrageous power imbalances and gender stereotypes (e.g., selling one's virginity online as a sex positive act; normalizing BDSM based on notions of consent rather than power implications; ignoring the fundamental economic imbalances of sex work, etc.). By fighting so hard against the specter of sexual repression, feminists no longer ask certain questions, particularly: *Do women want this kind of change? Do these forms of expression help to rectify and reverse the fundamental inequalities women face?* Collective visions for change have erupted into the prioritization of sexual freedom of expression at the expense of tough conversations about political solidarity. While the original intent of the sex-positive movement had goals in line with feminist politics, its cooptation by patriarchal forces leaves people in a bewildering state of wondering if, and where, certain political, social, and sexual lines can be drawn.

Thus, sexual politics progresses and then regresses; impulses toward liberation push forward and then pull back. The story of our mothers and grandmothers, while in many ways different than our story, has elements of the same dynamic at play. These seven chapters have relied upon the concept of 'performance' to address this particular cycle that repeatedly diminishes the impact of progressive social change: First, cultural, sexual, and social scripts often tell women to accept, endure, and resign themselves to a sexual life bound to traditional gender roles; second, disempowerment ensues, and grievances about some aspect of women's sexuality reaches a peak; third, feminists and their allies recognize the problem and mobilize against its existence; fourth, parts of this mobilization become successful while other parts fail; fifth, after challenging oppressive forces and creating some positive changes, the resulting shifts take hold and stay put for a short time; and sixth, those with explicit power to control discourse (e.g., antifeminist forces, drug companies, media, schools, the Christian Right, etc.) aided by those who remain complicit with such shifts (e.g., women, their partners, etc.) corrupt, co-opt, undermine, counteract, and distort that change in order to revert women's sexuality back to the status quo. Though not entirely linear in this way, and not equally effective for all groups of women (particularly along race and class lines), this cycle often leads to different performances that reveal conflicts between empowerment and disempowerment. Perhaps as a survival mechanism, or perhaps because performance helps women negotiate for power in the face of relative powerlessness, this cycle repeats itself again and again.

For example, during the second wave of feminism during the 1960s and 1970s, outrage about psychoanalytic constructions of vaginal orgasm as superior to clitoral orgasm, combined with the general 1950s suppression of women's sexuality, led to serious mobilization during the sexual revolution to value the clitoral orgasm. Consciousness-raising groups, public demonstrations, antipsychoanalysis groups, and prolesbian organizations raised the issue by discussing the mythology of the vaginal orgasm and its political implications as a mechanism to normalize vaginal intercourse (and, consequently, heterosexuality) as the primary, or "normal," sex act. Yet, as the clitoral orgasm gained power, shortly thereafter, some radical feminists noticed that *demand* for orgasm, particularly from men to their women partners, trumped those empowerment narratives. Suddenly, instead of the clitoral orgasm representing a marker of sexual liberation and empowerment, clitoral orgasm was inscribed as a *new mandate* that women *must* have in order to make their partners feel like sexually capable and potent lovers. Thus, what once served as a possible mechanism for subversiveness and empowerment later became coopted in the name of demonstrating men's sexual expertise at the expense of women's sexual pleasure. The mandate for a visible/audible orgasm marked men's sexual prowess while it overshadowed women's sexual pleasure, thus bringing the cycle back around to the starting point, where women have little control over their terms of sexual empowerment. Consequently, as discussed in chapter 1, women increasingly report that they fake orgasm or otherwise exaggerate pleasure. Looking prospectively (and this is purely a theoretical gesture), the next "round" of orgasm empowerment and disempowerment may prioritize *multiple* orgasms as the new sign of liberation, followed by negative attributions to those women who do not experience multiple orgasms.

As another example (addressed in chapters 2 and 6 with performative bisexuality and women's sexual fantasies), while women's same-sex eroticism and voluntary jaunts into bisexuality have at times subverted heteronormativity and heterosexism, the subversive potential of same-sex eroticism too often serves the interests of *preserving* the status quo. Even supposed violations of compulsory heterosexuality—something that evokes ideas of *taboo* and *illicitness*—only end up *reinforcing* the compulsory nature of heterosexuality. One only need look at the commodified representations of lesbian sex—mainstream pornography featuring faux lesbians, *Girls Gone Wild*, reality shows featuring "lesbian" contestants, TV shows where actors briefly dabble in same-sex eroticism only to compulsorily return to heterosexual relationships, and so on—along with the more immediate pressures women face (e.g., performative bisexuality, pressures for threesomes, etc.) to see the array of possible distortions to empowerment discourse people face. This treacherous cycle of coopting, commodifying, and distorting women's empowerment strategies is a cruel hoax that threatens the mental, physical, and sexual well-being of women (and, in all likelihood, men). This cycle constructs empowerment for women as a moving target vulnerable to a constant line of setbacks, making it especially important for feminists and social justice advocates to keep a watchful and strategic eye on the newer and more insidious forms of disempowerment that arise *in response to* and *in light of* empowering social advances.

The ongoing tension between liberatory and repressive forces raises these questions: What does it mean to resist if resistance is soon coopted and turned against those who resist? If *performances* of sex do not always constitute explicit forms of resistance—many of the performances discussed in this book reflect women's lower status, disempowerment, and the successful imposition of patriarchy onto women's internal sexual scripts—what kinds of *progressive* resistance are possible?

NARRATIVES OF RESISTANCE

> There are no relations of power without resistances; the
> latter are all the more real and effective because they are
> formed right at the point where relations of power are
> exercised; resistance does not have to come from elsewhere
> to be real, nor is it inexorably frustrated through being the
> compatriot of power. It exists all the more by being in the
> same place as power, hence, like power, resistance is multiple
> ... The binary division between resistance and non-resist-
> ance is an unreal one.
>   —Michel Foucault, *Power/Knowledge*

Much in line with James Scott's (1990) idea of hidden or private resistances (or, as he said, "a privileged peek backstage or a rupture in the
performance" [p. 4]), women consistently engage in resistance strategies
that undermine the legitimacy of power relations between men and
women, either explicitly via their overt actions or implicitly via their
words or clandestine actions. Though one can easily read any of these
resistances as themselves troubling, or perhaps even reinforcing of different dominant power dynamics, they nevertheless serve as relevant
commentaries on a collective vision for change. The women I interviewed offered skillful and strategic ideas about how to resist hegemonic definitions of their sexuality, whether via *speaking* about sex
(which Foucault has argued is itself a form of resistance), rejecting certain stereotypes or characterizations of women's sexuality, acting in
resistant ways, or articulating visions of change. Though I did not ask
them directly about resistance, collective action, or specific ways they
had challenged power, these stories nevertheless appeared frequently
and in a variety of moments throughout the interviews. Notably, the
versions of resistance portrayed here are more individualistic *gestures
toward change* rather than the more literal actions or collective activist
work that sociological and psychological literatures have characterized
as resistance (Hollander & Einwohner, 2004). Conflicts between ideologies of self, relations with others, and visions for broader cultural
change converge in women's resistance narratives.

For example, when women explained their ideas about what they
saw as the greatest sexual myths in this culture, they responded by

promptly and swiftly debunking many of the messages women internalize, particularly about their own passivity, receptivity, and lack of sexual
desire. This shows that women *can* and often *do* debunk various myths,
recognize efforts to disempower women, and respond by creating new
narratives of resistance. For example, roughly a third of women
described the vaginal orgasm as a myth—something that would have
been nearly unheard of four decades ago. Susan said,

> I think the biggest myth, and this would apply to me in partic-
> ular, is that women are supposed to come when they have
> penile intercourse alone, because I truly think most women
> don't, and then they feel guilty if they need either their partner
> or themselves to masturbate in order to get some more direct
> stimulation on the clitoris. The whole vaginal orgasm thing is
> really about telling women that they need to be perfect, and it
> fits with this whole notion that women have to be shaved and
> perfumed and have this tight little stomach and melon breasts
> or else men don't find us attractive.

Along these lines, many women commented about their frustration
with the way society constructs women as less sexual than men. Nora
said,

> The biggest myth is the fucking Hollywood myth, women not
> realizing that they can reclaim sex for themselves and define it
> however they want, and that they can have the kind of sex and
> sexuality that they want. Women can choose to express and feel
> whatever they want. We need to create our own definitions and
> experiences so that we can be proud of sex.

Women reacted particularly strongly to the false idea of the double
standard between men and women regarding sexual desire. Geena
voiced her opposition to these sexual double standards by saying,

> The biggest myth is that somehow sex is not okay for women,
> but it's okay for men. You know, that double standard that sex is
> not ladylike, or it's slutty. Even saying that makes me angry. It's

like 'sex light' for women, robust sex for men, but 'sex light' for women. You can have some sex but it has to be contained and measured and feminine. It has to be in a box.

Julie also expressed frustration at the denial of women as sexual beings:

It's a myth that women don't have strong sexual desire, that it's men who always want to have sex and have the strong sexual desire. Of all the women I know, it's just not the case. The consequence of that myth is that women can't feel open and honest about their desire because it's abnormal, or they'll be viewed as sluts or whores. It's that double standard, because men who want lots of sexual partners and are very sexual are looked upon as very masculine and conquerors, while women are looked upon as bad, dirty women.

Emily also talked about these gender stereotypes as troubling, again articulating a firm belief that women *possess their own desire*:

It really bothers me how people focus so much on saying that the guys are the gas, the girls are the brakes, or whatever, and like everything is this huge gender dichotomy where women are supposed to act this way about sex, and men are supposed to act this way about sex, that people are supposed to act a certain way based on what's between their legs.

In addition to critiquing sexual dichotomies and gender stereotypes, women also expressed the desire to resist the current system of sex education and dissemination of knowledge about sex, whether via abstinence-only education or, to a lesser degree, "comprehensive" sex education. Kate took issue with both:

I hate that women learn that there are certain benchmarks they have to reach, certain ideas about basic sexual health even. I wish we talked a lot more about sex in a social way, especially with young people. We learned the basic biological information about penetrative heterosexual intercourse, and that's it. Nothing about what men do together, what women do together, what the range of things that people can do together might be. Or even the bigger questions of, you know, what is sexuality? How does this relate to the way we feel about our bodies? How does this relate to society or culture or history? It's so important because sex does inform our sense of selves.

Dawn provided a more specific critique of the various kinds of misinformation promoted in this culture, saying that sex negativity has taken a serious toll on women's sexuality:

> I wish people had more information about sex, orgasm, birth control, STDs. I wish people had more accurate information about the fact that you can have pleasure without guilt, shame, or blame, that it's okay to be attracted to a member of your same sex, that it doesn't make you bad or wrong or condemned to hell . . . The myth that it's not okay to enjoy our bodies is a big one. Or that it's hard to have an orgasm. The general myth in our culture that sex is bad—what a heartbreak that is! Or that if you're not young and beautiful and don't look a certain way, then you won't have sexual experiences. It could be nothing more opposite of that.

Reacting to sexual mythology represents a way that women can label, and then resist, certain cultural narratives, particularly ones that inscribe sex as dirty and shameful or that promote ideologies of women as sexually inferior to, or less sexually motivated than, men. Other myths that women debunked included: oral sex not "counting" as real sex, older women not having sex after menopause, larger penises resulting in better sex, lack of orgasm resulting in lack of overall pleasure, women not masturbating (or masturbating less than men), and people's beliefs that homosexuality was sinful, troubling, or perverted. A few women also mentioned that they wanted to assert themselves as feminists while also engaging in sexual acts of submission. Jill said, "One thing that people are often misinformed about is that being a submissive in the bedroom does not necessarily mean that one is either not a feminist or a submissive in the rest of life. You can be a feminist and still want your boyfriend to handcuff you to the bed each night."

Women's descriptions of the positive and negative aspects of being "sexual women" in this particular cultural moment also represented another mode of potential resistance, as they outlined the specific challenges they saw themselves and other women facing right now. In particular, women expressed a keen awareness of the conflicts between inheriting a history of sexual repression while simultaneously feeling pressured to have a lot of sex with a lot of different partners. Jill articulated this "virgin/whore" theme directly:

> Sometimes it feels like there are a lot of forces in society that are trying to make it an either/or proposition, like either you are a pure, innocent virgin until marriage and then faithful to your husband until death do you part, or you're a slut who will sleep with anything that asks. It feels like in a lot of things people try to make issues black or white, either one way or another. Either you're straight, or you're gay. Either you're a virgin or a whore. Either you're a good girl or a bad girl. It makes it feel sort of awkward to be in an in-between state.

Emily argued a similar logic about the hazards of the "virgin/whore" paradigm, saying,

> I think we're all sexual beings, whether we admit it or not. I feel like being comfortable with my sexuality makes everything in my life seem so much easier. I mean, it's definitely hard always fighting against all of the stereotypes about women, who are supposed to be either really good or really bad, and the whole good girl/bad girl thing is definitely confusing. It's very frustrating at times, but I think that being open sexually is definitely rewarding enough to be worth it.

Lucy agreed, saying that these cultural dichotomies do not serve women and that they should be debunked: "I think that it is difficult either way, because if you're not a sexual woman in the culture nowadays, then you're seen as a prude. If you're not open to things, at least to a certain extent, you're going to be looked at by other people as being the odd one out."

Still, many women directly expressed that sex has dramatically improved for women in the last half century. In expressing such an assessment, some argued that sex felt less repressed, more open, and more full of possibilities compared to previous generations' experiences of sex. Shonda compared herself to her grandmother's generation: "At least we're more knowledgeable than we were back in the 20s and 30s, and women can practically do whatever they want. They're not considered a bad name because they're women. Everything is more or less coming out into the open." Brynn reveled in the idea that she could express her sexuality openly:

> There are a lot of people that are a little more accepting of sex now. You don't have to worry about being poked fun at, or told that you're different, or worrying about what other people think. You can just kind of go out there and be who you really are, love yourself for it, and not be ashamed of it. You can be prideful of it.

Themes of self-love and pride reverberated throughout women's stories of how their sexualities compared with previous generations' sexualities. Bonnie reveled in the sexual freedoms she saw for women today: "You get to be whatever you want or do whatever you want. You can wear and experience whatever you want. There's a real openness. I'm gonna do what I want to do and no one's gonna tell me what to do." These statements indicate that women perceived themselves as having the ability to express themselves sexually in a culture that historically suppressed women's sexuality.

Themes of direct empowerment through embracing women-only spaces and directly rebelling against patriarchy also appeared when women described being sexual women today. Dawn claimed that recognizing the *power* of women's sexuality represented an act of subversion and rebellion:

> Sex today is like being a subversive. There are many times I feel like I've gotten this secret key, and I am so powerful, but man,

our country doesn't want anyone to know that. It's hard being a feminist and womanist. I know that we are the creators of life, and we women really hold this space of sacredness and spirituality, that we are the *source*. But boy, my experience has been that our greater culture doesn't want to hear all of that stuff. It feels so beautiful to get to discuss it, talking amongst ourselves like we're doing together right now. I think there's another stratum of our culture that's very envious of women talking about their sexuality together. I definitely think that there's a part of the masculine dominant culture that is perhaps both in awe of women's power and also wants to take it away. I have taught other women how to have an orgasm, and to me, that's a powerful role to play.

The power of *talking* about sexuality also appeared in Maria's responses:

It's hard to talk about sex because people think we're sluts and hos, that just because we have sex, we're easy. I told my sister before I came here that I was participating in a sex study, and she said, "Oh my God, no!" and she's older than me! To edu-cate other women that don't really know anything about sex is powerful.

Geena argued that sex itself can empower women and help them reconnect with their bodies, saying,

Sex is fun, and it's empowering. It does wonders for your self-esteem, and I think physiologically it's a good thing for you to be a sexual person. I think it's good for stress, good for cramps, and I think that my attitude is generally better if I'm having some kind of active sex life, whether by myself or with other people. You have to like yourself to masturbate, I think.

From the perspective of younger women, Dorothy identified a progress narrative about sexuality in relation to having control and autonomy over her sexual self:

I think sex is a liberating thing. Maybe it's gone to an extreme with *Sex and the City* where Samantha has 75 partners, but I think it represents control over your life and your body and yourself in general. I think it's really important that we can negotiate how we have sex with our partners. To have the gender equality in a relationship with physical contact should be a defining feature of our culture as a progressive culture. I'm really lucky that I can be in this society, and I can do what I want to do.

While many women expressed feelings of empowerment and joy about their relationship to sex, other women expressed more reluctance about it, particularly related to themes of feeling "trapped" in a culture that enforces double standards and devalues women in general. Their resistance, therefore, came in the form of recognizing and criticizing these traps. For example, Kate provided some insightful claims about the pros and cons of sex as a political gesture:

Because I don't identify with the very right-wing, Christian definition of sexuality, or the very religious definition of sexuality, I almost feel like it's my duty to be oppositional to that, to identify as a strongly sexual person or at least a person that has sex generally, outside of marriage or outside of those kinds of things. It's confusing, though. Just to be a young woman now means to be sexually adventurous, to have a lot of partners, and attached to that, being fashionable and doing well financially for yourself and having all kinds of wonderful romantic and material experiences. I think that sex can sometimes feel like something you're supposed to do to be fashionable.

Geena, who said that she felt that her 1970s generation had a more healthy relationship to sex than younger generations, said, "I'm really concerned about young women. I imagine that women are having way more sex than they really want to have in order to connect with somebody. They're not really liking it or getting satisfaction from it, but that's the context that the men have created for them so they're kind of falling into that." Esther also expressed concern about young women: "I think that in this day and age women are coerced more than ever. I think that society has allowed or even almost demands that women have sex because this is what men want."

Building on the themes of resistance already described above—particularly the refutation of sexual double standards, recognition of the complexities of modern sexual life, and assertion of women's sexuality as a break with a repressive past—women also articulated ideas about what they would like to change about this culture's relationship to women's sexuality. Women addressed and diagnosed the grievances and injustices they saw for women as a whole. These prescriptive claims highlighted the importance of *imagined change* as a key component of social justice for women. Happily, women described a long list of things they wanted to change about the way their culture treats women's sexuality. This included, most prominently, the belief that women should be treated with more respect and should have more decision-making power over what happens to their bodies. For example, Lucy called for an end to objectification: "I think that men so often view women as sexual objects that I think that's taken to a whole new extreme. In porn, men can dissect women's bodies and then women learn not to feel comfortable with themselves because they're always being dissected like that. Men kind of need to step up and stop doing that." Jasmine also voiced her opinions that women needed to have more bodily integrity and more freedom from men making decisions for them:

> I think men should leave women alone. It's their body; let them decide who they want to sleep with, if they want to get pregnant, because if men get someone pregnant, they're not responsible for anything. Why can't men back women up and let them be strong? Because a man could be wrong 100%, and another man will back him up, but that never happens with women. Men gang up on women all the time.

Women also wanted to see women's sexuality constructed as less "dirty" and more positive and affirming. Edie wanted women to see their bodies differently: "I wish that women didn't have to look so badly upon themselves for having sex. It's such a widespread idea for sex to be seen as dirty. I wish people would change their minds about that." Similarly, Niko argued against treating women as asexual or less sexual than men: "I think females have a stronger sexual drive than most people believe, so I think maybe to change that we have to acknowledge that women want sex too, as much as men, or maybe sometimes even more than men, so it's not just something they only want. We want to be able to enjoy sex too, and we're active too." Ciara focused her critique more specifically on the stigma of the single woman, saying, "We should be more accepting of single women. You don't have to be married to have a good time and have sex with a partner, so people look at that as being maybe like a ho or a slut, but I don't believe that."

Many women wanted changes in other aspects of their sexual lives as well, particularly around homophobic culture, legal shifts, and educational improvements. Janet talked specifically about her distaste for the way homophobia affected her personal life as a lesbian:

> What gays and lesbians do with each other is just their business. It's nobody else's business. I really just wish that I could get married, and I wish that I had benefits like a straight couple would have if they got married. I care about this person, and I want to make sure that everything is okay with this person until the day I die, you know?

Brynn disliked the way that homophobia informed how others treated her in public, as she strongly disliked the culture of performative bisexuality:

> I'll be in a bar or a club or whatever, and they say, "Oh my God, there's two women that are kissing" and people will crowd around and watch and stare, like this is entertaining to them. It's not entertainment! It's people's true emotions or feelings, and I wish people wouldn't act that way just to get attention.

Desire for legal and education change also appeared prominently in women's wish lists for social change. For Dawn, this list covered a number of different entities:

I don't think we should condemn women that get pregnant and choose to not terminate or carry their pregnancies to term. I support abortion too, though. I support having the support of sex-positive sex education and available birth control. I want to take the shame and blame and judgment out of our mass culture and acknowledge that everyone is different, that every woman's sexuality is different, that women's sex histories are different. As a culture, I want us to stop the violence towards women, stop sexual abuse of women, stop rape of women. I have *no* tolerance for that. Also, wouldn't it be incredible if we had a culture where every person, not just females, but every person was honored for who they are and not judged?

Esther voiced her beliefs that legal change should be a major goal for improving women's lives:

I would like to see a little bit more respect for women and what they need and what they desire. Basically, our society is built around men and what they need. For it not to be a serious crime for a man to rape a woman, there's something wrong, and that is not something that people are willing to consider a serious crime. You can get more time for stealing than you can for raping a woman. I'd also like to see other things promoted for women's sexuality: health, love, and peace, rather than all the videos and all of the media that is centered on young people. We need more health and more joy, so I would like to see that change.

Finally, a few advocated a call for greater provisions for privacy and more solidarity among women. Jill said,

I'd like us to more strongly reinforce the idea that what I do in the bedroom with a consenting adult partner is my business, the consenting adult partner's business, and possibly the business of anyone I have legally or emotionally bound myself to, and nobody else's. Whether I choose to have sex, when I choose to have sex, and how I choose to have sex is me and my partner's business and pretty much no one else's.

Expanding on these themes of women claiming their sexuality, Emily argued for more political, social, and sexual solidarity and connection between women:

As far as women's sexuality, I think that it's such a unique personal thing that people have to decide what's best for themselves. I think that overall if women had more solidarity with each other and had better communication that it would help them individually figure out what's best for themselves. We need a lot more solidarity with each other on this stuff. I wish women didn't put so much emphasis on their appearances. I wish women refused to let others define for us what's sexy, what's attractive. I think if I could change anything, I would really just want women to be able to define that for themselves and erase whatever it is that they don't like. They could define that entirely for themselves.

CRITIQUE OF RESISTANCE AS A CONCEPT

The movements of deconstruction do not destroy structures from the outside. They are not possible and effective, nor can they take active aim, except by inhabiting those structures. Inhabiting them *in a certain way*, because one always inhabits, *and all the more when one does not suspect it.* Operating necessarily from the inside, borrowing all the strategic and economic resources of subversion from the old structure, borrowing them structurally, that is to say without being able to isolate their elements and atoms, the enterprise of deconstruction always *in a certain way* falls prey to its own work.

—Derrida, *Of Grammatology*

But I who am bound by mirror/as well as my bed/see
causes in color/as well as sex/and sit here
wondering/which me will survive/all these liberations.

—Lorde, "Who Said It Was Simple"

Though women's resistance narratives provide a compelling vision for ways that sexual culture can continue to evolve, the problem of articulating a concrete plan for resistance still arises. Can I, as the researcher, or you, as the reader, truly decide what *is* and *is not* resistance? If not, what are we left with? When speaking of this precise problem, Judith Butler (1990) argued,

> Just as metaphors lose their metaphoricity as they congeal through time into concepts, so subversive performances always run the risk of becoming deadening clichés through their repetition and, most importantly, through their repetition within commodity culture where "subversion" carries market value. The effort to name the criterion for subversiveness will always fail, and ought to. (p. xxi)

In women's narratives throughout the book, this becomes painfully clear, as the line between empowerment and disempowerment always shifts, moves, becomes colonized, and takes on new forms and shapes. Consequently, though the women I interviewed had a variety of "resistance narratives" (or, at the very least, narratives that implied unique and specific ways to subvert power and resist traditional sexual performances), I hesitate to unequivocally label anything women do or say as a *subversive performance* precisely for the reasons Butler has outlined: over time, all forms of resistance can—and often do—become even more deeply entrenched vehicles for oppression.

As a related question, the notion of deconstructing authenticity appeared throughout women's stories of their bodies and sexualities. How are women's orgasms, their same-sex experiences, their arousal and desire, their pleasures, their feelings about coercive experiences, and their fantasies all different versions of performance? If authenticity does not exist (as most social constructionists would say, since everything is already beholden to cultural scripts and performances of some sort), can people harness performance as a progressive force? While I do not pretend to answer these difficult questions, they nevertheless inform the center of the book. Performance may serve as *one of women's primary mechanisms for survival, empowerment, and resistance* in a sexual landscape dominated by discourses that favor men's desires, fantasies, and needs.

Further, performance, at times, undoubtedly brings women *pleasure*. In other words, if women learn to prioritize certain scripts about gender and power, they may also learn (much to the dismay of progressives) to *enjoy* the preservation of the status quo. Conversely, women may reject their expected performances by inventing new ways to perform as sexual women, thereby challenging the status quo. And, to complicate matters further, they may do both at the same time. Performance represents a real response to oppression while also promoting the competing interests of empowerment and disempowerment. By necessity, performance is living in reference to that which one cannot fully control. Women *make* and *unmake* their sexual lives, just as their sexual lives are *made* and *unmade* for them by larger forces of social control.

To more specifically address the problems of constructing women's sexual performances, one need only look at the recent debates within the sexology literatures about how to concretely measure what female orgasm actually is, when it occurs, and what it is for. Ongoing scientific and theoretical strife surrounds this tiniest of actions. Elizabeth Lloyd (2005) discussed competing accounts about what leads to—and represents the occurrence of—female orgasm, particularly surrounding the muscles and tissues involved in female orgasm. While most studies emphasize clitoral stimulation as important, others argue that "G-spot" stimulation provides an important or alternate source of input for orgasm to occur. Lloyd added, "Others have suggested that stimulation of the cervix and of the deep tissues surrounding the vagina and the uterus are important sources of stimulation, although there has been less experimental support for this claim" (p. 22). Lloyd also argued that sex researchers disagree on which muscle groups lead to orgasm, as there are roughly five muscle groups involved in women's orgasms. Added to that, some researchers have claimed that central brain activity, hormones, and neurotransmitters contribute to orgasm. And, of course, *social* aspects of sex profoundly influence the occurrence of orgasm as well, as safety, comfort, and arousal all respond to social contexts of sex. Given this, how can people mark the occurrence of female orgasm? Should they prioritize women's subjective accounts of its occurrence or the activity of certain muscle groups (not to mention *which* muscle groups)? Who should study this? Collectively, these disagreements reveal the difficulty in determining how to authentically measure the occurrence of orgasm and who is invested with the power to determine orgasm's occurrence. Even the so-called real orgasm has intense debates and disagreements surrounding it, pointing to the complexities of determining the causes, occurrences, and performances of women's sexuality.

This is not to suggest that discussions of performance should be abandoned simply because performances pervade people's lives and because everything relates to the social. Rather, people should more often interrogate the *consequences of performance*, the ways performance interacts with empowerment discourses, and what people *say* about the performances they enact. The fake orgasm (chapter 1) is itself a performance, just as the real orgasm is a performance. Women who fake orgasm may negotiate the terms of patriarchy so that they convey the real power imbalances between themselves and their partners; similarly, women who have real orgasms (however defined) may have internalized and *sexualized* power imbalances such that they eroticize the power-laden dynamics in their romantic partnerships. Both are performances, and both are *different* responses to the same cultural scripts.

Similarly, medically induced sexual arousal that occurs with the aid of women's Viagra (chapter 3) reflects multiple, simultaneous performances: first, the performance of the physiological state; second, the performances of the medical institution inducing that state; and third, the juxtaposition between the aroused body and the nonaroused mind. All are performances—the aroused body, the medical intrusions, and the mind/body interplay. Or, to take up a question from chapter 6, women invent sexual fantasies that reflect their experiences with sexual coercion (chapter 5) and their varied interpretations of pleasurable experiences (chapter 4). By inventing such fantasies, they draw from multiple scripts of empowerment and disempowerment, thus investing these fantasies with multiple layers of performance. Performances can be both subversive and oppressive, illuminating and disguising, a kind of truth-telling and a kind of posturing.

After progressing through a variety of themes and topics that emphasize women's conflicts about their sexual performances, the question remains: How should one proceed? If the labeling of resistance is fundamentally an impossible task—precisely because each time people label empowerment discourses, those who control discourse find ways to coopt and distort those discourses—and, further still, all actions are informed by multiple layers of simultaneously empowering and disempowering performances, thereby negating the idea that performance is *good* or *bad*, this question becomes complicated and convoluted. Within such a quandary, how does one move forward?

In light of this, I propose that the task is essentially to do three things: first, each time empowerment narratives become coopted, people need to, as a collective body, *create new discourses of empowerment* promptly and creatively; second, people must recognize that it keeps getting harder and harder for them (as feminists, as women, as those interested in social justice) to see the precise moment when empowerment turns into oppression, and as such, they must get better and more skillful at recognizing this transformation; and third, people need to learn how to build resistance narratives that are directed at a moving target while also not losing hope in light of the difficulty of this endeavor. As Foucault (1978) has argued, "There is no escaping from power . . . It is always-already present, constituting the very thing which one attempts to counter it with" (p. 82).

The complexity and intricacy of following these three steps cannot be overstated, as such actions presume that all solutions to the problem of women's sexual disempowerment are impermanent at best, futile at worst. So, instead of labeling resistance as such (and thus differentiating certain behaviors, attitudes, and ideologies into distinct categories of "good" and "bad"), one should instead focus on a set of related tasks that *keeps the question open*. Partly in the spirit of qualitative work, whose very definition relies upon the fundamental openness of the question, these six chapters have attempted to better illuminate the problems women face so that the question of resistance and how to respond can remain relatively open.

This book is a cautionary tale, one that shows the dangerous consequences of framing women's sexuality as liberated just because women no longer have to fight as hard to be sexual. If repression no longer reigns, this does not mean that the existing terms of sexual liberation are not equally, if not *more*, troubling indicators of oppression. We have our work cut out for us. The subjects considered in this book serve as a springboard to better understand the problems women face with their sexualities; as such, clearly delineated solutions, resistances to these problems, and reactions to the various injustices and inequalities illuminated here must be, for the time being, deferred.

Given the near total lack of research on women's conceptualizations of sexual pleasure, their subjective feelings about sex, and their ideas about the culture of sexuality, the field of sexuality research is clearly in its infancy. With few exceptions (Braun, Gavey, & McPhillips, 2003; Diamond, 2003; Fine, 1988; Tolman, 2002), research rarely addresses women's subjective accounts of sex. Going forward, I can imagine a number of different paths sex researchers could take to address some of the questions raised (but not answered) in this book. Future research could examine and inventory gender differences about sexual pleasure, women's subjective feelings about how their partnered relationships affect their sexual needs and desires, or how their fantasies correlate with their sexual practices. Scholars rarely *ask women* about their feelings about sex—why they enjoy certain actions, how they feel about their orgasms, how their sexual identities have changed over time, what they fear or dislike with sexuality, what they want from a sexual relationship, and so on—so qualitative research on these subjects is of paramount importance. Research could also address the potential benefits of collective resistance to patriarchal sexual norms, including how women use academic writing, art, street activism, group consciousness raising, protests, and other collective strategies as a means to combat increasingly rigid standards of what "good sex" means. Studies could examine how collective action beliefs might directly improve women's sexual lives, giving renewed vitality to the classic line, "the personal is political." Researchers could also examine the impact of feminist groups who already combat patriarchal norms, including groups such as The New View, Guerilla Girls, or feminist burlesque collectives; what tactics do they use that could translate to other kinds of activist work around sexuality?

Studies on men and masculinity, particularly the conditions within which men develop their feminist consciousness, ideologies about women's sexuality, and personal motives for changing hegemonic masculinity could prove especially interesting. Sexual performances, including demands placed both on women and on men, undoubtedly carry over into men's lives in ways that likely inspire some men to feel uneasy and alarmed. After all, "Men's power to *make* the world here is their power to make us make the world of their sexual interaction with us the way they want it" (MacKinnon, 1987, p. 58). One can imagine that men's control over women's sexuality does not sit well with men who

genuinely seek social change along gender lines, yet little is known
about how men concretely rebel against their control over sexual scripts
and norms.

Research could also address, much more specifically, the way
women's *many* social identities influence and construct their sexuality;
though this book includes women from diverse social backgrounds, far
more work is needed on the role of race, class, sexual identity, age,
cohort, size, disability, religious identification, political identification
(etc.) in women's experiences of sex. For women who already confront
stereotypes of hypersexualization and social/bodily "deviance," how
might social norms differently affect them? For women with less social
power, how might performance serve as an even *more* powerful form of
survival and resistance? How do various women traverse the space
between idealized femininity and their (imperfect) bodies and selves?
Interrogating people's *differences* and commonalities leads to more
nuanced understandings of sexuality, power, and embodiment.

At the more abstract level, we need to further interrogate the meaning of bodies and sexualities in a world that prioritizes the concerns of
men: What does it mean to occupy the female body, to live within a
body gendered as female? How can women understand themselves and
their sexualities in a culture that seeks to disconnect women from their
bodies, disconnect women from each other, and disconnect men from
anything that lessens their sociosexual power? Why do we construct
women's sexual power as a threat, yet fetishize their sexual powerlessness
as "sexy" or "hot"? Together, we must continue to ask questions—of
ourselves, of each other—even if the answers remain elusive.

Returning again to Foucault, two of his more substantial contributions to the study of sexuality—and to the politics of social justice and
resistance movements in general—are the following two arguments:
First, "we are much freer than we feel" (Martin, 1988, p. 9), and second,
that resistance must occur in small, multiple, strategic, decentered ways.
In *The History of Sexuality, Volume 1*, Foucault (1978) said,

> Hence, there is no single locus of great Refusal, no soul of
> revolt, source of all rebellions, or pure law of the revolutionary.
> Instead there is a plurality of resistances, each of them a special
> case: resistances that are possible, necessary, improbable; others

that are spontaneous, savage, solitary, concerted, rampant, or violent; still others that are quick to compromise, interested, or sacrificial; by definition, they can only exist in the strategic field of power relations . . . And it is doubtless the strategic codification of these points of resistance that makes a revolution possible, somewhat similar to the way in which the state relies on the institutional integration of power relationships. (p. 96)

Fusing these two points together, it becomes apparent that the former is made possible by the latter; in other words, *because* resistance (and by extension, revolution) is made possible by the plurality of ways people fight back, freedom and liberation are always already inscribed in those actions. Every challenge to power already renders the status quo less powerful. Every utterance already destabilizes the enforced silence around sexuality. Every performance of sex resists characterizations of sex as natural or essential. Every time people tell stories about sex, they have already begun to renarrate women's lives.

Women talk about this plurality of resistances—and, consequently, the moments of freedom found within those resistances—again and again. They resist by finding partners who break the mold, by speaking openly about sex in contexts that enforce silence (including, perhaps, in these interviews themselves), by debunking sexual myths, by doing things differently than previous generations. They resist by calling themselves "feminists" and embracing socially progressive political identities, by defining avenues to pleasure and satisfaction, by joining other women to enact collective social change, by changing the language of coercion ever so slightly. They take power back and give it away, or, more accurately, they notice and react when others have taken power from them. They try on performances of empowerment and performances of disempowerment, often simultaneously. They embrace sexual fluidity, choose same-sex partners, redefine their relationships with men, and invent new ways to be in marriages, all while juggling multiple roles as women. They shout back when sexually harassed on the street, work in solidarity with other women who face sexual mistreatment, and take charge of their own pleasure through masturbation. They work to change media images, redefine their home lives, and question the political implications of the "normal" and "natural" order.

Though women are surrounded on all sides by the potential for disempowerment, they find ways to navigate these dilemmas, even at the risk of contradiction and conflict. They work within the system and outside of it.

In this spirit, and in closing this book, we would do well to remember that we can outline problems without necessarily posing equally well-thought-out solutions. To illuminate, in more and more specific ways, the precise nature of problems and challenges as they exist in *this* time and space is itself a politically useful and strategic solution of its own. We need to know, in as much detail as possible, what women are up against. Of course, this is a book of *problems* far more than it is a book of solutions. By understanding the depths of internalized sexism that have permeated women's sexual lives, we can better anticipate the problems that may arise when women cannot work (or are prevented from working) in unison to address these problems, in part due to class, race, sexual identity, and age fissures. Similarly, resistance need not be labeled in a fixed sense, but rather, we can advocate for resistance at the same time that we embrace the impossibility of *consistency* and *permanence* within resistance narratives. And in the spirit of Foucault, we can state the impossibility of full escape from oppression while still arguing that people have more freedom than they realize, that there is much discursive space within which to strategize, resist, rebel, and revolt.

It is up to each of us to decide whether performing sex—particularly in the ways outlined here—constitutes a multifaceted kind of resistance or a further entrenchment of troubling gender norms and patriarchal sexual fantasies (or maybe both?). Performance may well be a subversive act, or it may reinforce the worst aspects of power and privilege. As individuals and as a collective body, we have a responsibility to come up with our own solutions in response to these performances. As women fight to gain recognition socially, politically, and interpersonally, questions of how to define sexual empowerment will continue in full force. There is no escape from power, and the resulting clashes and conflicts it creates within the realm of sexuality—indeed, there is no "out" from oppression—and yet this lack of escape creates new possibilities for nuancing the gendered politics of sex. In sorting through the conflicts about what will lead to a better and more just sexual world for women, we will undoubtedly be forced to ask some difficult questions, to hear answers we might not like, and to work passionately against numbness, self-negation, and despair. Each of these contradictions and conflicts opens up a space for conversation, for opposition, for a unique dialectic that the study of sexuality demands. Let us be careful and purposeful in creating our visions of freedom, convicted about what we will *not* stand for, cautious and reflective about the many layers of complicity we combat, and resolutely open to changing our minds—frequently, strategically, shamelessly, and with vigor and vitality.

APPENDICES

PARTICIPANT DEMOGRAPHIC INFORMATION

Name	Age	Race	Sexual Identity
Margaret	54	White	Heterosexual
Aya	25	Chinese-American	Heterosexual
Ophelia	56	White	Lesbian
Susan	45	White	Heterosexual
Fiona	24	White	Bisexual
Mitra	29	Indian-American	Heterosexual
Geena	51	White	Heterosexual
Courtney	23	White	Heterosexual
Kate	25	White	Heterosexual
Leigh	21	White	Lesbian
Nora	23	White	Bisexual
Maria	21	Mexican-American	Lesbian
Priya	23	Indian-American	Heterosexual
Dorothy	19	Chinese-American	Heterosexual
Julie	23	White	Bisexual
Charlene	44	Native American	Bisexual
Melanie	21	White	Heterosexual
Pam	42	African-American	Heterosexual
Anita	46	Mexican-American	Heterosexual
Lori	33	White	Bisexual
Esther	44	African-American	Heterosexual
Janet	21	White	Lesbian
Brynn	25	White	Lesbian
Shonda	44	African-American	Heterosexual
Dawn	43	White	Bisexual
Bonnie	51	White	Heterosexual
Marilyn	54	White	Heterosexual

PARTICIPANT DEMOGRAPHIC (CONTINUED)

Name	Age	Race	Sexual Identity
Lucy	25	Mexican-Am./Filipina	Bisexual
Diana	50	White	Lesbian
Charlotte	34	African-Am./Indian-Am.	Heterosexual
Ruth	46	White	Heterosexual
Jasmine	37	Mexican-American	Lesbian
Sally	20	White	Heterosexual
Edie	19	White	Heterosexual
Jill	32	White	Heterosexual
Niko	23	Asian-American	Heterosexual
Ciara	24	White	Bisexual
Sonja	24	White	Heterosexual
Emily	22	White	Bisexual
Carol	38	White	Bisexual

Note: The first 20 participants were interviewed in Ann Arbor, Michigan, in 2005. The second 20 participants were interviewed in Phoenix, Arizona, in 2007.

Note: Demographics are self-reported. In the case of sexual identity, their reported behavior, attitudes, and attraction did not always align with their self-reported sexual identities.

SUMMARY TABLE:
PARTICIPANT DEMOGRAPHIC INFORMATION

Demographic	Percentage	# Participants
Age		
18–31	52%	21
32–45	28%	11
46–59	20%	8
Race		
White	65%	26
Women of Color	35%	14
—African American	7.5%	3
—Chicana/Latina	7.5%	3
—Indian American	5%	2
—Asian American	7.5%	3
—Native American	2.5%	1
—Biracial	5%	2
Sexual Identity		
Heterosexual	58%	23
Bisexual	24%	10
Lesbian	18%	7
Total	100%	40

APPENDIX 2. SAMPLING INFORMATION

This book utilized two waves of qualitative data from a sample of 40 women recruited over the span of three years (2005–2007). While 40 women can hardly represent the entirety of women's sexual experiences, this number was chosen in order to accommodate a diverse sample and to prioritize labor-intensive qualitative transcriptions and data analysis. Because I conducted this research first as a graduate student at the University of Michigan and then as a professor at Arizona State University, half of these participants (wave 1) were interviewed in Ann Arbor, MI, and the other half (wave 2) of these participants were interviewed in Phoenix, AZ. Participants in wave 1 were found through local entertainment and arts listings (N=20) distributed free to the community of Ann Arbor, MI. These listings were a common way for researchers to recruit potential participants, as they reached out to the larger community and did not simply exclusively recruit people from the university setting. Only five of the Ann Arbor participants had any affiliation to the university. This method of sampling allowed access to a wider range of women from different age, education, racial, and social class backgrounds. That said, participants from the Ann Arbor sample reported having higher paying jobs and more education than the Phoenix sample. Building on the interviews from wave 1 in Ann Arbor, participants in wave 2 were recruited both through local entertainment and arts listings (N=12) distributed free to the Phoenix, AZ, community and through the volunteers section on the Phoenix, AZ, online section of Craigslist (http://phoenix.craigslist.org) (N=8).

I asked participants to agree to a two-hour face-to-face semistructured interview with me about their sexual histories, sexual practices, and feelings and attitudes about sexuality. I conducted all of the interviews myself and typically completed each wave over the course of two months. Interviews in Ann Arbor were conducted at a psychological clinic in a room designed to maximize comfort and relaxation (e.g., plants, large windows, soft lighting, etc.). Interviews in Phoenix were conducted in private at the Women's Resource Center on Arizona State University's West campus, a space also designed for comfort, relaxation, and conversation. In order to choose participants, I asked only for their gender, racial/ethnic background, sexual identity, and age. I then chose the women based on these demographic characteristics. Sexual minority women and racial/ethnic minority women were oversampled, and a diverse range of ages was represented in the sample. I received many more requests for participation than I could accommodate, as each wave brought in more than 100 women stating their interest in the project. To create a diverse sample, I typically chose participants who responded earliest and who met the various demographic characteristics I was looking for in terms of age, race, gender, and sexual identity. I wanted a minimum of 30% women of color, at least 8 women in each of the three age brackets I identified, and at least 25% sexual minority women. All of these procedures were in compliance with the University of Michigan (wave 1) and Arizona State University (wave 2) Institutional Review Boards. Participants were paid $20.00 for doing the interview, and they were asked to give consent to have their interviews audiotaped, though they were not excluded if they did not agree to be audiotaped. All of the participants agreed to have their interviews audiotaped. All interviews were fully transcribed, identifying data (e.g., place of work, names of partners, etc.) was removed, and each participant was assigned a pseudonym to ensure anonymity.

In terms of demographic characteristics, participants came from a variety of backgrounds. For sexual identity, 58% identified as heterosexual (N=23), 18% as lesbian (N=7), and 24% as bisexual (N=10). For racial and ethnic backgrounds, 65% identified as white (N=26), and 35% identified as women of color (N=14). Participants' racial/ethnic backgrounds included white, African American, Asian American, Latina/Chicana, Indian American, Native American, and biracial. Further, a diverse group of ages was represented in the sample, including 52% ages 18–31 (N=21), 28% ages 32–45 (N=11), and 20% ages 46–59 (N=8). Participants reported a range of socioeconomic backgrounds, educational backgrounds, employment histories, presence/absence of children, and relationship statuses, though this information was not collected in advance of the interviews and was instead gleaned during the interviews. In terms of sexual frequency, I interviewed women that ranged from completely celibate since the 1980s to a working pornography actress (who reportedly had already had sex with hundreds of men and women), along with mostly everything in between (e.g., highly sexed newlyweds, women who reported feeling "bored" by sex, those who occasionally dated, those with multiple partners, etc.).

Because all of the women mentioned their occupation, it was possible to determine that there was diversity in socioeconomic class as well. While there were a few college students in the study, most participants worked outside the home and were not college students. Some women had high-paying jobs (e.g., administrator, engineer), while others had low-paying jobs (e.g., receptionist, waitress), indicating diversity of incomes. That said, the group of women I interviewed was more educated than the general population, particularly for the Ann Arbor participants, who essentially lived in an intellectual research center of the country. As such, the women I interviewed seemed unusually articulate and verbal in their responses and were able to give elaborate answers to questions ranging from concrete to quite abstract. As the less educated women gave shorter and less elaborate answers, chapters may skew toward participants with more education, and the results should therefore be interpreted with caution and attention to these biases for educational background. Because recruitment took place primarily through entertainment and arts listings, this may have also skewed the sample toward women with more interest in cultural and educational experiences such as arts, music, and film. If recruitment had taken place through other avenues (e.g., domestic violence shelters, church bulletins, listservs, etc.), the results might have been different.

Partnering and reasons for participation also differed greatly among the sample. There was a lot of diversity in terms of current relationship statuses, as some women were married, while others were single (some with no sexual partners, some with one partner, some with multiple partners), cohabitating, or divorced. Most women had had multiple sexual partners in the past, yet most currently reported having one primary sexual partner at the present time. In addition, most of the women explicitly told me their stated reasons for participating in the study, and this too represented a substantial range of motivations. For example, some women said that participating in a sex research study helped them to rebel against their repressed upbringings, while others said that they wanted to support sex positive research. Some women said they felt it was an opportunity to talk about aspects of their sexuality they usually

kept to themselves, while other women said they participated just for
the money and because they were "broke." Some women enjoyed vol-
unteering while others wanted a space to think intellectually about sexuality. Nearly all participants mentioned that they were glad they had
participated once the interview had finished, and some happily accepted
their $20.00 payment, while others tried to reject the payment. This sug-
gests that self-selection for the study did not yield a particular type of
woman who participated, but rather, that many different women participated for many different reasons.

As with any qualitative project, the qualities of the researcher may
affect the findings of the study. While it is impossible to definitively
determine how my identities as the interviewer were perceived, and
responded to, by interview participants, there was some indication that
my gender, age, race, marital status, and class were salient during the
interviews. Some women commented specifically on our shared traits
in this regard (e.g., noting that I would likely know certain cultural references because of my age or commenting on my lack of wedding ring
as a sign of uncertainty about whether I identified as lesbian or heterosexual), while others either implicitly or explicitly marked our differences as women during the interviews (e.g., speaking about Latina
women as a category that I did not belong to or commenting about
how they had never visited a college campus before). Similarly, it is
notable that I conducted the first round of interviews while I completed my predoctoral internship in clinical psychology, and I conducted the second round of interviews while working as a postdoctoral
clinical psychologist. While I made every effort to conduct these interviews *as a researcher* and not as a clinician, my background as a therapist
may have influenced the style, tone, facial expressions, and methods of
communication during these interviews.

I interviewed all 40 women using a semistructured list of interview
questions, with interviews lasting for approximately two hours on average. Participants were asked 30 open-ended questions about their
sexual histories, practices, and beliefs. Questions extended existing
research in a variety of areas, including sexual satisfaction, sexual behavior, political socialization, body image, partner relationships, sexual
identity fluidity, and generational/cohort differences between women
(see appendix for full interview protocol). Taking seriously both the

advantages and limitations of feminist qualitative research, the interviews were designed as a way for women to construct their own narratives about sexuality without the constraints of the researcher superimposing categories or "frames" as much as possible. For example, when asking about sexual identity, I specifically probed for their *stories* of how they came to understand themselves as bisexual, lesbian, or heterosexual, as well as their history of (possible) sexual fluidity. Questions were designed to allow women to discuss social and cultural norms in a variety of ways, for example, the way these norms affected their sexual fantasies, attitudes about other women, or ideas about masturbation. During our conversations, I made every effort not to interrupt or interject with affirmations, negations, or value judgments; instead, I let the women speak about each question until they had exhausted their thought processes.

To give a specific example of one of the questions, I asked the women, "Many women report that their feelings about their own bodies greatly affect their experience of sex. How do you feel your body image affects your sexual experiences?" Some questions included follow-up probing questions depending on the information they provided. For example, in the body image question mentioned above, if the women did not discuss comfort with nudity or comfort with having sex while menstruating, I asked about these issues during our conversation about that question. This method allowed for rich and vivid descriptions of women's thoughts and feelings about their sexualities.

In terms of processing the data, I did not convert the data to quantitative categories, and I primarily used a qualitative thematic analysis when interpreting the data. I grouped and distilled a list of common interpretations that gave expression to the commonalities across participants. In doing so, I reviewed lines, sentences, and paragraphs of the transcripts, looking for patterns in their ways of discussing each sexual theme (Braun and Clarke, 2006). I selected and generated themes through the process of identifying logical links and overlaps between participants. After creating these themes, I compared them to previous themes in order to identify similarities, differences, and general patterns. This type of thematic analysis relied upon a data-driven inductive approach (Boyatzis, 1998) in which themes were generated prior to interpretation. As such, initial themes were identified, codes were applied and then connected back to the themes, and these themes were then corroborated and legitimized, per Fereday and Muir-Cochrane's (2006) method of inductive thematic analysis. Throughout this process, I relied upon a critical realist framework that contextualized themes and patterns found within the transcripts. While sorting and naming themes required some level of interpretation, I generally did not delve into covert, implicit, or subtextual meanings in the transcripts. The book relies upon a combination of their words along with my analysis and framing in order to illuminate the concepts and themes presented in each chapter.

Subjectively, I can attest to my own perceptions that the interviews were characterized, on the whole, by great ease and rapport between the participants and me and that most women seemed comfortable and open to sharing stories about their intimate lives during the interview. There were only a few occasions when anyone decided not to answer a question, and I was impressed by the forthright and honest answers I seemed to get from participants. Many women (close to a third) cried during the interviews, particularly when discussing sexual violence and/or abuse or when discussing an expartner no longer in their lives, and many said that the interviews "brought things up" for them that they wanted to think more about or even seek therapy for. The interviews were designed to situate women's lived experiences of their bodies into an open-ended conversational framework. In all, I felt, and continue to feel, incredibly fortunate to have had such an interesting, diverse, forthcoming, and insightful group of women to speak with in such intensity and detail.

APPENDIX 3. INTERVIEW PROTOCOL

Opening Script

During this interview, I am going to ask you several questions about the course of your sexual life. Some of these questions will be quite broad and will ask you about your opinions, beliefs, and attitudes about your sexuality. Other questions will be more specific in nature and will ask you to talk about your sexuality in more detailed ways. Please remember that you can choose not to answer any of the questions I ask during the interview. These questions are intended to be open-ended and will hopefully allow us a chance to reflect together about your sexual experiences throughout your lifetime. I will start by asking you about your past experiences with sexuality and will then ask you about your current experiences with sex. I will then ask you about some of your political attitudes and whether or not these affect your sexuality, and I will conclude the interview by asking you about how your sexuality fits into the broader context of contemporary culture. Please remember that you must not tell me any identifying information about your past or current sexual partners, as they have not consented to provide such information. Please also do not refer to yourself directly by name, and do not provide the name of your employer or workplace during the interview.

Questions

1. I want to start by asking you some questions about your sexual past, including your experiences with sex as a child and as a teenager. Many women report that they had many experiences with sex growing up, possibly through reading or looking at magazines and books, masturbation, conversations with friends, and early sexual experiences. Can you tell me about your first experiences with sexuality?
   Probe for:
   How did your parents' views of sexuality influence your sexuality?
   Did sex feel prohibited and secretive, or more open?
   What was your first sexual experience like? How did it affect your later life experiences with sexuality?
2. Sometimes women report that they think about their sexuality in terms of "highs" and "lows." In other words, many women remember their best and worst sexual experiences as defining experiences of their lives. Can you talk first about what you consider to be the best sexual experience you've had in your life? This could include a sexual experience that felt particularly arousing or exciting or an

experience that involved a loving interaction with a partner. It could also include a private experience with masturbation or even a sexual dream. Talk about anything that comes to mind.

Probe for:

What emotions do you have when thinking about this experience?

3. Can you talk about what you consider to be the worst sexual experience you've had in your life? This could include an experience that felt coercive or painful or an emotionally difficult sexual interaction. It could also include an experience that felt embarrassing or shameful. Talk about anything that comes to mind.

Probe for:

What emotions do you have when thinking about this experience?

4. Women often report different reasons for having sex. There are many reasons why you might have sex with someone. What do you feel are the primary reasons you have sex?

5. I now want to talk about sexual satisfaction and pleasure. Many women describe sexual satisfaction and pleasure in different ways. How would you define sexual satisfaction for yourself?

Probe for:

What are the most important aspects of physical pleasure for you?

What, if any, is the connection between physical pleasure and emotional satisfaction?

6. Along these lines, what emotions do you typically feel when having sex with your partner?

Probe for:

What other [positive, negative] emotions do you feel? (probe for opposite if not mentioned)

Do you ever feel "checked out" or absent during sex? If so, what is this like?

7. Some women report that they sometimes cry during or after sex. Can you talk about whether this has ever happened to you and if so, why you think you cried.

8. Many women report pleasurable experiences with masturbation. Can you describe your experiences with masturbation?

Probe for:

How often do you masturbate? How often do you orgasm while masturbating? What emotions do you have about masturbation?

What experiences have you had, if any, with sex toys during masturbation?

9. I want to open up the conversation a little further now. Many women report that their desire to have sex and their actual sexual activity (or the amount they have sex) sometimes differ. Some women report that they agree to have sex with a partner because their partner wants them to. Others say their own desire is much more intense than their partner's desire. Women often negotiate this in different ways. Can you talk about your experience with this?

Probe for:

Have you ever been forced or coerced into having sex when you did not want to?

Have you ever felt pressured to have sex?

What kinds of sexual acts feel uncomfortable?

How do you negotiate sexual positions? What are your favorite and least favorite positions?

10. Some women report that they feel very strongly that they cannot have sex with someone unless they are in love with that person. Other women say that they like to have sex strictly for physical pleasure and without emotional attachments. How do you feel about this?

Probe for:

How do you feel about women who are "promiscuous" or who have a lot of sex with or without emotions attached to it?

11. Related to my last question, I also want to talk with you about the kinds of partners you're attracted to. Women differ greatly in their descriptions of attractive sexual partners. Many women find that they are only attracted to men, while other women find that they are sometimes or always attracted to women. Can you describe your preferences for sexual partners and the way this has been negotiated in your life?

Probe for:

[If heterosexual identified] Have you ever experienced same-sex attraction or had a same-sex sexual encounter? [If so], what was that like?

Do you identify as heterosexual, bisexual, or lesbian now? Has that changed over time for you?

12. Many women report that their feelings about their own bodies greatly affect their experience of sex. How do you feel your body image affects your sexual experiences?

    Probe for:

    Do you alter your body in any way before having sex, such as shaving, showering, or otherwise preparing for sex?

    How do you feel about having sex while menstruating?

    How do you feel about nudity, either alone or with a partner?

13. Related to the topic of your body, I want to bring up the topic of orgasm as a specific and important feature of women's sexuality. Many women report that they engage in sex but that they don't always orgasm. What are your experiences with orgasm?

    Probe for:

    How often do you typically orgasm, either alone or with a partner?

    How long does it take to orgasm, alone or with a partner?

    How important is it to you to have an orgasm during sex?

    Do you feel pressured to orgasm during sex, either internally from yourself or externally from a partner?

    Do you feel like you can have good sex without having an orgasm?

14. Many women report that they have faked orgasm during their lives. What are your experiences with faking orgasm or with faking your experience of pleasure?

15. It is very common for women to report that their sexual experiences are affected by circumstances in their lives, such as health problems, stress, emotional problems, or sexual dysfunction. What kinds of things have interfered with your sex life?

    Probe for:

    (If reporting interferences) Did you seek help for this problem?

    Have you ever discussed sexuality in the context of therapy? (If yes) What was this like for you? Did it help you?

16. As a more specific question related to this topic, have you heard anything about the development of female Viagra, a drug intended to boost women's sexual responsiveness? (If yes) How would you make the decision about whether or not to take such a drug? Under what conditions would you be interested in taking the drug?

17. Women often report that fantasy is a big part of their sexual life and that fantasies can be intensely arousing and exciting. The content of women's fantasies tends to include a wide range of different

scenarios. Some women are turned on by the idea of a threesome, while others might find the idea of being forced to have sex appealing. What are your experiences with sexual fantasy?

Probe for:

Which sexual fantasy is most recurrent for you?

What has stopped you from acting on your fantasies?

What emotions do you have about your sexual fantasies, positive and/or negative?

Who do you share your sexual fantasies with?

18. I now want to ask you about your ideas about other women's sexuality and its relationship to your own. Specifically, I am interested to hear your views about whether you feel like your sexuality is "normal" compared to other women and whether you feel like there are any sex acts that you consider to be "wrong"?

19. Women differ greatly in their knowledge about sexuality, and many claim there are many things related to sexuality that they wish they knew but are too embarrassed to ask. Consequently, there are many myths circulating about sex. What do you think is the biggest myth about sexuality?

20. There are many influences on our sexual lives, both in terms of particular people who have influenced our beliefs about sexuality and in terms of cultural, popular, or societal influences. Who (or what) in your life has had the most impact on your feelings, beliefs, and attitudes about sexuality?

Who has had the most positive impact? Who has had the most negative impact?

Do you feel affected by sexual norms in popular culture?

21. As a broader question, what is it like to be a sexual woman in the context of contemporary culture?

Probe for:

Do you feel like this has changed over time?

22. Many women believe that there is a strong generational difference in the way that sexuality is viewed and experienced. How do you feel that your generation is different in its relationship to female sexuality than previous generations or younger generations?

23. When thinking broadly about sexuality—both in relationship to your own sexuality and to other women's sexuality—what do wish was different about the way our culture treats female sexuality? In

other words, what do you hope we can work to collectively change about the social construction of female sexuality?

24 Are you at all familiar with the *Girls Gone Wild* franchise of advertisements and movies, which portray college-aged women stripping on camera while receiving no financial compensation?

[If yes] What are your thoughts about *Girls Gone Wild* and its meaning for young women's sexuality?

25. It is increasingly common for women to report that they feel pressure to engage in sexual acts with other women, usually in the context of being in front of men. Have you ever had experiences like this?

[If yes] What was this like for you?

What are your feelings about women performing as "bisexual" in front of male audiences? Have you ever felt pressure to perform as bisexual in front of men?

26. Most women report that they have had the experience of being treated as a sexual object. For example, many women have been sexually harassed at work or have been whistled at on the street, stared at inappropriately, etc. What are your experiences with being treated as a sexual object?

Probe for:

How did you respond? How did it feel?

27. I want to conclude our interview by asking you some questions about your political attitudes, as these beliefs can sometimes be related to sexuality. I am particularly interested to hear your views on feminism and whether you feel feminists have made it easier to be sexual in our culture.

28. I am also interested to hear your political beliefs about abortion. Can you tell me more about your feelings on these issues and how these beliefs related to your sexuality?

29. I am also interested to hear your political beliefs about homosexuality. Can you tell me more about your feelings on the way homosexuality is constructed in the larger political culture, particularly as it relates to legal and social rights?

30. As a related question, I am also interested to hear your personal and political beliefs about pornography, as many women report having conflicted feelings about the consumption and circulation of

pornography. What are your thoughts about pornography as it relates to your life and as it relates to the culture at large?
Probe for:
Do you personally use pornography? [If yes] How do you feel about using pornography?
Do you personally use sex toys? [If yes] How do you feel about using sex toys?

NOTES

INTRODUCTION

1. In a related way, J. L. Austin's (1962) work on "speech act performatives" nuanced these analyses by offering that speech itself constitutes performances, that utterances have within them various *actions*; Eve Sedgwick (2003) and Jacques Derrida (1979) further argued that, because speech is performative, meanings can shift depending on the speaker, listener, and context, but speech itself *always* exists within the sphere of (gendered) performances.

2. All women were assigned a pseudonym (i.e., if her real name was "Cindy," she was named "Alicia") in order to ensure anonymity.

CHAPTER 1. GETTING, GIVING, FAKING, HAVING

1. We can see the residue of such conflicts in many of our customs today, including, for example, young women's insistence upon wearing a white dress at their weddings despite that fact that the vast majority of women are technically not virgins at the time of marriage.

2. "Hysteria" is currently defined by Merriam-Webster's dictionary as "a nervous disorder marked especially by defective emotional control, unmanageable fear, and outbursts of emotion." Hysteria also has many common uses, most notably "hysterical," "hysterics," and the DSM-IV-adopted "histrionic personality disorder."

3. Note that, according to the National Institute of Mental Health, women are 2–3 times more likely to be diagnosed with depression, 10 times more likely to be diagnosed with an eating disorder, 2–3 times more likely to

attempt suicide, and twice as likely to receive an anxiety disorder diagnosis (APA, 1994).

4. The significance of Freud himself should also be noted. He characterized his work by saying he had "disturbed the sleep of the world" (Robinson, 1993, p. 9). He may have been correct, as his is the second most cited work in the world, after the Bible. In a poem commemorating Freud's death, W. H. Auden wrote, "To us he is no more than a person/Now but a whole climate of opinion" (Bloom, 1986).

5. A key element of Kinsey's work focused on the relationship of "biological potential" to that of the social and cultural world (Laumann, 1994). Other social scientists later echoed Kinsey's claim that sexual expression is deeply tied to biological characteristics (Jones & Kelly, 1984; Udry & Campbell, 1994; Rossi, 1994; Posner, 1992). This biological emphasis was later countered by those who constructed sexuality as a social phenomenon (Foucault, 1978; Gagnon & Simon, 1973; Janus & Janus, 1993; Laumann, 1994, Tiefer, 2004).

6. This may have been particularly true given that the book about men (1948) was released a full five years before the book about women (1953), likely sparking interest and anxiety about normative female sexuality.

7. Deutsch, however, agreed with Freud's ideas about the primacy of the vaginal orgasm, saying that vaginal orgasm produced an "essential heterosexuality" and that it trained women to accept a naturally masochistic posture in their sexual relationships. Deutsch also had much to say about the natural qualities of women's arousal in the face of domination, arguing, "The 'undiscovered' vagina is—in favorable instances—eroticized by an act of rape" (Gerhard, 2000, p. 455).

8. Freud declared, "The feminists . . . are anxious to force us to regard the two sexes as completely equal in position and worth" (p. 13). Kofman (1980) posits that Freud himself knew that feminists would criticize his work as inadequate in its analysis of women. Freud may have intentionally done so in order to generate publicity and prestige.

9. Gay and lesbian studies also critiqued psychoanalysis and sexological research by questioning categories (e.g., straight versus gay), challenging the relationship of personal identity and sexual behavior, and recognizing incongruent patterns of fantasy, desire, identity, and behavior.

10. Fisher was, however, particularly puzzled by the fact that schizophrenic women, as a group, seemed to have a higher capacity for orgasm than "mature and adjusted" women.

11. Notably, however, not all feminists accepted the link between advancing women's rights and deconstructing the primacy of heterosexuality in women's sexual lives; indeed, many resisted the unification of gay and lesbian rights movements with the feminist movement.

12. Ellison (2001) questioned participants about recent sexual concerns with their previous partners, and found that 34% reported low sexual desire or desire discrepancy, 28.5% reported difficulties with physical responsiveness (e.g. female arousal and orgasm, male partners' erectile difficulties, ejaculatory control), 16% disliked their sexual technique, 7.5% had difficulty finding a consistent sexual partner, and the remaining 5% included such difficulties as fertility issues, pregnancy concerns, STDs, women's body/health, infidelity, and shifts in sexual orientation.

13. For a more thorough discussion of Marxist critiques of sex, see Delphy (1984), Folbre (1982), and Ferguson (1989).

CHAPTER 3. THE RISE OF VIAGRA FOR WOMEN

1. Note that there has been widespread evidence that diagnoses of Attention Deficit Disorder have risen substantially during the past decade, particularly for adults, as the pharmaceutical industries have attempted to further medicalize many symptoms of modern consumerist lifestyles: boredom, restlessness, insomnia, and the like (Conrad & Potter, 2000).

2. This is similar to the drug treatments for PMDD, as these drugs are most basically a repackaging of Prozac in a pink package so that it will appeal to women patients. Many of the women involved in the clinical trials for other sexual pharmaceuticals report the same thing, as doctors give them pink pills.

3. I asked women if they had heard anything about the development of Viagra for women, a drug intended to boost women's sexual responsiveness, and, regardless of their response, I asked them, "How would you make the decision about whether or not to take such a drug?"

CHAPTER 4. ON THE MANY JOYS OF SEX

1. Recent work about the complications of being a "feminist slut" or an "ethical slut" speak to these complexities as well, as women seek out ways to embrace pleasure and resist patriarchy, all while claiming identities typically denigrated by contemporary culture (Easton & Liszt, 2009). The claiming of "slut" as a positive or affirming identity presents an interesting spin on the problem of how sex and power overlap.

2. Though subaltern studies has not typically been applied to women as a category, the concepts of 'subalterity' illuminate a compelling vision for what happens when the dominant narratives of one group suppress and speak for the secondary narratives of the oppressed group. As such, and in light of what

Gayatri Spivak calls "gendered subaltern" (1989), I use subalterity loosely enough to apply broadly to the study of women even though that formulation goes against the precise intent of how Spivak originally used the term in her 1988 essay, "Can the Subaltern Speak?"

CHAPTER 5. THE CULTURE OF DOMINATION

1. W. E. B. Du Bois (1994) was the first to coin the term *double consciousness*. In *The Souls of Black Folk*, he wrote about "this sense of always looking at one's self through the eyes of others, of measuring one's soul by the tape of a world that looks on in amused contempt and pity . . . two warring ideals in one dark body, whose dogged strength alone keeps it from being torn asunder" (p. 2).

2. Indeed, when women demonstrate greater freedom and more sexual autonomy, this directly violates the tenants of hegemonic masculinity, which asserts that men should use force toward women who challenge male ascendancy.

CHAPTER 6. IMAGERY AND IMAGINATION

1. Dworkin (1989) wrote that "pornography is the orchestrated destruction of women's bodies and souls; rape, battery, incest, and prostitution animate it; dehumanization and sadism characterize it; it is war on women, serial assaults on dignity, identity, and human worth; it is tyranny" (p. xxvii). According to Dworkin, pornography advocated a world where "the woman is hole, hot wet fuck tube . . . Where huge, monster, atom-smashing cock is god and master" (1997, p. 157).

2. Other scholars (including men) agreed with this assertion. For example, Robert Jensen (2004) argued, "In this culture, rape is normal. That is, in a culture where the dominant definition of sex is the taking of pleasure by women, rape is an expression of the sexual norms of the culture, not a violation of those norms" (p. 57).

3. Divides between white feminists and feminists of color and between heterosexual feminists and queer feminists are notable.

REFERENCES

Adams, C. (2003). *The pornography of meat.* New York: Continuum. *Aggression and Violent Behavior, 1*(1), 27–45.

Ahrens, C. E., Campbell, R., Ternier-Thames, K. N., Wasco, S. M., & Sefl, T. (2007). Deciding whom to tell: Expectations and outcomes of rape survivors' first disclosures. *Psychology of Women Quarterly, 31*(1), 38–49.

Alfonso, V. C., Allison, D. B., & Dunn, G. M. (1992). Sexual fantasy and satisfaction: A multidimensional analysis of gender differences. *Journal of Psychology & Human Sexuality, 5*(3), 19–37.

Alison, L., Santtila, P., Sandnabba, N. K., & Nordling, N. (2001). Sadomasochistically oriented behavior: Diversity in practice and meaning. *Archives of Sexual Behavior, 30*(1), 1–12.

Allina, A. (2001). Orgasms for sale: The role of profit and politics in addressing women's sexual satisfaction. *Women & Therapy, 24*(1–2), 211–218.

American Psychiatric Association. (1994). *Diagnostic and statistical manual of mental disorders (4th Ed.).* Washington, DC: Author.

Angelides, S. (2001). *A history of bisexuality.* Chicago: University of Chicago Press.

Angier, N. (2007, April 10). The search for the female equivalent of Viagra. Retrieved August 28, 2008, from *The New York Times.* Website: http://www.nytimes.com/2007/04/10/science/10wome.html.

Antecol, H., & Cobb-Clark, D. (2006). The sexual harassment of female active-duty personnel: Effects on job satisfaction and intentions to remain in the military. *Journal of Economic Behavior & Organization, 61*(1), 55–80.

Aosved, A. C., & Long, P. J. (2006). Co-occurrence of rape myth acceptance, sexism, racism, homophobia, ageism, classism, and religious intolerance. *Sex Roles, 55*(7–8), 481–492.

Armstrong, E. A., Hamilton, L., & Sweeney, B. (2006). Sexual assault on campus: A multilevel, integrative approach to party rape. *Social Problems, 53*(4), 483–499.

Arndt, B. (2008, November 6). Viagra disappointment as erectile dysfunction persists. Retrieved on August 29, 2008, from *Courier mail*. Website: http://www.news.com.au/couriermail/story/0,23739,24612080–953,00.html.

Atkinson, T. (1974). *Amazon odyssey: The first collection of writings by the political pioneer of the women's movement.* New York: Links Books.

Attwood, F. (2005). What do people do with porn? Qualitative research into the consumption, use, and experience of pornography and other sexually explicit media. *Sexuality & Culture: An Interdisciplinary Quarterly, 9*(2), 65–86.

Austin, J. L. (1962). *How to do things with words.* Oxford: Clarendon.

Baldwin, J. (1993). *Another Country.* New York: Vintage Books.

Baldwin, J., & Giovanni, N. (1973). *A dialogue.* Philadelphia: Lippincott Williams & Wilkins.

Bancroft, J. (2002). The medicalization of female sexual dysfunction: The need for caution. *Archives of Sexual Behavior, 31*(5), 451–455.

Bancroft, J., Loftus, J., & Long, S. J. (2004). Distress about sex: A national survey of women in heterosexual relationships. *Archives of Sexual Behavior, 13*(3), 193–208.

Barrett, A. (2004). Oral sex and teenagers: A sexual health educator's perspective. *Canadian Journal of Human Sexuality, 13*(3–4), 197–200.

Barry, K. (1979). *Female sexual slavery.* Englewood Cliffs, NJ: Prentice Hall.

Barton, B. (2006). *Stripped: Inside the lives of exotic dancers.* New York: New York University Press.

Baumeister, R. F. (2000). Gender differences in erotic plasticity. *Psychological Bulletin, 126*(3), 347–374.

Baumeister, R., & Tice, D. (1998). *The social dimension of sex.* Boston: Allyn & Bacon.

Baumgardner, J. (2007). *Look both ways: Bisexual politics.* New York: Farrar, Straus, & Giroux.

Bay-Cheng, L. Y., & Eliseo-Arras, R. K. (2008). The making of unwanted sex: Gendered and neoliberal norms in college women's unwanted sexual experiences. *Journal of Sex Research, 45*(4), 386–397.

Berdahl, J. L. (2007). The sexual harassment of uppity women. *Journal of Applied Psychology, 92*(2), 425–437.

Berdahl, J. L., & Moore, C. (2006). Workplace harassment: Double jeopardy for minority women. *Journal of Applied Psychology, 91*(2), 426–436.

Berkowitz, A. (1992). College men as perpetrators of acquaintance rape and sexual assault: A review of recent research. *Journal of American College Health, 40*(4), 175–181.

Berman, L., Berman, J., Miles, M., Pollets, D., & Powell, J. A. (2003). Genital self-image as a component of sexual health: Relationship between genital self-image, female sexual function, and quality of life measures. *Journal of Sex & Marital Therapy, 29*(1), 11–21.

Bhabha, H. K. (1996). Unsatisfied: Notes on vernacular cosmopolitanism. In L. Garcia-Moreno & P. C. Pfeiffer (Eds.), *Text and nation: Cross-disciplinary essays on cultural and national identities* (pp. 191–207). Columbia, SC: Camden House.

Birnbaum, G. E. (2007). Beyond the borders of reality: Attachment orientations and sexual fantasies. *Personal Relationships, 14*(2), 321–342.

Bleecker, T. E., & Murnen, S. K. (2005). Fraternity membership, the display of degrading sexual images of women, and rape myth acceptance. *Sex Roles, 53*(7–8), 487–493.

Bloom, H. (1986, March 23). Freud, the greatest modern writer. *The New York Times Book Review*, p. 27.

Blumstein, P., & Schwartz, P. (1990). Intimate relationships and the creation of sexuality. In D. P. McWhirter, S. A. Sanders, & J. M. Reinisch (Eds.), *Homosexuality/heterosexuality: Concepts of sexual orientation* (pp. 307–320). New York: Oxford University Press.

Bobo, L., Kluegel, J. R., Smith, R. A. (1997). Laissez-faire racism: The crystallization of a kinder, gentler, antiblack ideology. In S. Tuch & J. K. Martin (Eds.), *Racial attitudes in the 1990s: Continuity and change* (pp. 15–44). Santa Barbara, CA: Greenwood.

Bondurant, B. (2001). University women's acknowledgment of rape. *Violence against Women, 7*(3), 294–314.

Bostock, D. J., & Daley, J. G. (2007). Lifetime and current sexual assault and harassment victimization rates of active-duty United States Air Force women. *Violence against Women, 13*(9), 927–944.

Bowman C. G. (1993). Street harassment and the informal ghettoization of women. *Harvard Law Review, 106*(3), 517–580.

Boyatzis, R. (1998). Transforming qualitative information: Thematic analysis and code development. Thousand Oaks, CA: Sage.

Boyle, K. (2000). The pornography debates: Beyond cause and effect. *Women's Studies International Forum, 23*(2), 187–195.

Braun, V., & Clarke, V. (2006). Using thematic analysis in psychology. *Qualitative Research in Psychology, 3*(1), 77–101.

Braun, V., Gavey, N., & McPhillips, K. (2003). The "fair" deal? Unpacking accounts of reciprocity in heterosex. *Sexualities, 6*(2), 237–261.

Brickell, C. (2005). Masculinities, performativity, and subversion: A sociological reappraisal. *Men and Masculinities, 8*(1), 24–43.

Bridges, S. K., Lease, S. H., & Ellison, C. R. (2004). Predicting sexual satisfaction in women: Implications for counselor education and training. *Journal of Counseling & Development, 82*(2), 158–166.

Brown, J. D., Steele, J. R., & Walsh-Childers, K. (2002). *Sexual teens, sexual media: Investigating media's influence on adolescent sexuality.* New York: Erlbaum.

Browning, J. R., Hatfield, E., Kessler, D., & Levine, T. (2000). Sexual motives, gender, and sexual behavior. *Archives of Sexual Behavior, 29*(2), 135–153.

Brownmiller, S. (1975). *Against our will: Men, women, and rape.* New York: Simon & Schuster.

Bryan, T. S. (2002). Pretending to experience orgasm as a communicative act: How, when, and why some sexually experienced college women pretend to experience orgasm during various sexual behaviors. *Dissertation Abstracts International, 63,* 2049.

Buchanan, N. T., & Ormerod, A. J. (2002). Racialized sexual harassment in the lives of African American women. *Women & Therapy, 25*(3–4), 107–124.

Bufkin, J., & Eschholz, S. (2000). Images of sex and rape: A content analysis of popular film. *Violence against Women, 6*(12), 1317–1344.

Buhle, M. J. (1998). *Feminism and its discontents: A century of struggle with psychoanalysis.* Cambridge: Harvard University Press.

Bullough, V. L. (1999). *The wandering womb: A cultural history of outrageous beliefs about women.* Amherst: Prometheus Books.

Burch, B. (1998). Lesbian sexuality/female sexuality: Searching for sexual subjectivity. *Psychoanalytic Review, 85*(1), 349–372.

Burgess, G. H. (2007). Assessment of rape-supportive attitudes and beliefs in college men: Development, reliability, and validity of the rape attitudes and beliefs scale. *Journal of Interpersonal Violence, 22*(8), 973–993.

Butler, C. A. (1976). New data about female sexual response. *Journal of Sex & Marital Therapy, 2*(1), 40–46.

Butler, J. (1990). *Gender trouble: Feminism and the subversion of identity.* New York: Routledge.

Butler, J. (1997). *Excitable speech: A politics of the performative.* New York: Routledge.

Byers, S., Purdon, C., & Clark, D. A. (1998). Sexual intrusive thoughts of college students. *Journal of Sex Research, 35*(4), 359–369.

Byrne, D., & Osland, J. A. (2000). Sexual fantasy and erotica/pornography: Internal and external imagery. In L. T. Szuchman & F. Muscarella (Eds.), *Psychological perspectives on human sexuality* (pp. 283–305). Toronto, ON: Wiley.

Campbell, R., & Wasco, S. M. (2005). Understanding rape and sexual assault: 20 years of progress and future directions. *Journal of Interpersonal Violence, 20*(1), 127–131.

Campbell, R., Sefl, T., & Ahrens, C. E. (2004). The impact of rape on women's sexual health risk behaviors. *Health Psychology, 23*(1), 67–74.

Caputi, J. (2006). Everyday pornography. In G. Dines & J. M. Humez (Eds.), *Gender, race, and class in media: A text reader* (pp. 434–450). Thousand Oaks, CA: Sage.

Carey, B. (2005, July 5). Gay, straight, or lying? Bisexuality revisited. Retrieved July 5, 2005, from *The New York Times*. Website: http://www.nytimes.com/2005/07/05/health/05sex.html.

Carroll, J. S., Padilla-Walker, L. M., Nelson, L. J., Olson, C. D., Barry, C. M., & Madsen, S. D. (2008). Generation XXX: Pornography acceptance and use among emerging adults. *Journal of Adolescent Research, 23*(1), 6–30.

Césaire, A. (2000). *Discourse on colonialism*. (J. Pinkham, Trans.). New York: Monthly Review Press.

Chapleau, K. M., Oswald, D. L., & Russell, B. L. (2008). Male rape myths: The role of gender, violence, and sexism. *Journal of Interpersonal Violence, 23*(5), 600–615.

Charmaz, K. (2003). Grounded theory: Objectivist and constructivist methods. In N. K. Denzin & Y. S. Lincoln (Eds.), *Strategies for qualitative inquiry* (pp. 249–291). Thousand Oaks, CA: Sage.

Christopher, S. F. (1988). An initial investigation into a continuum of premarital sexual pressure. *The Journal of Sex Research, 25*(2), 255–266.

Clarke, S. B., Rizvi, S. L., & Resick, P. A. (2008). Borderline personality characteristics and treatment outcome in cognitive-behavioral treatments for PTSD in female rape victims. *Behavior Therapy, 39*(1), 72–78.

Collins, I. (2008, November 3). If you suffer from any kind of sexual dysfunction, do something about it! Retrieved December 2, 2008, from *eFluxMedia*. Website: http://www.efluxmedia.com/news_If_You_Suffer_From_Any_Kind_Of_Sexual_Dysfunction_Do_Something_About_It_28010.html.

Conoscenti, L. M., & McNally, R. J. (2006). Health complaints in acknowledged and unacknowledged rape victims. *Journal of Anxiety Disorders, 20*(3), 372–379.

Conrad, P., & Potter, D. (2000). From hyperactive children to ADHD adults: Observations on the expansion of medical categories. *Social Problems, 47*(4), 559–582.

Cook, L. C. (2005, September 20). Meeting women's desire for desire: Testosterone fix risky, some experts say. *The Washington Post*, HE01.

Cooley, C. (1902). *Human nature and the social order.* New York: Charles Scriber's Sons.

Cooper, A., McLoughlin, I. P., & Campbell, K. M. (2000). Sexuality in cyberspace: Update for the 21st Century. *CyberPsychology & Behavior, 3*(4), 521–536.

Copenhaver, S., & Grauerholz, E. (1991). Sexual victimization among sorority women: Exploring the link between sexual violence and institutional practices. *Sex Roles, 24*(1–2), 31–41.

Costa, R. M., & Brody, S. (2007). Women's relationship quality is associated with specifically penile-vaginal intercourse orgasm and frequency. *Journal of Sex & Marital Therapy, 33*(4), 319–327.

Cowan, G. (2000). Beliefs about the causes of four types of rape. *Sex Roles, 42,* 807–823.

Critelli J. W., & Bivona, J. M. (2008). Women's erotic rape fantasies: An evaluation of theory and research. *Journal of Sex Research, 45*(1), 57–70.

Cushman, P. (1996). *Constructing the self, constructing America: A cultural history of psychotherapy.* Cambridge, MA: Da Capo.

Daneback, K., Cooper, A., & Månsson, S. A. (2005). An Internet study of cybersex participants. *Archives of Sexual Behavior, 34*(3), 321–328.

Darling, C. A., & Davidson, J. K. (1987). The relationship of sexual satisfaction to coital involvement: The concept of technical virginity revisited. *Deviant Behavior, 8*(1), 27–46.

Davidson, J. K., & Hoffman, L. E. (1986). Sexual fantasies and sexual satisfaction: An empirical analysis of erotic thought. *Journal of Sex Research, 22*(2), 184–205.

Davidson, J. K., & Moore, N. B. (1994). Guilt and lack of orgasm during sexual intercourse: Myth versus reality among college women. *Journal of Sex Education & Therapy, 20*(3), 153–174.

Davis, C. M., Blank, J., Lin, H. Y., & Bonillas, C. (1996). Characteristics of vibrator use among women. *Journal of Sex Research, 33*(4), 313–320.

Davis, K. C., Morris, J., George, W. H., Martell, J., & Heiman, J. R. (2006). Men's likelihood of sexual aggression: The influence of alcohol, sexual arousal, and violent pornography. *Aggressive Behavior, 32*(6), 581–589.

de Beauvoir, S. (1953). *The second sex.* New York: Knopf Books.

de Beauvoir, S. (1989). *The second sex.* (H. M. Parshley, Trans.). New York: Vintage.

De Bruijn, G. (1982). From masturbation to orgasm with a partner: How some women bridge the gap—and why others don't. *Journal of Sex & Marital Therapy, 8*(2), 151–167.

De Solenni, P. D. (2003). Girls gone wild. Retrieved November 16, 2008, from *National Review.* Website: http://findarticles.com/p/articles/mi_m1282/is_8_55/ai_100202167/.

DeCarlo, T. (2009). What lies beneath. Retrieved February 12, 2009, from *Brooklyn rail: Critical perspectives on arts, politics, and culture.* Web site: http://www.brooklynrail.org/2009/02/film/what-lies-beneath-feb-09.

Deci, E. L., & Ryan, R. M. (2008). Hedonia, eudaimonia, and well-being: An introduction. *Journal of Happiness Studies, 9*(1), 1–11.

Deleuze, G. (1989). *Cinema 2: The time machine.* (H. Tomlinson & R. Galeta, Trans.) Minneapolis: University of Minnesota Press.

Delphy, C. (1984). *Close to home: A materialist analysis of women's oppression.* Amherst, MA: University of Massachusetts.

Densmore, D. (1973). Independence from the sexual revolution. In A. Koedt, E. Levine, & A. Rapone (Eds.), *Radical feminism* (pp. 107–118). New York: Quadrangle Books.

Denzin, N. K. (2002). Much ado about Goffman. *The American Sociologist, 33*(2), 105–117.

Derrida, J. (1974). *Of Grammatology.* (G. C. Spivak, Trans.) Baltimore: John Hopkins University Press.

Derrida, J. (1979). *Speech and phenomena, and other essays on Husserl's theory of signs.* (D. B. Allison, Trans.). Evanston: Northwestern University Press. (Original work published 1973).

Deutsch, H. (1944). *The psychology of women.* New York: Gruen and Stratton.

Diamond, L. M. (2003). Was it a phase? Young women's relinquishment of lesbian/bisexual identities over a 5-year period. *Journal of Personality and Social Psychology, 84*(2), 352–364.

Diamond, L. M. (2008). Female bisexuality from adolescence to adulthood: Results from a 10-year longitudinal study. *Developmental Psychology, 44*(1), 5–14.

Dilorio, C., Pluhar, E., & Belcher, L. (2003). Parent-child communication about sexuality: A review of the literature from 1980–2002. *Journal of HIV/AIDS Prevention & Education for Adolescents & Children, 5*(3–4), 7–32.

Dines, G., Jensen, R., & Russo, A. (1998). Dirty business: *Playboy* magazine and the mainstreaming of pornography. In G. Dines, R. Jensen, & A. Russo (Eds.), *Pornography: The production and consumption of inequality* (pp. 37–64). New York: Routledge.

Doane, M. A. (1990). Technophilia: Technology, representation, and the feminine. In M. Jacobus, E. Fox-Keller, & S. Shuttleworth (Eds.), *Body/Politics: Women and the discourses of science* (pp. 163–176). New York: Routledge.

Dove, N. L., & Wiederman, M. W. (2000). Cognitive distraction and women's sexual functioning. *Journal of Sex & Marital Therapy, 26*(1), 67–78.

Du Bois, W. E. B. (1994). *The souls of black folk.* New York: Gramercy Books.

Dubner, S. J. (2008, January 24). What don't we know about the pharmaceutical industry? A freakonomics quorum. Retrieved February 15, 2008, from *Freakonomics.* Website: http://www.freakonomics.blogs.nytimes.com/ 2008/01/24/what-dont-we-know-about-the-pharmaceutical-industry-a-freakonomics-quorum/?scp-2&sq=female%20sexual%20dysfunction &st=cse.

Duenwald, M. (2003, March 25). Effort to make sex drug for women challenges experts. Retrieved December 2, 2008, from *The New York Times.* Website: http://query.nytimes.com/gst/fullpage.html?res=9B02E3DD15 30F936A15750C0A9659C8B63&sec=&spon=&pagewanted=1.

Duffy, M. (1994). Getting out of the wrecking ball. Retrieved on March 20, 2009, from *Time Magazine.* Website: http://www.time.com/time/maga-zine/article/0,9171,982008,00.html.

Dunbar, R. (1969). Sexual liberation: More of the same thing. *No More Fun and Games, 3,* 49–56.

Dworkin, A. (1989). *Pornography: Men possessing women.* New York: Plume Books.

Dworkin, A. (1997). *Intercourse.* New York: Free Press.

Easton, D., & Hardy, J. W. (2009). *The ethical slut: A practical guide to polyamory, open relationships, & other adventures.* Berkeley: Celestial Arts.

Ellis, B. J., & Symons, D. (1990). Sex differences in sexual fantasy: An evolutionary psychological approach. *Journal of Sex Research, 27*(4), 527–555.

Ellison, C. R. (2001). A research inquiry into some American women's sexual concerns and problems. *Women & Therapy, 24*(1–2), 147–159.

Emmers-Sommer, T. M., Pauley, P., Hanzal, A., & Triplett, L. (2006). Love, suspense, sex, and violence: Men's and women's film predilections, exposure to sexually violent media, and their relationship to rape myth acceptance. *Sex Roles, 55*(5–6), 311–320.

Fahs, B., & Swank, E. (2011). Social identities as predictors of women's sexual satisfaction and sexual activity. *Archives of Sexual Behavior.*

Fallon, M. (1995). Sextec: Excerpt from working hot. In E. A. Grosz, & E. Probyn (Eds.), *Sexy bodies: The strange carnalities of feminism* (pp. 42–85). London: Routledge.

Faravelli, C., Giugni, A., Salvatori, S., & Ricca, V. (2004). Psychopathology after rape. *American Journal of Psychiatry, 161*(8), 1483–1485.

Fasting, K., Brackenridge, C., & Walseth, K. (2007). Women athletes' personal responses to sexual harassment in sport. *Journal of Applied Sport Psychology, 19*(4), 419–433.

Fereday, J., & Muir-Cochrane, E. (2006). Demonstrating rigor using thematic analysis: A hybrid approach of inductive and deductive coding and theme development. *International Journal of Qualitative Methods, 5*(1), 1–11.

Ferguson, A. (1989). *Blood at the root: Motherhood, sexuality, and male domination.* New York: Pandora/Unwin and Hyman.

Findlay, H. (1992). Freud's "fetishism" and the lesbian dildo debates. *Feminist Studies, 18*(3), 563–579.

Fine, M. (1988). Sexuality, schooling, and adolescent females: The missing discourse of desire. *Harvard Educational Review, 58*(1), 29–53.

Fingerson, L. (2005). Do mother's opinions matter in teens' sexual activity? *Journal of Family Issues, 26*(7), 947–974.

Fisher, S. (1973). *The female orgasm: Psychology, physiology, fantasy.* New York: Basic Books.

Fishman, J. R., & Mamo, L. (2001). What's in a disorder: A cultural analysis of medical and pharmaceutical constructions of male and female dysfunction. *Women & Therapy, 24*(1–2), 179–193.

Flowe, H. D., Ebbesen, E. B., & Putcha-Bhagavatula, A. (2007). Rape shield laws and sexual behavior evidence: Effects of consent level and women's sexual history on rape allegations. *Law and Human Behavior, 31*(2), 159–175.

Folbre, N. (1982). Exploitation comes home: A critique of the Marxian theory of family labor. *Cambridge Journal of Economics, 6*(4), 317–329.

Fonow, M. M., Richardson, L., & Wemmerus, V. A. (1992). Feminist rape education: Does it work? *Gender and Society, 6*(1), 108–121.

Foucault, M. (1978). *The history of sexuality, Volume 1.* New York: Vintage Books.

Foucault, M., & Gordon, C. (1980). *Power/Knowledge.* New York: Pantheon Books.

Franiuk, R., Seefelt, J. L., Cepress, S. L., & Vandello, J. A. (2008). Prevalence and effects of rape myths in print journalism: The Kobe Bryant case. *Violence against Women, 14*(3), 287–309.

Franklin, K. (2004). Enacting masculinity: Antigay violence and group rape as participatory theater. *Sexuality Research & Social Policy, 1*(2), 25–40.

Freud, S. (2000). *Three essays on the theory of sexuality.* New York: Basic Books.

Friedan, B. (1963). *The feminine mystique.* New York: Norton Books.

Frith, H., & Kitzinger, C. (2001). Reformulating sexual script theory: Developing a discursive psychology of sexual negotiation. *Theory & Psychology, 11*(2), 209–232.

Fugl-Meyer, K. S., OBerg, K., Lundberg, P. O., Lewin, B., & Fugl-Meyer, A. (2006). On orgasm, sexual techniques, and erotic perceptions in 18- to 74-year-old Swedish women. *Journal of Sexual Medicine, 3*(1), 56–68.

Gagnon, J. H., & Simon, J. (1973). *Sexual conduct: The social origins of human sexuality*. Chicago: Aldine.

Gallagher, C. & Laqueur, T. W. (1987). *The making of the modern body: Sexuality and society in the nineteenth century*. Berkeley: University of California Press.

Ganahl, J. (2006, May 7). Sex could be just a sniff away. Retrieved August 28, 2008, from *San Francisco Chronicle*. Website: http://www.sfgate.com/cgi-bin/article.cgi?f=/c/a/2006/05/07/LVGNOIJDBE1.DTL.

Garber, M. (1995). *Vice versa: Bisexuality and the eroticism of everyday life*. New York: Simon & Schuster.

Gardner, A. (2008, October 31). Almost half of women have sexual problems. Retrieved August 28, 2008, from *U.S. News & World Report*. Website: http://health.usnews.com/articles/health/healthday/2008/10/31/almost-half-of-women-have-sexual-problems.html.

Gardner, C. B. (1995). *Passing by: Gender and public harassment*. Berkeley: University of California Press.

Gellene, D. (2008, July 23). Viagra helpful for women on antidepressants, study finds. Retrieved August 28, 2008, from *The Los Angeles Times*. Website: http://articles.latimes.com/2008/jul/23/science/sci-viagra23.

Gerhard, J. (2000). Revisiting "The myth of the vaginal orgasm": The female orgasm in American sexual thought and second wave feminism. *Feminist Studies, 26*(2), 449–476.

Get revved for great sex. (2009). Retrieved March 1, 2009, from *Cosmopolitan*. Website: http://www.cosmopolitan.com/sex-love/sex/revved-great-sex-2.

Gidycz, C. A., Orchowski, L. M., King, C. R., & Rich, C. L. (2008). Sexual victimization and health-risk behaviors: A prospective analysis of college women. *Journal of Interpersonal Violence, 23*(6), 744–763.

Gilbert, S. M., & Gubar, S. (1984). *The madwoman in the attic: The woman writer and the nineteenth-century literary imagination*. New Haven: Yale University Press.

Gilfoyle, J., Wilson, J., & Own, B. (1992). Sex, organs, and audiotape: A discourse analytic approach to talking about heterosexual sex and relationships. *Feminism & Psychology, 2*(2), 209–230.

Glascock, J. (2005). Degrading content and character sex: Accounting for men and women's differential reactions to pornography. *Communication Reports, 18*(1), 43–53.

Goffman, E. (1956). *The presentation of self in everyday life*. Edinburgh: University of Edinburgh Press.

Gold, S. R. (1991). History of child sexual abuse and adult sexual fantasies. *Violence and Victims, 6*(1), 75–82.

Golden, J. H., Johnson, C. A., & Lopez, R. A. (2001). Sexual harassment in the workplace: Exploring the effects of attractiveness on perception of harassment. *Sex Roles, 45*(11–12), 767–784.

González, M., Viáfara, G., Caba, F., Molina, T., & Ortiz, C. (2006). Libido and orgasm in middle-aged woman. *Maturitas, 53*(1), 1–10.

Grady, D. (1999, February 14). The nation: Better loving through chemistry; Sure, we've got a pill for that. Retrieved August 28, 2008, from *The New York Times.* Website: http://query.nytimes.com/gst/fullpage.html?res=9C01E7DA143AF937A25751C0A96F958260&sec=&spon=&page-wanted=2.

Greene, E. (1999). *Reading Sappho: Contemporary approaches.* Berkeley: University of California Press.

Greer, G. (1972). *The female eunuch.* New York: Bantam Books.

Grossman, A. J. (2008). Catcalling: Creepy or a compliment? Retrieved May 14, 2008, from CNN. Website: http://www.cnn.com/2008/LIVING/personal/05/14/lw.catcalls/index.html.

Grosz, E. (1991). *Sexual subversions: Three French feminists.* Sydney: Allen & Unwin.

Grosz, E. (1994). *Volatile bodies: Toward a corporeal feminism.* Bloomington: Indiana University Press.

Grosz, E. (1995a). Animal sex: Libido as desire and death. In E. Grosz & E. Probyn (Eds.), *Sexy bodies: The strange carnalitles of feminism* (pp. 278–299). London: Routledge.

Grosz, E. (1995b). Introduction. In E. Grosz & E. Probyn (Eds.), *Sexy bodies: The strange carnalitles of feminism* (pp. ix–xv). London: Routledge.

Gruber, J. E., & Fineran, S. (2007). The impact of bullying and sexual harassment on middle and high school girls. *Violence against Women, 13*(6), 627–643.

Guerette, S. M., & Caron, S. L. (2007). Assessing the impact of acquaintance rape: Interviews with women who are victims/survivors of sexual assault while in college. *Journal of College Student Psychotherapy, 22*(2), 31–50.

Haavio-Mannila, E., & Kontula, O. (1997). Correlates of increased sexual satisfaction. *Archives of Sexual Behavior, 26*(4), 399–419.

Hald, G. M. (2006). Gender differences in pornography consumption among young heterosexual Danish adults. *Archives of Sexual Behavior, 35*(5), 577–585.

Hald, G. M., & Malamuth, N. M. (2008). Self-perceived effects of pornography consumption. *Archives of Sexual Behavior, 37*(4), 614–625.

Harding, A. (2008, November 6). Testosterone patch may kick-start sex drive in women. Retrieved November 23, 2008, from CNN Website:

http://www.cnn.com/2008/HEALTH/conditions/11/06/healthmag.test osterone.patch.sex/index.html.

Harned, M. S., & Fitzgerald, L. F. (2002). Understanding a link between sexual harassment and eating disorder symptoms: A mediational analysis. *Journal of Consulting and Clinical Psychology, 70*(5), 1170–1181.

Harris, G. (2004, February 28). Pfizer gives up testing Viagra on women. *The New York Times*, C–1.

Hartley, H. (2006). The "pinking" of Viagra culture: Drug industry efforts to create and repackage sex drugs for women. *Sexualities, 9*(3), 363–378.

Hartley, H., & Coleman, C. L. (2008). News media coverage of direct-to-consumer pharmaceutical advertising: Implications of countervailing powers theory. *Health: An Interdisciplinary Journal for the Social Study of Health, Illness, and Medicine, 12*(1), 107–32.

Haugh, A. (2005). Bukkake: When did it get to this? Sad men doing sadder things. *Craccum, 19*(1), 16–18.

Haywood, H., & Swank, E. (2008). Rape myths among Appalachian college students. *Violence and Victims, 23*(3), 373–389.

Hegarty, P., & Pratto, F. (2001). Sexual orientation beliefs: Their relationship to anti-gay attitudes and biological determinist arguments. *Journal of Homosexuality, 41*(1), 121–135.

Helliwell, C. (2000). "It's only a penis": Rape, feminism, and difference. *Signs, 25*(3), 789–816.

Hicks, T. V., & Leitenberg, H. I. (2001). Sexual fantasies about one's partner versus someone else: Gender differences in incidence and frequency. *Journal of Sex Research, 38* (1), 43–50.

Hill-Collins, P. (1997). Pornography and black women's bodies. In J. R. Schiffman & L. L. O'Toole (Eds.), *Gender violence: Interdisciplinary perspectives* (pp. 395–399). New York: New York University Press.

Hill-Collins, P. (2005). *Black sexual politics: African Americans, gender, and the new racism.* New York: Routledge.

Hilt, J. (2000, February 20). The second sexual revolution. Retrieved August 28, 2008, from *The New York Times*. Website: http://query.nytimes.com/gst/fullpage.html?res=9F07E5DC1531F933A15751C0A9669C8B63&sec=&spon=&pagewanted=1.

Hirsch, E. D., Kett, J. F., & Trefil, J. (2002). *The new dictionary of cultural literacy* (3rd edition). New York: Houghton Mifflin.

Hite, S. (1976). *The Hite report: A nationwide study on female sexuality.* Oxford: Macmillan.

Hitlan, R. T., Schneider, K. T., & Walsh, B. M. (2006). Upsetting behavior: Reactions to personal and bystander sexual harassment experiences. *Sex Roles, 55*(3–4), 187–195.

Hoburg, R., Konik, J., Williams, M., & Crawford, M. (2004). Bisexuality among self-identified heterosexual college students. *Journal of Bisexuality, 4*(1), 25–36.

Hochschild, A. R., & Machung, A. (2003). *The second shift.* New York: Penguin.

Hollander, J. A., & Einwohner, R. L. (2004). Conceptualizing resistance. *Sociological Forum, 19,* 533–554.

hooks, b. (1996). Tough talk for tough times. *On the Issues: The progressive Women's Quarterly, 5*(1), 47–51.

Horney, K. (1942). *The collected works of Karen Horney: Volume II.* New York: Norton.

Hsu, B., Kling, A., Kessler, C., Knapke, K., Diefenbach, P., & Elias, J. E. (1994). Gender differences in sexual fantasy and behavior in a college population: A ten-year replication. *Journal of Sex & Marital Therapy, 20*(2), 103–118.

Hunt, M. (1974). *Sexual behavior in the 1970s.* Oxford: Playboy.

Hurlbert, D. F., & Apt, C. (1993). Female sexuality: A comparative study between women in homosexual and heterosexual relationships. *Journal of Sex & Marital Therapy, 19*(4), 315–327.

Hurlbert, D. F., Apt, C., & Rabehl, S. M. (1993). Key variables to understanding female sexual satisfaction: An examination of women in nondistressed marriages. *Journal of Sex & Marital Therapy, 19*(2), 154–165.

Hyde, J. S., & DeLamater, J. D. (1997). *Understanding human sexuality.* New York: McGraw-Hill.

Irigaray, L. (1985). *This sex which is not one.* Ithaca, NY: Cornell University Press.

Irvine, J. M. (2002). *Talk about sex: The battles over sex education in the United States.* Berkeley: University of California Press.

Jackson, S., & Scott, S. (2001). Embodying orgasm: Gendered power relations and sexual pleasure. *Women & Therapy, 24*(1–2), 99–110.

Janssen, E., Carpenter, D., & Graham, C. A. (2003). Selecting films for sex research: Gender differences in erotic film preference. *Archives of Sexual Behavior, 32*(3), 243–251.

Janus, S. S., & Janus, C. L. (1993). *The Janus report on sexual behavior.* New York: Wiley & Sons.

Jeffreys, S. (1990). *Anticlimax: A feminist perspective on the sexual revolution.* New York: New York University Press.

Jensen, R. (1995). Pornographic lives. *Violence against Women, 1*(1), 32–54.

Jensen, R. (2004, Spring). A cruel edge: The painful truth about today's pornography—and what men can do about it. *Ms. Magazine, 14*(1), 54–58.

Jensen, R. (2007). *Getting off: Pornography and the end of masculinity.* Cambridge, MA: South End.

336   REFERENCES

Jochen, P., & Valkenburg P. M. (2007). Adolescents' exposure to a sexualized media environment and their notions of women as sex objects. *Sex Roles, 56*(5), 381–395.

Johansson, T., & Hammarén, N. (2007). Hegemonic masculinity and pornography: Young people's attitudes toward and relations to pornography. *Journal of Men's Studies, 15*(1), 57–70.

Johnston, J. (1973). *Lesbian nation: The feminist solution.* New York: Simon & Schuster.

Jones, F. L., & Kelley, J. (1984). Decomposing differences between groups: A cautionary note on measuring discrimination. *Sociological Methods and Research, 12*(3), 323–343.

Jones, S. L., & Hostler, H. R. (2002). Sexual script theory: An integrative exploration of the possibilities and limits of sexual self-definition. *Journal of Psychology & Theology, 30*(2), 120–130.

Jordan, J. (2004). Beyond belief? Police, rape and women's credibility. *International Journal of Policy and Practice, 4*(1), 29–59.

Kahlor, L., & Morrison, D. (2007). Television viewing and rape myth acceptance among college women. *Sex Roles, 56*(11–12), 729–739.

Kahn, A. S. (2004). 2003 Carolyn Sherif award address: What college women do and do not experience as rape. *Psychology of Women Quarterly, 28*(1), 9–15.

Kahn, A. S., Jackson, J., Kully, C., Badger, K., & Halvorsen, J. (2003). Calling it rape: Differences in experiences of women who do or do not label their sexual assault as rape. *Psychology of Women Quarterly, 27*(3), 233–242.

Kahr, B. (2008). *Who's been sleeping in your head? The secret world of sexual fantasies.* New York: Basic Books.

Kelly, J. R., Murphy, J. D., Craig, T. Y., & Driscoll, D. M. (2005). The effect of nonverbal behaviors associated with sexual harassment proclivity on women's performance. *Sex Roles, 53*(9–10), 689–701.

Kelly, L. (1996). "It's everywhere": Sexual violence as a continuum. In S. Jackson, & S. Scott (Eds.), *Feminism and sexuality: A reader.* Edinburgh: Edinburgh University Press.

Kermode, F. (1995, July 9). Beyond category. Retrieved August 25, 2008, from *The New York Times.* Website: http://www.nytimes.com/1995/07/09/books/beyond-category.html.

Kerner, I. (2008). It is ok to fantasize about my ex? Retrieved December 1, 2008, from *Cosmopolitan.* Website: http://www.cosmopolitan.com/sex-love/advice/expert/ex-fantasies?click=main_sr.

Kiefer, A. K., & Sanchez, D. T. (2007). *Scripting sexual passivity: A gender role perspective.* Personal Relationships, 14(2), 269–290.

Kiefer, A. K., Sanchez, D. T., Kalinka, C. J., & Ybarra, O. (2006). How women's nonconscious association of sex with submission relates to their subjective sexual arousability and ability to reach orgasm. *Sex Roles, 55*(1–2), 93–94.

Kilbourne, J. (2007). "You talkin' to me?" In M. Anderson and P. Hill-Collins (Eds.), *Race, class, and gender: An anthology* (pp. 228–233). Belmont, CA: Wadsworth.

Kimes, L. A. (2002). "Was it good for you too?" An exploration of sexual satisfaction. *Dissertation Abstracts International, 62,* 4791.

Kimmel, M., & Plante, R. F. (2002). The gender of desire: The sexual fantasies of women and men. *Advances in Gender Research, 6,* 55–77.

Kimmel, M. S., & Plante, R. F. (2005). The gender of desire: The sexual fantasies of women and men. In M. S. Kimmel (Ed.), *The gender of desire: Essays on male sexuality.* Albany: State University of New York Press.

Kingsberg, S. (2002). The impact of aging on sexual function in women and their partners. *Archives of Sexual Behavior, 31*(5), 431–437.

Kingsberg, S. (2008). A commentary on sexual well-being, happiness, and satisfaction in women: The case for a new conceptual paradigm. *Journal of Sex & Marital Therapy, 34*(4), 302–304.

Kinsey, A. C., Pomeroy, W. B., & Martin, C. E. (1948). *Sexual behavior in the human male.* Philadelphia: Saunders.

Kinsey, A. C., Pomeroy, W. B., & Martin, C. E. (1953). *Sexual behavior in the human female.* Philadelphia: Saunders.

Kinsey, A. C., Pomeroy, W. B., Martin, C. E., & Gebhard, P. H. (1953). *Sexual behavior in the human female.* Philadelphia: Saunders.

Kirkey, S. (2008, October 30). Only 12% of women bothered by low sex drive: study. Retreived November 14, 2008, from *The National Post.* Website: http://www.nationalpost.com/news/world/story.html?id=920739.

Kissling, E. A. (1991). Street harassment: The language of sexual terrorism. *Discourse & Society, 2*(4), 451–460.

Kite, M. E., & Whitley, B. R., Jr. (2003). Do heterosexual women and men differ in their attitudes toward homosexuality? A conceptual and methodological analysis. In L. Garnets & D. C. Kimmel (Eds.), *Psychological perspectives on lesbian, gay, and bisexual experiences* (pp. 165–187). New York: Columbia University Press.

Klusmann, D. (2002). Sexual motivation and the duration of partnership. *Archives of Sexual Behavior, 31*(3), 275–287.

Koedt, A. (1973). The myth of the vaginal orgasm. In A. Koedt, E. Levine, & A. Rapone (Eds.), *Radical feminism* (pp. 199–207). New York: Quadrangle Books.

Kofman, S. (1980). *The enigma of woman: Woman in Freud's writings*. Ithaca: Cornell University Press.

Kohn, D. (2008, August 28). Viagra may work for women, too: In matters of desire, however, not much help. *Baltimore Sun*, C–1.

Kolata, G. (1998, April 25). Doctors debate use of drug to help women's sex lives. Retrieved August 28, 2008, from *The New York Times*. Website: http://query.nytimes.com/gst/fullpage.html?res=9C04E5DA133FF936A1 575760A96F958260&scp=14&sq=female=sexual=dysfunction&st=nyt.

Koss, M. P. (1985). The hidden rape victim: Personality, attitudinal, and situational characteristics. *Psychology of Women Quarterly, 9*(2), 193–212.

Koss, M. P., Gidycz, C. A., & Wisniewski, N. (1987). The scope of rape: Incidence and prevalence of sexual aggression and victimization in a national sample of higher education students. *Journal of Clinical and Consulting Psychology, 55*(2), 162–170.

Koss, M. P., Heise, L., Russo, N. F. (1994). The global health burden of rape. *Psychology of Women Quarterly, 18*(4), 509–537.

Kwan, N. (2008, October 23). "Pink Viagra" gel may boost desire: Testosterone is secret to love drug trial. Retrieved November 14, 2008, from *NBC Chicago*. Website: http://www.nbcchicago.com/health/women/Pink_ Viagra_could_be_a_gel_that_boosts_desire_.html.

Laqueur, T. (1990). *Making sex: Body and gender from the Greeks to Freud*. Cambridge: Harvard University Press.

Laqueur, T. (2002). *Solitary sex: A cultural history of masturbation*. New York: Zone Books.

Laumann, E., Paik, A., & Rosen, R. C. (1999). Sexual dysfunction in the United States. *Journal of the American Medical Association, 281*(6), 537–544.

Laumann, E. O., Gagnon, J. H., Michael, R. T., & Michaels, S. (1994). *The social organization of sexuality: Sexual practices in the United States*. Chicago: University of Chicago Press.

Le Doeuff, M. (1989). *L'Imaginaire Philosophique*. Paris: Payot.

Leitenberg, H., & Henning, K. (1995). Sexual fantasy. *Psychological Bulletin, 117*(3), 469–496.

Levitt, E. E., & Moser, C. (1987). An exploratory-descriptive study of a sadomasochistically oriented sample. *Journal of Sex Research, 23*(3), 322–337.

Levy, A. (2005). *Female chauvinist pigs: Women and the rise of raunch culture*. New York: Free Press.

Lindberg, S. M., Grabe, S., & Hyde, J. S. (2007). Gender, pubertal development, and peer sexual harassment predict objectified body consciousness in early adolescence. *Journal of Research on Adolescence, 17*(4), 723–742.

Littleton, H., & Breitkopf, C. R. (2006). Coping with the experience of rape. *Psychology of Women Quarterly, 30*(1), 106–116.

Littleton, H. L., Rhatigan, D. L., & Axsom, D. (2007). Unacknowledged rape: How much do we know about the hidden rape victim? *Journal of Aggression, Maltreatment & Trauma, 14*(4), 57–74.

Lloyd, E. (2005). *The case of the female orgasm: Bias in the science of evolution.* Cambridge: Harvard University Press.

Loe, M. (2004a). *The rise of Viagra: How the little blue pill changed sex in America.* New York: New York University Press.

Loe, M. (2004b). Sex and the senior woman: Pleasure and danger in the Viagra era. *Sexualities, 7*(3), 303–326.

Lonsway, K. A., & Fitzgerald, L. F. (1994). Rape myths: In review. *Psychology of Woman Quarterly, 18*(2), 133–164.

Lonsway, K. A., & Fitzgerald, L. F. (1995). Rape myth acceptance and sociodemographic characteristics: A multidimensional analysis. *Sex Roles, 36*(11–12), 693–707.

Lorber, J. (1994). *Paradoxes of gender.* New Haven, CT: Yale University Press.

Lorde, A. (1993). The uses of the erotic: The erotic as power. In H. Abelove, M. A. Barale, & D. M. Halperin (Eds.), *The lesbian and gay studies reader* (pp. 339–343).

Lorde, A. (n.d.). Who said it was simple. Retrieved January 31, 2010, from New York State Writer's Institute. Website: http://www.albany.edu/writers-inst/webpages4/archives/lorde.html.

Lottes, I. L. (1993). Nontraditional gender roles and the sexual experiences of heterosexual college students. *Sex Roles, 29*(9–10), 645–669.

Lottes, I. L., & Weinberg M. S. (1997). Sexual coercion among university students: A comparison of the United States and Sweden. *Journal of Sex Research, 34*(1), 67–76.

Love advice: Am I gay if I have thoughts about other women? (2009). Retrieved March 1, 2009, from *Cosmopolian.* Website: http://www.cosmopolitan.com/sex-love/advice/questions/gay-if-thoughts-about-women?click=main_sr.

Lyon, L. (2008, July 22). For women, four alternatives to Viagra: The iconic drug is not the only way to fix sexual dysfunction. Retrieved July 30, 2008, from *U.S. News and World Report.* Website: http://health.usnews.com/articles/health/sexual-reproductive/2008/07/22/for-women-4-alternatives-to-viagra.html.

Lyon, L. (2008, March 27). Women lacking libido aren't sick: Birth of "pink Viagra" would wrongly medicalize low sex drive, says Lenore Tiefer. Retrieved August 28, 2008, from *U.S. News and World Report.* Website:

http://health.usnews.com/articles/health/sexual-reproductive/
2008/03/27/women-lacking-libido-arent-sick.html.

MacKinnon, C. A. (1987). Desire and power. In C. A. MacKinnon (Ed.), *Feminism unmodified: Discourses on life and law* (pp. 48–62). Cambridge: Harvard University Press.

Macmillan, R., Nierobisz, A., & Welsh, S. (2000). Experiencing the streets: Harassment and perceptions of safety among women. *Journal of Research in Crime and Delinquency, 37*(3), 306–322.

MacNeil, S., & Byers, S. E. (2005). Dyadic assessment of sexual self-disclosure and sexual satisfaction in heterosexual dating couples. *Journal of Social and Personal Relationships, 22*(2), 169–181.

Mah, K. (2002). Development of a multidimensional model of the psychological experience of male and female orgasm. *Dissertation Abstracts International, 62*, 5947.

Mah, K., & Binik, Y. M. (2001). The nature of human orgasm: A critical review of major trends. *Clinical Psychology Review, 21*(6), 823–856.

Maines, R. P. (1999). *The technology of orgasm: "Hysteria," the vibrator, and women's sexual satisfaction.* Baltimore: Johns Hopkins University Press.

Malamuth, N. M., Addison, T., & Koss, M. (2000). Pornography and sexual aggression: Are there reliable effects and can we understand them? *Annual Review of Sex Research, 11*, 26–91.

Martin, E. (2001). *The woman in the body: A cultural analysis of reproduction.* Boston: Beacon.

Martin, E. K., Taft, C. T., & Resick, P. A. (2007). A review of marital rape. *Aggression and Violent Behavior, 12*(3), 329–347.

Martin, K., Vieraitis, L. M., & Britto, S. (2006). Gender equality and women's absolute status: A test of the feminist models of rape. *Violence against Women, 12*(4), 321–339.

Martin, R. (1988). Truth, power, self: An interview with Michel Foucault, October 25, 1982. In L. Martin, H. Gutman, & P. Hutton (Eds.), *Technologies of the self: A seminar with Michel Foucault* (pp. 9–15). Amherst: University of Massachusetts Press.

Marx, B. P., Van Wie, V., & Gross, A. M. (1996). Date rape risk factors: A review and methodological critique of the literature. Masters, W. H., & Johnson, V. E. (1966). *Human sexual response.* Boston, MA: Little, Brown.

Masters, W. H., & Johnson, V. E. (1966). *Human sexual response.* New York: Bantam Books.

McCauley, C., & Swann, C. P. (1978). Male-female differences in sexual fantasy. *Journal of Research in Personality, 12*(1), 76–86.

McClelland, S. I., & Fine, M. (2008). Embedded science: Critical analysis of abstinence-only evaluation research. *Cultural Studies <=> Critical Methodologies, 8*(1), 50–81.

McClelland, S. I., & Fine, M. (2008). Writing *on* cellophane: Studying teen women's sexual desires; Inventing methodological release points. In K. Gallagher (Ed.), *The methodological dilemma: Critical and creative approaches to qualitative research* (pp. 232–260). London: Routledge.

McKee, A. (2007). The relationship between attitudes towards women, consumption of pornography, and other demographic variables in a survey of 1,023 consumers of pornography. *International Journal of Sexual Health, 19*(1), 31–45.

McMaster, L. E., Connolly, J., Pepler, D., & Craig, W. M. (2002). Peer to peer sexual harassment in early adolescence: A developmental perspective. *Development and Psychopathology, 14*(1), 91–105.

McMullin, D., & White, J. W. (2006). Long-term effects of labeling a rape experience. *Psychology of Women Quarterly, 30*(1), 96–105.

McNulty, J. K., & Fisher, T. D. (2008). Gender differences in response to sexual expectancies and changes in sexual frequency: A short-term longitudinal study of sexual satisfaction in newly married couples. *Archives of Sexual Behavior, 37*(2), 229–240.

Mead, G. H. (1934). *Mind, self, and society.* (C. W. Morris, Trans.). Chicago: University of Chicago Press.

Means, M. C. (2001). An integrative approach to what women really want: Sexual satisfaction. *Dissertation Abstracts International, 61*, 4417.

Miller, B. (2007, November 6). A billion-dollar romance novel industry, and its lonely black author: The Fabio business finds itself short on diversity. Retrieved November 8, 2008, from *Seattle Weekly*. Website: http://www.seattleweekly.com/2007-11-07/news/a-billion-dollar-romance-novel-industry-and-its-lonely-black-author.php?page=full.

Millet, K. (1970). *Sexual politics.* New York: Simon & Schuster.

Miner-Rubino, K., & Cortina, L. M. (2004). Working in a context of hostility toward women: Implications for employees' well-being. *Journal of Occupational Health Psychology, 9*(2), 107–122.

Miner-Rubino, K., & Cortina, L. M. (2007). Beyond targets: Consequences of vicarious exposure to misogyny at work. *Journal of Applied Psychology, 92*(5), 1254–1269.

Mitchell, D., Angelone, D. J., Hirschman, R., Lilly, R. S., & Hall, G. C. (2002). Peer modeling and college men's sexually impositional behavior in the laboratory. *Journal of Sex Research, 39*(4), 326–333.

Mitchell, J. (1975). *Psychoanalysis and feminism.* New York: Vintage.

Mitchell, K. J., Finkelhor, D., & Wolak, J. (2007). Online requests for sexual pictures from youth: Risk factors and incident characteristics. *Journal of Adolescent Health, 41*(2), 196–203.

Mitchell, K. J., Wolak, J., & Finkelhor, D. (2007). Trends in youth reports of sexual solicitations, harassment, and unwanted exposure to pornography on the internet. *Journal of Adolescent Health, 40*(2), 116–126.

Mitchell, K. J., Wolak, J., Finkelhor, D. (2008). Are blogs putting youth at risk for online sexual solicitation or harassment? *Child Abuse & Neglect, 32*(2), 277–294.

Mohler-Kuo, M., Dowdall, G. W., Koss, M. P., & Wechsler, H. (2004). Correlates of rape while intoxicated in a national sample of college women. *Journal of Studies on Alcohol, 65*(1), 37–45.

Moore, D. (2005). Empirical investigation of the conflict and flexibility models of bisexuality. *Journal of Bisexuality, 5*(1), 5–25.

Morgan, D. (2007, October 18). Birth control foe to head family planning: Bush picks for contraceptive program called birth control part of "culture of death." Retrieved February 2, 2009, from *CBS News.* Website: http://www.cbsnews.com/stories/2007/10/18/health/main3380290.shtml.

Mosher, D. L., & MacIan, P. (1994). College men and women respond to X-rated videos intended for male or female audiences: Gender and sexual scripts. *Journal of Sex Research, 31*(2), 99–113.

Mosher, W. D., Chandra, A., & Jones, J. (2005). Sexual behavior and selected health measures: Men and women 15–44 years of age, United States, 2002. *Advanced Data, 15*(1), 1–55.

Moynihan, R. (2003). The making of a disease: Female sexual dysfunction. *BMJ, 326*, 45–47.

Munson, M., & Stelboum, J. P. (1999). Introduction. In M. Munson & J. Stelboum (Eds.), *The lesbian polyamory reader: Open relationships, non-monogamy, and casual sex* (pp. 1–10). London: Routledge.

Murdoch, M., Polusny, M. A., Hodges, J., & O'Brien, N. (2004). Prevalence of in-service and post-service sexual assault among combat and noncombat veterans applying for Department of Veterans Affairs posttraumatic stress disorder disability benefits. *Military Medicine, 169*(5), 392–395.

Nagle, J. (1997). First ladies of feminist porn: A conversation with Candida Royalle and Debi Sundahi. In J. Nagle (Ed.), *Whores and Other Feminists* (pp. 156–166). New York: Routledge.

Napolitano, M. (2005, August). Just looking: A view of street harassment of women. Retrieved August 4, 2008, from *The Villager.* Website: http://www.thevillager.com/villager_118/justlookingaviewof.html.

Nicolson, P. (2004). Reproductive success and the social construction of "frigidity": Do women "go off" sexual intercourse because they are "ill?" *Sexualities, Evolution, & Gender, 6*(1), 55–57.

Nicolson, P., & Burr, J. (2003). What is "normal" about women's (hetero)sexual desire and orgasm? A report of an in-depth interview study. *Social Science & Medicine, 57*(9), 1735–1745.

Nurnberg, G. H., Hensley, P. L., Gelenberg, A. J., Fava, M., Lauriello, J., & Paine, S. (2003). Treatment of antidepressant-associated sexual dysfunction with sildenafil: A randomized controlled trial. *JAMA*, 289, 56–64.

Nutter, D. E., & Condron, M. K. (1983). Sexual fantasy and activity patterns of females with inhibited sexual desire versus normal controls. *Journal of Sex & Marital Therapy, 9*(4), 276–282.

O'Connor, A. (2004, March 16). Sex and the brain: Researchers say, "Vive la différence!" *The New York Times*, F–5.

O'Reilly, S., Knox, D., & Zusman, M. (2007). College student attitudes toward pornography use. *College Student Journal, 41*(2), 402–406.

Odede, R., & Asghedom, E. (2001). The continuum of violence against women in Eritrea. *Development, 44*(3), 69–73.

Oliver, K. (2007). *Women as weapons of war: Iraq, sex, and the media*. New York: Columbia University Press.

Packer, J. (1986). Sex differences in the perception of street harassment. *Women & Therapy, 5*(2–3), 331–338.

Pain, R. H. (1997). Social geographies of women's fear of crime. *Transactions of the Institute of British Geographers, 22*(2), 231–244.

Palmer, J. S. (2007, January 8). A little blue pill for women? A German drug-maker has stumbled on a substance that increases female arousal. Retrieved August 28, 2008, from *Business Week*. Website: http://www.businessweek.com/magazine/content/07_02/b4016050.htm.

Parillo, K. M., Freeman, R. C., & Young, P. (2003). Association between child sexual abuse and sexual revictimization in adulthood among women sex partners of injection drug users. *Violence and Victims, 18*(4), 473–484.

Parvez, Z. F. (2006). The labor of pleasure: How perceptions of emotional labor impact women's enjoyment of pornography. *Gender & Society, 20*(5), 605–631.

Paul, E. L., & Hayes, K. A. (2002). The casualties of "casual" sex: A qualitative exploration of the phenomenology of college students' hookups. *Journal of Social and Personal Relationships, 19*(5), 635–661.

Paul, E. L., McManus, B., & Hayes, A. (2000). "Hookups": Characteristics and correlates of college students' spontaneous and anonymous sexual experiences. *Journal of Sex Research, 37*(1), 76–88.

Pazak, S. J. (1998). Predicting sexual satisfaction and marital satisfaction. *Dissertation Abstracts International, 58*, 6244.

Pearson, S. E., & Pollack, R. H. (1997). Female response to sexually explicit films. *Journal of Psychology & Human Sexuality, 9*(2), 73–88.

Pedersen, W., & Blekesaune, M. (2003). Sexual satisfaction in young adulthood: Cohabitation, committed dating or unattached life? *Acta Sociologica, 46*(3), 179–193.

Pelletier, L. A., & Herold, E. S. (1988). The relationship of age, sex guilt, and sexual experience with female sexual fantasies. *Journal of Sex Research, 24*(27), 250–256.

Pendleton, E. (1997). Love for sale: Queering heterosexuality. In J. Nagle (Ed.), *Whores and Other Feminists* (pp. 73–82). New York: Routledge.

Penley, C. (2004). Crackers and whackers: The white trashing of porn. In L. Williams (Ed.), *Porn studies* (pp. 309–331). Durham, NC: Duke University Press.

Pepler, D. J., Craig, W. M., Connolly, J. A., Yuile, A., McMaster, L., & Jiang, D. (2006). A developmental perspective on bullying. *Aggressive Behavior, 32*(4), 376–384.

Peterson, Z. D., & Muehlenhard, C. L. (2004). Was it rape? The function of women's rape myth acceptance and definitions of sex in labeling their own experiences. *Sex Roles, 51*(3–4), 129–144.

Peterson, Z. D., & Muehlenhard, C. L. (2007). Conceptualizing the "wantedness" of women's consensual and nonconsensual sexual experiences: Implications for how women label their experiences with rape. *Journal of Sex Research, 44*(1), 72–88.

Pinkerton, S. D., Bogart, L. M., Cecil, H., & Abramson, P. R. (2002). Factors associated with masturbation in a collegiate sample. *Journal of Psychology and Human Sexuality, 14*(2/3), 103–121.

Pinkerton, S. D., Cecil, H., Bogart, L. M., & Abramson, P. R. (2003). The pleasures of sex: An empirical investigation. *Cognition and Emotion, 17*(2), 341–353.

Pinney, E. M., Gerrard, M., & Denney, N. W. (1987). The Pinney Sexual Satisfaction Inventory. *Journal of Sex Research, 23*(2), 233–251.

Pitchford, N. (1997). Reading feminism's pornography conflict. In T. Foster, C. Siegel, & E. E. Berry (Eds.), *Sex positives? The cultural politics of dissident sexualities* (pp. 3–38). New York: New York University Press.

Plante, R. F. (2006a). *Sexualities in context: A social perspective.* Boulder, CO: Westview.

Plante, R. F. (2006). Sexual spanking, the self, and the construction of deviance. *Journal of Homosexuality, 50*(2–3), 59–79.

Plummer, K. (2002). *Sexualities: Critical concepts in sociology.* London: Taylor & Francis.

Posner, R. (1992). *Sex and reason.* Cambridge: Harvard University Press.

Price, J. H., & Allensworth, D. D. (1985). Comparison of sexual fantasies of homosexuals and of heterosexuals. *Psychological Reports, 57*(3), 871–877.

Procter & Gamble to license Noven's hormone skin patch designed to boost women's sex drive (2008, August 21). Retrieved August 28, 2008, from

The Los Angeles Times. Website: http://libigelfemaleviagra.blogspot. com/2008/02/libigel.html.

Purdon, C., & Holdaway, L. (2006). Non-erotic thoughts: Content and relation to sexual functioning and sexual satisfaction. *Journal of Sex Research, 43*(2), 154–162.

Quackenbush, D. M., Strassberg, D. S., & Turner, C. W. (1995). Gender effects of romantic themes in erotica. *Archives of Sexual Behavior, 24*(1), 21–35.

Queen, C. (1997). *Real live nude girl: Chronicles of sex-positive culture.* Pittsburgh: Cleis.

Quinn, B. A. (2002). Sexual harassment and masculinity: The power and meaning of "girl watching." *Gender & Society, 16*(3), 386–402.

Raboch, J., & Raboch, J. (1992). Infrequent orgasms in women. *Journal of Sex & Marital Therapy, 18*(2), 114–120.

Raffaelli, M., & Ontai, L. L. (2001). "She's 16 years old and there's boys calling over to the house": An exploratory study of sexual socialization in Latino families. *Culture, Health & Sexuality, 3*(3), 295–310.

Réage, P. (1965). *Story of O.* New York: Grove.

Rederstorff, J. C., Buchanan, N. T., & Settles, I. H. (2007). The moderating roles of race and gender-role attitudes in the relationship between sexual harassment and psychological well-being. *Psychology of Women Quarterly, 31*(1), 50–61.

Reid, S. A., Byrne, S., Brundidge, J. S., Shoham, M. D., & Marlow, M. L. (2007). A critical test of self-enhancement, exposure, and self-categorization explanations for first- and third-person perceptions. *Human Communication Research, 33*(2), 143–162.

Renaud, C. A., & Byers, E. S. (1999). Exploring the frequency, diversity, and content of university students' positive and negative sexual cognitions. *Canadian Journal of Human Sexuality, 8*(1), 17–30.

Rich, A. C. (1980). Compulsory heterosexuality and the lesbian existence. *Signs, 5*(3), 631–660.

Riordan, T. (1999, April 26). Patents: Viagra's success has brought to light a second big market for sexual dysfunction therapies: Women. Retrieved August 28, 2008, from *The New York Times.* Website: http://query. nytimes.com/gst/fullpage.html?res=980CE3D91F3AF935A15757C0A96 F958260&scp=1&sq=female+sexual+dysfunction&st=nyt.

Risman, B., & Schwartz, P. (2002). After the sexual revolution: Gender politics in teen dating. *Contexts, 1*(1), 16–24.

Risman, B. J., & Johnson-Family, D. (1998). Doing it fairly: A study of postgender marriages. *Journal of Marriage and Family, 60*(1), 23–40.

Roberts, C., Kippax, S., Waldby, C., & Crawford, J. (1995). Faking it: The story of 'Ohh!' *Women's Studies International Forum, 18*(5–6), 523–532.

Robinson, J. D., & Parks, C. W. (2003). Lesbian and bisexual women's sexual fantasies, psychological adjustment, and close relationship functioning. *Journal of Psychology & Human Sexuality, 15*(4), 185–203.

Robinson, P. (1993). *Freud and his critics.* Berkeley: University of California Press.

Rodkin, P. C., & Fischer, K. (2003). Sexual harassment and the cultures of childhood: Developmental, domestic violence, and legal perspectives. *Journal of Applied School Psychology, 19*(2), 177–196.

Rose, J. (2005). *Sexuality in the field of vision.* London: Verso.

Rospenda, K. M., Richman, J. A., Ehmke, J. L., & Zlatoper, K. W. (2005). Is workplace harassment hazardous to your health? *Journal of Business and Psychology, 20*(1), 95–110.

Rossi, A. S. (1994). Eros and caritas: A biosocial approach to sexuality and reproduction. In A. S. Rossi (Ed.), *Sexuality across the life course* (pp. 3–36). Chicago: University of Chicago Press.

Roth, L. M. (2007). Women on Wall Street: Despite diversity measures, Wall Street remains vulnerable to sex discrimination charges. *Academy of Management Perspectives, 21*(1), 24–35.

Rozee, P. D. (2005). Rape resistance: Successes and challenges. In A. Barnes (Ed.), *The handbook of women, psychology, and the law* (pp. 265–279). Hoboken, NJ: Wiley & Sons.

Rozee, P. D., Biaggio, M., & Hersen, M. (2000). Sexual victimization: Harassment and rape. In M. Biaggio & M. Hersen (Eds.), *Issues in the psychology of women* (pp. 93–113). Dordrecht, Netherlands: Kluwer.

Ruggiero, K. J., Smith, D. W., Hanson, R. F., Resnick, H. S., Saunders, B. E., Kilpatrick, D. G., & Best, C. L. (2004). Is disclosure of childhood rape associated with mental health outcome? Results from the National women's study. *Child Maltreatment, 9*(1), 62–77.

Russell, D. E. H. (1993). *Against pornography: The evidence of harm.* Berkeley: Russell.

Russo, A. (1987). Conflicts and contradictions among feminists over issues of pornography and sexual freedom. *Women's Studies International Forum, 10*(2), 103–112.

Rust, P. C. R. (1992). The politics of sexual identity: Sexual attraction and behavior among lesbian and bisexual women. *Social Problems, 39*(4), 366–386.

Ryan, T. (2007). *Sexuality in Greek and Roman literature and society.* Oxford: Taylor & Francis.

Rye, B. J., & Meaney, G. J. (2007). The pursuit of sexual pleasure. *Sexuality & Culture, 11*(1) 28–51.

Sable, M. R., Danis, F., Mauzy, D. L., & Gallagher, S. K. (2006). Barriers to reporting sexual assault for women and men: Perspectives of college students. *Journal of American College Health, 55*(3), 157–162.

Sanchez, D. T., & Kiefer, A. K. (2007). Body concerns in and out of the bedroom: Implications for sexual pleasure and problems. *Archives of Sexual Behavior, 36*(6), 808–820.

Sanchez, D. T., Crocker, J., & Boike, K. R. (2005). Doing gender in the bedroom: Investing in gender norms and the sexual experiences. *Personality and Social Psychology Bulletin, 31*(10), 1445–1455.

Sanday, P. R. (2007). *Fraternity gang rape: Sex, brotherhood, and privilege on campus* (2nd ed.). New York: New York University Press.

Sandnabba, N. K., Santtila, P., & Nordling, N. (1999). Sexual behavior and social adaptation among sadomasochistically-oriented males. *Journal of Sex Research, 36*(3), 273–282.

Sarkar, N. N., & Sarkar, R. (2005). Sexual assault on woman: Its impact on her life and living in society. *Sexual and Relationship Therapy, 20*(4), 407–419.

Savin-Williams, R. C. (2005). *The new gay teenager.* Cambridge: MA: Harvard University Press.

Scarry, E. (1985). *The body in pain: The making and unmaking of the world.* Oxford: Oxford University Press.

Schauer, T. (2005). Women's porno: The heterosexual female gaze in porn sites "for women." *Sexuality & Culture, 9*(2), 42–64.

Scott, J. (1990). *Domination and the arts of resistance: Hidden transcripts.* New Haven, CT: Yale University Press.

Scott, J. W. (1988). Deconstructing equality-versus-difference: Or, the uses of poststructuralist theory for feminism. *Feminist Studies, 14*(1), 33–50.

Sedgwick, E. K. (2003). *Touching feeling: Affect, pedagogy, performativity.* Durham, NC: Duke University Press.

Seto, M. C., Maric, A., & Barbaree. H. E. (2001). The role of pornography in the etiology of sexual aggression. *Aggression and Violent Behavior, 6*(1), 35–53.

Sherfey, M. J. (1970). A theory on female sexuality. In R. Morgan (Ed.), *Sisterhood is powerful: An anthology of writings from the Women's Liberation movement* (pp. 220–230). New York: Vintage Books.

Shifren, J. L., Monz, B. U., Russo, P. A., Segreti, A., & Johannes, C. B. (2008). Sexual problems and distress in United States women: Prevalence and correlates. *Obstetrics & Gynecology, 112*(5), 970–978.

Shim, J. W. (2007). Online pornography and rape myth acceptance: Sexually degrading content, anonymous viewing conditions, and the activation of antisocial attitudes. *Dissertation Abstracts International Section A: Humanities and Social Sciences, 67*(12–A), 4378.

Shrier, D. K., Zucker, A. N., Mercurio, A. E., Landry, L. J., Rich, M., & Shrier, L. A. (2007). Generation to generation: Discrimination and harassment experiences of physician mothers and their physician daughters. *Journal of Women's Health, 16*(6), 883–894.

Shulman, J. L., & Horne, S. G. (2006). Guilty or not? A path model of women's sexual force fantasies. *Journal of Sex Research, 43*(4), 368–377.

Siebler, F., Sabelus, S., & Bohner, G. (2008). A refined computer harassment paradigm: Validation, and test of hypotheses about target characteristics. *Psychology of Women Quarterly, 32*(1), 22–35.

Silberstein, L. R., Striegel-Moore, R. H., Timko, C., & Rodin, J. (1988). Behavioral and psychological implications of body dissatisfaction: Do men and women differ? *Sex Roles, 19*(3–4), 219–232.

Singer, J., & Singer, I. (1972). Types of female orgasm. *The Journal of Sex Research, 8,* 255–267.

Smith, C. (2007). *One for the girls: The pleasures and practices of reading women's porn.* Bristol, UK: Intellect.

Smith, J. C., & Ferstman, C. J. (1996). *The castration of Oedipus: Feminism, psycho-analysis, and the will to power.* New York: New York University Press.

Smith-Rosenberg, C. (1985). *Disorderly conduct: Visions of gender in Victorian America.* New York: Oxford University Press.

Smith-Rosenberg, C. (1985). *Disorderly conduct: Visions of gender in Victorian America.* New York: Knopf.

Snow, I. (n.d.). Top 10: Female sex fantasies. Retrieved October 17, 2008, from Ask Men. Website: http://www.askmen.com/dating/vanessa/27_love_secrets.html.

Spivak, G. C. (1988). Can the subaltern speak? In C. Nelson, & L. Gross (Eds.), *Marxism and the Interpretation of Culture* (pp. 271–313). Urbana: University of Illinois Press.

Sprecher, S. (2002). Sexual satisfaction in premarital relationships: Associations with satisfaction, love, commitment, and stability. *Journal of Sex Research, 39*(3), 190–196.

Sprecher, S., & Regan, P. C. (1996). College virgins: How men and women perceive their sexual status. *Journal of Sex Research, 33*(1), 3–15.

Sprecher, S., Barbee, A., & Schwartz, P. (1995). "Was it good for you too?" Gender differences in first sexual intercourse experiences. *Journal of Sex Research, 32*(1), 3–15.

Strassberg, D. S., & Locker, L. K. (1998). Force in women's sexual fantasies. *Archives of Sexual Behavior, 27*(4), 403–414.

Strauss, A., & Corbin, J. (1990). *Basics of qualitative research: Grounded theory procedures and techniques.* Newbury Park, CA: Sage.

Street, A. E., Gradus, J. L., Stafford, J., & Kelly, K. (2007). Gender differences in experiences of sexual harassment: Data from a male-dominated environment. *Journal of Consulting and Clinical Psychology, 75*(3), 464–474.

Strong Viagra sales boost Pfizer. (2008, October 21). Retrieved November 14, 2008, from *City A.M.* Website: http://www.cityam.com/index.php?news=23271.

Sweeney, C. (2005, June 5). Not tonight: The search for desire. Retrieved August 28, 2008, from *The New York Times*. Website: http://www.nytimes.com/2005/06/05/health/womenshealth/05sweeney.html?pagewanted=1&_r=1&sq=intrinsa&st+cse&scp=5.

Szabo, L. (2008, July 25). Study: Viagra may help women on antidepressants. Retrieved August 28, 2008, from *USA Today*. Website: http://www.usatoday.com/news/health/2008–07–22-viagra_N.htm.

Tellis, K. M., & Spohn, C. C. (2008). The sexual stratification hypothesis revisited: Testing assumptions about simple versus aggravated rape. *Journal of Criminal Justice, 36*(3), 252–261.

The New View Campaign (2008). Retrieved November 15, 2008, from *The New View Campaign*. Website: www.fsd-alert.org.

Thomas, M. (2007). Treatment of family violence: A systemic perspective. In J. Hamel & T. L. Nicholls (Eds.), *Family interventions in domestic violence* (pp. 417–436). New York: Springer.

Thompson, E. M. (2007). Girl friend or girlfriend? Same-sex friendship and bisexual images as a context for flexible sexual identity among young women. *Journal of Bisexuality, 6*(3), 47–67.

Tiefer, L. (2001). Arriving at a "new view" of women's sexual problems: Background, theory, and activism. *Women & Therapy, 24*(1–2), 63–98.

Tiefer, L. (2003). Female sexual dysfunction (FSD): Witnessing social construction in action. *Sexualities, Evolution, & Gender, 5*(1), 33–36.

Tiefer, L. (2004). *Sex is not a natural act and other essays*. Boulder, CO: Westview.

Tiefer, L. (2006a). Sex therapy as a humanistic enterprise. *Sexual & Relationship Therapy, 21*(3), 359–75.

Tiefer, L. (2006b). Female sexual dysfunction: A case study of disease mongering and activist resistance. *PLoS Med, 3*, e178.

Tiefer, L. (2007). Beneath the veneer: The troubled past and future of sexual medicine. *Journal of Sex & Marital Therapy, 33*(5), 473–477.

Tjaden, P., & Thoennes, N. (2000). Extent, nature, and consequences of intimate partner violence: Findings from the National Violence against Women survey. Retrieved June 18, 2008, from *Department of Justice*. Website: www.ojp.usdoj.gov/nij/pubs-sum/181867.htm.

Tjaden, P., & Thoennes, N. (2000). Prevalence and consequences of male-to-female and female-to-male intimate partner violence as measured by the National Violence against Women Survey. *Violence against Women, 6*(2), 142–161.

Toll, B., & Ling, P. (2005). Virginia Slims identity crisis: An inside look at tobacco industry marketing to women. *Tobacco Control, 14*(3), 172–180.

Tolman, D. L. (2002). *Dilemmas of desire: Teenage girls talk about sex*. Cambridge, MA: Harvard University Press.

U.S. Department of Health and Human Services, Food and Drug Administration. (2000, May). Guidance for industry female sexual dysfunction: Clinical development of drug products for treatment. Retrieved April 20, 2009, from *U. S. Department of Health and Human Services*. Website: http://www.fda.gov/CDER/GUIDANCE/3312dft.htm.

UCSC rape prevention education: rape statistics. Retrieved on January 1, 2008, from UCSC. Website: www2.ucsc.edu.

Udry, J. R., & Campbell, B. C. (1994). Getting started on sexual behavior. In A.S. Rossi (Ed.), *Sexuality across the life course* (pp. 187–208). Chicago: University of Chicago Press.

Ullman, S. E. (2007). A 10-year update of "Review and critique of empirical studies of rape avoidance." *Criminal Justice and Behavior, 34*(3), 411–429.

Ullman, S. E., & Knight, R. A. (1992). Fighting back: Women's resistance to rape. *Journal of Interpersonal Violence, 7*, 31–43.

Ullman, S. E., Townsend, S. M., Filipas, H. H., & Starzynski, L. L. (2007). Structural models of the relations of assault severity, social support, avoidance coping, self-blame, and PTSD among sexual assault survivors. *Psychology of Women Quarterly, 31*(1), 23–37.

Valentine, G. (1989). The geography of women's fear. *Area, 21*(4), 385–390.

Van House, N. A. (2009). Collocated photo sharing, story-telling, and the performance of self. *International Journal of Human-Computer Studies, 67*(12), 1073–1086.

Vance, C. (1984). *Pleasure and danger: Exploring women's sexuality*. London: Routledge.

Vares, T., & Braun, V. (2006). Spreading the word, but what word is that? Viagra and male sexuality in popular culture. *Sexualities, 9*(3), 315–332.

Venkataraman, B. (2008, July 29). Nostrums: Viagra may benefit some women. Retrieved August 28, 2008, from *The New York Times*. Website: http://www.nytimes.com/2008/07/29/health/research/29nost.html?scp=7&sq=female%20sexual%20dysfunction&st=cse.

Viki, G. T., Abrams, D., & Masser, B. (2004). Evaluating stranger and acquaintance rape: The role of benevolent sexism in perpetrator blame and recommended sentence length. *Law and Human Behavior, 28*(3), 295–303.

Vogt, D., Bruce, T. A., Street, A. E., & Stafford, J. (2007). Attitudes toward women and tolerance for sexual harassment among reservists. *Violence against Women, 13*(9), 879–900.

Wade, L. D., Kremer, E. C., & Brown, J. (2005). The incidental orgasm: The presence of clitoral knowledge and the absence of orgasm for women. *Women & Health, 42*(1), 117–138.

Walker, A. (2004). *You can't keep a good woman down*. New York: Harcourt Trade.

Walker-Hill, R. (2000). An analysis of the relationship of human sexuality knowledge, self esteem, and body image to sexual satisfaction in college and university students. *Dissertation Abstracts International, 60,* 4560.

Wallin, P. (1960). A study of orgasm as a condition of women's sexual enjoyment of intercourse. *Journal of Social Psychology, 5*(1), 191–198.

Ward, L. M. (2003). Understanding the role of entertainment media in the sexual socialization of American youth: A review of empirical research. *Developmental Review, 23*(3), 347–388.

WebMD. (2007, March 30). Getting close to a female Viagra? Retrieved April 15, 2007, from *Fox News.* Website: http://www.foxnews.com/story/0,2933,262784,00.html.

Weeks, J. (1990). *Coming out: Homosexual politics in Britain from the nineteenth century to the present.* London: Quartet Books.

Welsh, S. (1999). Gender and sexual harassment. *Annual Review of Sociology, 25,* 169–190.

West, C., & Zimmerman, D. H. (1987). Doing gender. *Gender and Society, 1*(2), 125–151.

Whealin, J. M., Zinzow, H. M., Salstrom, S. A., & Jackson, J. L. (2007). Sex differences in the experience of unwanted sexual attention and behaviors during childhood. *Journal of Child Sexual Abuse, 16*(3), 41–58.

Wiederman, M. W. (1997). Pretending orgasm during sexual intercourse: Correlates in a sample of young adult women. *Journal of Sex & Marital Therapy, 23*(2), 131–139.

Wiederman, M. W. (2005). The gendered nature of sexual scripts. *Family Journal, 13*(4), 496–502.

Wilson, F. (2000). The subjective experience of sexual harassment: Cases of students. *Human Relations, 53*(8), 1081–1097.

Wilson, G. D. (1987). Male-female differences in sexual activity, enjoyment, and fantasies. *Personality and Individual Differences, 8*(1), 125–127.

Wilson, G. D., & Lang, R. J. (1981). Sex differences in sexual fantasy patterns. *Personality and Individual Differences, 2*(4), 343–346.

Witte, F. M., Stratton, T. D., & Nora, L. M. (2006). Stories from the field: Students' descriptions of gender discrimination and sexual harassment during medical school. *Academic Medicine, 81*(7), 648–654.

Wolitzky-Taylor, K. B., Ruggiero, K. J., Danielson, C. K., Resnick, H. S., Hanson, R. F., Smith, D. W., Saunders, B. E., & Kilpatrick, D. G. (2008). Prevalence and correlates of dating violence in a national sample of adolescents. *Journal of the American Academy of Child and Adolescent Psychiatry, 47*(7), 755–762.

Wood, E. A. (2000). Working in the fantasy factory: The attention hypothesis and the enacting of masculine power in strip clubs. *Journal of Contemporary Ethnography, 29*(1), 5–31.

Workman, J. E., & Orr, R. L. (1996). Clothing, sex of subject, and rape myth acceptance as factors affecting attributions about and incident of acquaintance rape. *Clothing and Textile Research Journal, 14*(4), 276–284.

Wynter, S. (1987). Whisper: Women hurt in systems of prostitution engaged in revolt. In P. Alexander, & F. Delacoste (Eds.), *Sex work: Writings by women in the sex industry* (pp. 266–270). Pittsburgh: Cleis.

Yarab, P. E., & Allgeier, E. R. (1998). Don't even think about it: The role of sexual fantasies as perceived unfaithfulness in heterosexual dating relationships. *Journal of Sex Education & Therapy, 23*(3), 246–254.

Ybarra, M. L., Espelage, D. L., & Mitchell, K. J. (2007). The co-occurrence of Internet harassment and unwanted sexual solicitation victimization and perpetration: Associations with psychosocial indicators. *Journal of Adolescent Health, 41*(6 Supplement), S31–S41.

Yost, M. R., & Zurbriggen, E. L. (2006). Gender differences in the enactment of sociosexuality: An examination of implicit social motives, sexual fantasies, coercive sexual attitudes, and aggressive sexual behavior. *Journal of Sex Research, 43*(2), 163–173.

Young, M., Luquis, R., Denny, G., & Young, T. (1998). Correlates of sexual satisfaction in marriage. *The Canadian Journal of Human Sexuality, 7*(2), 115–127.

Zurbriggen, E. L., & Yost, M. R. (2004). Power, desire, and pleasure in sexual fantasies. *Journal of Sex Research, 41*(3), 288–300.

INDEX

Symons, Donald, 238, 239
Szabo, Liz, 125

Taft, Casey T., 2, 190
"Technophilia: Technology, Representation, and the Feminine," 158
Tellis, Katharine, 190
Testosterone, 124, 125–126, 127
Therapeutic sex, 163–164
Thomas, Nancy, 200
Thompson, Lana, 35
This Sex Which Is Not One, 48, 71, 115, 133
Therapy, sex, 13, 130, 131
Thoennes, Nancy, 188, 189
Thompson, Elisabeth Morgan, 78
Threesomes, 2, 12, 24, 75, 86–87, 90, 172–173, 207, 212, 235, 246–248, 273
Tiefer, Leonore, 57, 95, 120, 129, 130–131
Timko, Christine, 2
Tjaden, Patricia, 188, 189
Tolman, Deborah L., 245, 297
Toll, Ben, 81
"Tough Talk for Tough Times," 227
Trauma bonds, 200
Triplett, Laura, 192

University of Michigan, 305–306
Ullman, Sarah E., 19, 195

Vacation sex, 160, 175–178. *See also* Pleasure
Vaginal tiredness, 147
Van House, Nancy A., 9
Van Wie, Victoria, 188
Valentine, Gill, 224
Vance, Carole S., 10, 261
Valkenburg, Patti M., 234
Vares, Tiina, 122
Venkataraman, Bina, 125
Viáfara, Gloria, 154

Viagra. *See* Pharmaceuticals
Victorian sexuality, 32–35, 153, 277–278
Viki, G. Tendayi, 188
Violence, sexual, 16, 26, 64, 71–72, 98, 185, 200, 201, 205, 208, 213, 221–224, 234, 237, 261, 273. *See also* Rape; Coercion
Virginity, 152, 169, 278
Vogt, Dawne, 196
Volatile Bodies, 275

Waldby, Catherine, 47, 48
Walker, Alice, 241
Walker-Hill, R., 45
Wallin, Paul, 45
Walsetha, Kristin, 196
Walsh-Childers, Kim, 180
Wandering womb, 35. *See also* Victorian sexuality
War Zone, 195
Ward, L. Monique, 234
Wasco, Sharon M., 188
Weeks, Jeffrey, 76–77
Welsh, Sandy, 195
Wemmerus, Virginia A., 192
West, Candace, 7, 8
West, Maggie Hadleigh, 195
"What Don't We Know about the Pharmaceutical Industry? A Freakonomics Quorum," 115
Whealin, Julia M., 196
White, Jacquelyn W., 189
Whitley, Bernard E., 224
"Who Said It Was Simple," 292
Wiederman, Michael, 2, 10, 45, 46, 59
Williams, Michelle, 75
Wilson, Fiona, 2
Wilson, Glenn D., 75, 236
Wilson, Jonathan, 50
Witte, Florence M, 196
Wolak, Janis, 197
Wolf whistling. *See* Street harassment